Top 40 Herbs
Of North America

Angela Harris
Fifth Generation Herbalist

Ranier LLC, Panguitch, Utah USA

Ranier LLC
P.O. Box 625
Panguitch, Utah 84759
United States of America
https://herbu.org

Copyright © 2022 Ranier LLC

All rights reserved. No part of this book may be reproduced or utilized in any form or by any means, electronic or mechanical, including photocopying, recording, or by any information storage and retrieval system, without permission in writing from the publisher. Contact the publisher in writing to request permission to use select quotes in reviews or in an educational context.

Published by Ranier LLC

Angela Harris reserves the right to be identified as the author of this work.

ISBN: 978-1-957198-00-2

Includes bibliographical references and indexes.

Printed and bound in the United States of America.

10 9 8 7 6 5 4 3 2 1

Disclaimer:

The information contained in this writing is for educational purposes only and is not recommended as a means of diagnosing or treating illness. Neither the publisher nor the author shall assume responsibility or liability for any loss, injury or damage allegedly arising from opinions, ideas or information contained in this book. The publisher or author neither directly nor indirectly prescribes or dispenses medical advice, remedies, or assumes responsibility for those who choose to treat themselves. All matters concerning physical and mental health should be supervised by a healthcare practitioner.

Correspondence to the author can be sent care of the publisher at the address shown above.

INTRODUCTION

While the United States and other developed countries systematically outlaw curative herbs, many beloved by my family, I have wondered why no one else seems to notice or care. Why *should you* care that herbs like Comfrey or Chaparral have been banned if you don't know anything about them? I am convinced if you knew about the fabulous medicinal value of these God given plants, they would never have been taken off the market.

As I have witnessed the proscription of many precious herbs used and loved by my family for generations, I prayed with all my heart for inspiration on how to save them. The answer came suddenly and powerfully to me, "Teach them about the herbs that grow on this, the American continent." The download of information that followed was detailed, specific, and is still vivid in my mind. I grabbed a piece of paper and wrote down all of my favorite herbs of North America, electrified by every herb I wrote down; each herb well known and loved like an intimate friend to me. There were over 120! I tried to narrow the list down to a manageable 40, but each herb I removed was like giving up one of my precious children. Then I realized there need to be more books…

The **Top 40 Herbs of North America** is a well-rounded compilation of herbs that address just about any situation that may arise, from staunching blood flow to balancing hormones to supporting serotonin levels and improving your outlook on life. Herbs help nourish and support your body in amazing ways! Discovering the magic of herbs will benefit your family for generations to come. Pick one that tickles your fancy and let your love of herbs grow.

DEDICATION

I dedicate this book to each of my beloved children:

Collette

Rachelle

Curtiss Jr.

Camilla

Emma

Abbigail

Eliza

Hannah

Graciella

May the sacred knowledge of these miraculous healing plants be passed down to your children's children's children.

CONTENTS

1	Alfalfa	1	25	Licorice	221
2	Aloe Vera	12	26	Lobelia	231
3	Barley	26	27	Milk Thistle	242
4	Bilberry	37	28	Mullein	249
5	Black Cohosh	43	29	Peppermint	257
6	Blessed Thistle	50	30	Red Clover	267
7	Brigham Tea	55	31	Red Raspberry	274
8	Burdock	61	32	Saw Palmetto	280
9	Catnip	72	33	Slippery Elm	287
10	Cayenne	78	34	St. John's Wort	297
11	Chamomile	91	35	Uva Ursi	308
12	Chaparral	99	36	Valerian	316
13	Chaste Tree	108	37	Wild Lettuce	325
14	Comfrey	112	38	Wild Yam	330
15	Dandelion	122	39	Yarrow	339
16	Echinacea	130	40	Yellow Dock	349
17	Eyebright	141	41	References	356
18	Flaxseed	148	42	Bibliography	360
19	Garlic	159	43	Glossary	367
20	Ginger	176	44	Index	376
21	Goldenseal	188	45	Common Names	416
22	Hawthorn	200	46	Latin Names	421
23	Juniper	207	47	Key Components	422
24	Kelp	214	48	Studies	427

Alfalfa

Latin Name: *Medicago sativa*

Also known as: Buffalo Herb, Buffalo Grass, Lucerne, Lucerne Grass, Chilean Clover, Father of All Foods, Purple Medic

This herb is known as Lucerne in the United Kingdom, Australia, and New Zealand, and as Lucerne Grass in South Asia

Scientific Classification

Family: Fabaceae – legume, pea family
Genus: Medicago – alfalfa
Species: M. sativa – alfalfa

Influence on the Body	(PRINCIPAL ACTIONS are listed in CAPITAL LETTERS)
Autoimmune	ARTHRITIS • RHEUMATISM • systemic lupus
Blood and Circulatory System	BLOOD PURIFIER • ANEMIA (supplies iron) • thin blood • BLOOD CLOTTING NORMALIZATION • HEMORRHAGE • hemophilia • scurvy • nosebleeds • high blood pressure • hypertension • heart • heart disease • varicose veins • vascular system
Body System	ACIDITY • toxemia • counteracts toxins • body building • chronic weakness • endurance • energy • vitality • tonic (increases energy and strength throughout the body)
Bones and Teeth	teeth • TOOTH DECAY • tooth surgery • fractures
Cancer	COLON CANCER PREVENTION • tumor regression
Cleansing	BLOOD PURIFIER • depurative (cleanses blood by promoting eliminative functions) • kidney cleanser • toxemia • DEODORANT (for breath and body odors)
Blood Sugar	DIABETES • HYPOGLYCEMIA
Digestive Tract	NUTRITIVE (full of nutrients for the body) • IMPROVES APPETITE • DIGESTIVE DISORDERS • NAUSEA • stomachic (strengthens stomach function) • stomach inflammation • PEPTIC ULCERS • colon • sluggish bowels • constipation • INTESTINAL SCRUB • hemorrhoids

ALFALFA — 1

Endocrine System	hormone imbalance • PITUITARY GLAND • Cushing's disease (adrenal gland disorder)
First Aid	Wounds
Infections and Immune System	ALLERGIES • hay fever • colds • whooping cough • fever • tonsillitis • bacterial infections • flu • fungal infections • yeast infections
Inflammation	inflammation • stomach inflammation • joint inflammation/swelling • ARTHRITIS • RHEUMATISM • BURSITIS • GOUT • uric acid retention
Liver	liver conditions • hepatitis • jaundice • alcoholic liver
Lungs and Respiratory System	NASAL DOUCHE • sinus • ASTHMA • whooping cough
Mouth and Throat	pyorrhea (gum disease) • gargle • tonsillitis
Muscles	muscle spasms • muscle tone • physical FATIGUE
Nervous System	nerves • nervousness • mental FATIGUE • BELL'S PALSY (facial nerve paralysis) • stroke • senility
Pain	minor pain • headache
Reproductive System	*Female:* uterus • vaginal douche • MENSTRUATION • MORNING SICKNESS • NURSING • LACTATION (increases quality and quantity of mother's milk)
Skin, Tissues and Hair	acne • skin • tissue repair • boils
Sleep	Insomnia
Urinary Tract	kidneys • kidney stones • kidney cleanser • bladder • dysuria (painful urination) • diuretic (increases urine flow)
Weight	normalizes weight (gain or loss, as needed)

Key Properties:

BLOOD CLEANSER • **BLOOD BUILDER**
DIGESTIVE AID *increases appetite, supplies bulk, stabilizes blood sugar*
NUTRITIVE *full of nutrients for the body, improves lactation*

Primarily affecting: *BLOOD • DIGESTION*

ALFALFA — 2

History	Alfalfa was discovered by the Arabs, who called it the "Father of All Foods." The herb is also known as the "King of Plants" because it is extremely rich in vitamins, minerals, and other nutrients.

Darius, King of Persia, reportedly brought alfalfa to Greece when he was in a battle over Athens. In early Chinese medicines, physicians used young alfalfa leaves to treat disorders related to the digestive tract and the kidneys. In Hindu societies, Ayurvedic physicians used the leaves for treating poor digestion and for the pain relief brought to arthritic patients. They also made a cooling poultice from the seeds for boils.

The Columbians used alfalfa for coughs, while the Costanoan Indians applied it as a poultice for earaches. As early as 1597, the English herbalist John Gerard recommended alfalfa for upset stomachs.

North American Indians adapted alfalfa quickly for human use, as well as for animals. Early Americans also found it useful for treating scurvy, urinary problems, and menstrual symptoms. Frank Bouer, noted author and biologist, discovered that the leaves of alfalfa contain all eight essential amino acids.

As long as I can remember, my Mom has had jars of sprouts on her kitchen window sill. It was an inexpensive and effective way to get good nutrients into us kids. I appreciate her wisdom and thriftiness now that I am a mother.

If you were to ask me if there was one herb that was most important to take on a daily basis, it would have to be alfalfa grass. The nutrients are off the chart in this little plant. People notice the biggest difference in their health when they begin or increase the amount they consume of chlorophyll-rich plants like alfalfa grass and barley grass. |
| **Attributes** | Alfalfa contains all the known vitamins and minerals for life, some in trace amounts, yet many in substantial quantities. Alfalfa permits rapid absorption of plant elements into the body. This is one of the reasons alfalfa is used as a base in many herb combinations and vitamin formulas.

Key Components: *(including, but not limited to)* |

ALFALFA — 3

Vitamins A • B1 (thiamine) • B2 (riboflavin) • B3 (niacin) • B5 (pantothenic acid) • B6 (pyridoxine) • B9 (folic acid) • B12 (cobalamin, a rich source) • Biotin • Choline • Inositol • PABA (Para-Amino Benzoic Acid) • C (four times that found in citrus juice) • D • E • K (found in high quantities, Vitamin K is a clotting factor and a friend to women suffering from morning sickness)

Calcium (the ashes of alfalfa leaves are 99 percent pure calcium) • Fluorine (Helps prevent tooth decay and strengthens bones naturally. It should be noted that the fluorine in alfalfa is not the same as the artificially made 'sodium fluoride' found in some community water treatments. Sodium fluoride is an aluminum manufacturing by-product that can be toxic to the body) • Iron • Magnesium • Phosphorus • Potassium • Silicon • Sodium • Sulfur • other Trace Minerals

Minerals figure in the formation and function of all body enzymes and keep the proper alkaline electrical charge in all body cells, guarding them against acidic degeneration and invasion from harmful microbes that live on acidic substances in the body.

• Chlorophyll (One of the highest concentrations in a plant known to man and accounts for many of the health benefits attributed to alfalfa. Among other things, chlorophyll helps regulate and maintain calcium levels in the blood.)

• High in Fiber (provides bulk which carries intestinal wastes out of the body)

• High Enzyme content of fresh, freeze-dried and sprouted alfalfa. Enzymes help the body balance its systems, ward off infectious diseases, and restore the immune system's ability to defeat many degenerative diseases such as cancer and arthritis.

• All eight Essential Amino Acids • Saponins • Isoflavones • Sugars • Sterols • Coumarins • Alkaloids • Porphyrins

Digestion

The chlorophyll and enzymes in alfalfa stimulate the appetite and aid in the digestion and absorption of proteins, fats, and carbohydrates. Very ill patients often need foods that are rich in nutrients which the body can easily assimilate. Alfalfa may be used for debilitated and weak individuals.

Ulcers

Alfalfa promotes digestive health and the healing of a damaged and ulcerated stomach and intestinal lining. The chlorophyll in the herb helps neutralize acids in the body which produce putrefaction in the bowel. Enzymes aid food digestion, relieving the damaged tissues of the stomach and intestines. Less acid is needed to break down food in the stomach. Chlorophyll lubricates the ileocecal valve (between the small and large intestines) and keeps it functioning properly.

Bioflavonoids found in alfalfa build capillary strength and reduce inflammation of the digestive tract lining. Chlorophyll accelerates the replacement of damaged bowel tissue and helps to eliminate mucus. It also destroys toxins and disease-causing bacteria. Nutrients in alfalfa help heal and maintain the entire digestive tract.

Cleansing

Chlorophyll in alfalfa is a natural healer and cleanser for chronic conditions both internally and externally. It acts as a detergent in the body. Using chlorophyll in a cleansing diet progressively cleans the blood, cells, tissues, and organs while providing nutrients for new cell life. It has been called 'liquid sunshine' because it absorbs energy from the sun.

Taking greens deodorizes the bowel and is a natural antiseptic to the intestinal tract. Chlorophyll neutralizes acid and poisons and is an excellent blood purifier. It has even been used to remove toxic metals from children and stops the growth and development of toxic bacteria. Disease-causing bacteria find it difficult to live in the presence of chlorophyll. Fewer bacteria result in fewer odors. Chlorophyll is a natural deodorizer, eliminating bad breath, smelly feet, and body odors of all types, because it works at the cellular level.

Liver

Greens like alfalfa help purify the liver and eliminate stored drug deposits, old toxic material, chemical sprays on food, artificial flavoring, colors, and coal tar buildup. Bile function and circulation is also enhanced.

Fights Infection

Alfalfa is a natural infection fighter, largely due to its high level of Vitamin A. It inhibits the metabolic action of carcinogens (cancer causing elements).

When used topically, the herb acts as an astringent. It has been used to heal infections at surgery wound sites and infected bed sores. Chlorophyll is a great gargle for tonsillitis and helps to reduce fevers.

ALFALFA — 5

Tooth Decay	Alfalfa contains a natural fluoride and helps prevent tooth decay, even rebuilding decayed teeth.
Pituitary Gland	Alfalfa has a natural ability to stimulate and feed the pituitary gland, which has a major role in the regulation of many endocrine functions.
Diabetes and Hypoglycemia	Alfalfa helps the body normalize blood sugar problems in diabetics and hypoglycemics. The condition of people with diabetes who fail to respond to insulin has been shown to greatly improve when they take alfalfa plus manganese. (1)
Blood	The green pigment 'chlorophyll' is found in most plants. Its molecular structure is almost exactly the same as human red blood cell 'hemoglobin'. The only difference is the substitution of a magnesium molecule in place of the iron found in the 'heme' group making up hemoglobin. Chlorophyll in the blood has the same effect as iron, making it a natural blood builder and cleanser. This strengthens and may temporarily thicken the blood. As the body adjusts to the nutrients and cleanses the body of toxins and wastes, the blood ultimately thins to its natural level.
Cholesterol	Saponins found in alfalfa help lower blood cholesterol by impeding intestinal absorption, without affecting heart-healthy HDL (high-density lipoproteins) cholesterol. This effectively slows the progress of atherosclerosis and begins to reverse the plaque buildup already lining arterial walls. (2)
Skin and Tissue	Chlorophyll accelerates healing of damaged tissues by cleansing out dead cell matter and providing nutrients to the cells, increasing cell activity and the re-growth of cells. Chlorophyll has been applied topically in salves and ointments for this purpose.
Women	*Menstruation:* Due to alfalfa's numerous estrogenic qualities, women over the years have used the herb to relieve discomfort and other symptoms associated with hormonal imbalance. Alfalfa, like other leguminous crops, is a known source of phyto-estrogens (plant derived estrogens). These provide a gentle substitute for estrogen after menopause. (3) Alfalfa contains plant-world equivalents of human estrogens, so a woman, whether she is going through menopause or

breastfeeding a baby, may derive some benefit from it. (4)

Female Cancers:
Hot flashes and other menopausal symptoms are rare among women who consume a lot of legumes (such as black beans, mung beans, soybeans and alfalfa) which have mild estrogenic activity.

In addition to acting like estrogen in women whose own sex hormone production has declined, phytoestrogens also appear to reduce the risk of estrogen-linked cancers such as breast cancer. Laboratory experiments show that phytoestrogens are effective in preventing tumors in breast tissue. (1)

Osteoporosis:
Clinical studies in Japan have found that Vitamin K (found in alfalfa and in green leafy vegetables such as kale and spinach) can help prevent some bone loss caused by estrogen deficiency. Vitamin K interacts with Vitamin D to increase the formation of new bone. The combination is not sufficient, however, to completely compensate for osteoporosis caused by estrogen-depleting medications. (1)

Lactation:
Chlorophyll increases iron in the milk of nursing mothers.

Alfalfa Sprouts

All the energy and life of a plant goes toward making seeds. Each seed holds vitamins, minerals, proteins, fats, and carbohydrates (starches) in reserve, waiting for a suitable environment to begin growing. When the seed germinates (begins to sprout), an incredible flow of energy is released. Enzymes are produced to convert the concentrated nutrients into those needed by the growing plant.

As the sprouting process continues, carbohydrates, proteins, and fats are broken down into sugars, amino acids, and fatty acids. Vitamins are produced and additional minerals are pulled from the water used in the germinating process. Sprouting alfalfa seeds provides a highly digestible, live food that aids digestion and absorption of nutrients.

Some scientists believe that the highest potency of nutrients in sprouts is released just before the seed germinates completely and produces chlorophyll (the green part of the leaf on the sprout itself). Vitamin C and other vitamins found only in trace amounts

ALFALFA — 7

Nutrients	in the seed are produced in larger quantities during the sprouting process.

Found in Alfalfa Sprouts

Key Components: *(including, but not limited to)*

Vitamins A (in the form of carotene) • B-complex vitamins are abundant • B1 (thiamine) • B2 (riboflavin) • B3 (Niacin) • C • E • K

Calcium • Magnesium • Potassium • Iron (a good source) • Selenium • Zinc (an especially rich source) Zinc is essential for the synthesis of protein, many liver functions, and the healing of cuts and wounds.)

In addition to the minerals found in the seeds, sprouts absorb minerals from the water used to grow and rinse them, becoming bound to amino acids that are easily assimilated by the human body. (5)

Chlorophyll: When sprouting seeds in sunlight, chlorophyll is developed. Direct sun will wither tender sprouts and destroy enzymes. Indirect light is sufficient for chlorophyll production.

Enzymes: Minutes after seeds are placed in water to soak, enzymes begin making the young sprouts into easy-to-digest food. These same enzymes can assist food digestion in the body. |
| **Herb Parts Used** | The above-ground parts are used medicinally, including the leaves, flowers, stems, and sprouted seeds. |
| **Preparations and Remedies**

Powdered Form | Young alfalfa grass may be juiced for a fresh, wholesome, green drink or to have the chlorophyll extracted. The plant may be dried, powdered, and put into capsules, and the seeds may also be germinated and eaten as sprouts.

Vitamin and Mineral Supplement
Taking 4-12 capsules or 1 tablespoon powder daily is recommended as one of the best vitamin, mineral, and health supplements you can buy.

Cholesterol:
For cholesterol or diabetes, take four capsules or one teaspoon of alfalfa grass powder with each meal. |

ALFALFA — 8

Tea

The cut and sifted form of this herb is a popular tea, having a very soft, delicate flavor. It is often prepared with mint and lemon. Use one to two teaspoons of dried alfalfa leaves in a cup of boiling water.

Liquid Chlorophyll

Liquid chlorophyll may be purchased as a prepared supplement, usually derived from alfalfa. It is often extracted in a way that makes it high in copper content. In my opinion, taking green young alfalfa grass in a whole form whenever possible is superior in health-giving results.

Green Drink:
One tablespoon powdered alfalfa or barley grass to one cup of water, or one tablespoon liquid chlorophyll either taken straight or in water or juice, makes a nutritious green drink.

Gargle for Tonsillitis:
One teaspoon liquid chlorophyll in a half cup of water.

Sprout Use

Use fresh sprouts in salads, sandwiches, green drinks, soups, and sprout loaves. Heating or drying sprouts over 105° F will destroy their living enzymes.

Infections:
Use blender to liquefy raw alfalfa spouts and drink four to six ounces or apply directly to the site of the infection.

Sprouting Seeds

Seeds and beans may be sprouted in jars, sprout bags, trays, or automatic sprouting appliances. Whichever method you select, the basic steps are the same: Wash, initial soak, drain, rinse periodically, and harvest.

Choosing and Preparing the Seeds:
Alfalfa seeds are small, about the size of a pinhead, and tan in color. Not all seeds are created equal. Organically grown alfalfa seed is easily found in most natural food stores. When choosing seeds for sprouting, look for uniformity of shape, color, and perfection. Avoid broken, chipped, or damaged seeds. Organically grown seeds will often look less clean and polished, but a quick wash before sprouting will remove any grime on them. Remove any sticks, stones, or dirt from the seeds.

The Jar Method:
Small seeds like alfalfa should just cover the bottom of the jar (larger seeds and beans can fill the jar one-eighth to one-quarter

ALFALFA — 9

full). Cover the jar with cheesecloth or screen, then fill jar halfway with water. Allow seeds to soak four to six hours for smaller seeds, and twelve hours for larger seeds and beans, and then drain. Place jar at a 45-degree angle, mouth down, in a place where it can drain, and air can circulate freely.

For best results, rinse the sprouts 2-3 times each day. Rinsing removes waste produced by the sprouts. The water coming out may appear a little foamy. After rinsing, replace the jar of sprouts again to a 45-degree angle to drain excess water. Place in light to develop chlorophyll the last couple of days before harvesting.

Harvest when sprouts are one to one and a half inches long. After four to six days, they are ready to eat or store. Removing the hulls may improve the taste, but is not necessary with lentils like alfalfa, as the hulls are soft and do not readily detach from the seeds.

Sprout Storage:
Keep thoroughly drained sprouts in a glass jar or sealable plastic bag and store in the refrigerator for up to seven to ten days. Alfalfa sprouts will expand up to eight times the initial size of the seeds.

Safety	No health hazards or adverse side effects are known.
	Taking alfalfa greens may temporarily alter blood thickness as the body adjusts to available nutrients and blood cleansing actions. Dosage requirements for individuals taking blood thinning medications may be affected. Contact your health care professional to correctly monitor blood thickness and adjust medications if needed.
Plant Profile	*Natural Habitat:* Indigenous to the Mediterranean region, alfalfa has been widely cultivated elsewhere for thousands of years and now is grown worldwide. Spanish explorers brought alfalfa to the New World, and gold prospectors carried it from South America into California.
	Alfalfa is hardy and easy to grow. It thrives in varied climates throughout the world from the temperate agricultural regions of the Mediterranean to the extremes of the very cold northern plains, high mountain valleys, and searing hot deserts.

Description

Alfalfa is a green, herbaceous legume living for three to twelve years, depending on the seed variety and environmental conditions. It has bluish-purple or yellow flowers that grow from a tall, erect, and smooth stem. The seed pods appear spiraled. Alfalfa is usually harvested in the summertime once it has grown one to three feet. Alfalfa exhibits auto-toxicity and resists reseeding in existing alfalfa fields. Plant rotation is required to maintain a consistent yield.

As one of the earliest cultivated plants, alfalfa has been used for centuries for feeding livestock. The cattle readily digest the nutritious, high-protein fodder. However, the human digestive tract cannot break down the fiber in the alfalfa plant as animals do, making it less appealing as a viable food source. The nutrient and medicinal benefits we derive from the plant are made available to us when prepared as an herb remedy (as described above).

Deep Roots:
Alfalfa has an extensive and deep root system, stretching up to 50 feet. This makes it very resilient, especially to droughts. It also accounts for the abundance of minerals, vitamins, and nutrients found in the herb. In the right conditions, alfalfa roots can pull and absorb valuable nutrients from surrounding soil up to 125 feet below the earth's surface. Alfalfa also has the ability to draw on nitrogen from the air in which it grows, yielding a high-protein plant that literally feeds the soil nitrogen.

Aloe

Latin Name: *Aloe Vera*
Aloe barbadensis

Also known as: Barbados Aloe, Medicine Plant, Lily of the Desert, True Aloe, Burn Aloe, First Aid Plant, Wand of Heaven, Elephant's Gall

Scientific Classification

There are more than 300 species of the aloe plant. There are three principal varieties: Barbados (or Curacao aloes), Socotrine aloes, and Cape aloes.

Family: Asphodelaceae

also Family: Liliaceae, lily family – Used by earlier classification systems. The lily family was formerly a 'catch-all' group that included a great number of genera now classified in other families. We include it here, as so much of our knowledge about herbs is founded on earlier manuals and literature that use this nomenclature.

Subfamily: Aloeaceae – aloe family

Genus: Aloe – aloe

Species:
- A. *vera*, also known as *A. barbadensis* – barbados or curacao in earlier literature. Stronger than Socotrine aloes in purgative action, of West Indies.
- B. *perryi* – Perry's aloe. Socotrine aloes including Zanzibar, of East Africa.
- C. *ferox* – Cape aloes. More powerfully purgative than any other variety and preferred in Europe. Chiefly employed in the United States for veterinary purposes, of South Africa.

True aloes are natives of the Old World and are not to be confused with the so-called New World 'American Aloe' plant, known better as the Agave Americana. In practicality, there is no likeness between aloes and agave plants

Influence on the Body	(PRINCIPAL ACTIONS are listed in CAPITAL LETTERS)
Blood and Circulatory System	heart (increases oxygen) • anemia • BLEEDING • CIRCULATION • BLOOD CLEANSING • reduces high blood pressure • varicose veins • thins blood
Body System	DEMULCENT (softens and soothes inflammation of mucous membranes) • stimulant (increases internal heat, dispels internal

ALOE — 12

	chill, and strengthens metabolism and circulation) • tonic (increases energy and strength throughout the body)
Cleansing	DEODORANT • BLOOD CLEANSING • topical cleanser • detoxifying • DEPURATIVE (cleanses blood by promoting eliminative functions)
Diabetes	Diabetes (blood sugar)
Digestive Tract	bitter (stimulates digestive juices and improves appetite) • HEARTBURN • HYPER ACIDITY • DIGESTION • INDIGESTION • SOOTHES STOMACH • peptic ulcers • regulates bowels • constipation • colic • COLITIS • GASTRITIS • COLON CLEANSER • PURGATIVE (causes watery evacuation of intestinal contents) • ENEMAS • Diverticulitis • dysentery • HEMORRHOIDS • EXPELS PIN WORMS • tapeworm
Ears	tinnitus • ear infection
Eyes	eyesight circulation • pink eye
First Aid	abrasions • cuts • WOUNDS • SCAR TISSUE • calluses •corns • WARTS • BED SORES • ULCERATED SORES •leg ulcers • bruises • TISSUE REPAIR • BURNS • SCALDS •THERMAL BURNS • SUNBURN • RADIATION BURNS •FROST BITE • INSECT BITES or STINGS • POISON IVY •POISON OAK
Infections and Immune System	• AIDS • ALLERGIES • antibacterial • antifungal • antimicrobial • antiviral • antiseptic • athlete's foot • FLU • fever blisters • HERPES • RINGWORM
Inflammation	inflammation • arthritis • rheumatism • bursitis
Liver	jaundice • liver disorders • gallbladder (bile flow)
Lungs	asthma • tuberculosis
Mouth and Throat	CANKER SORES • DENTURE SORES • tonsillitis
Nervous System	nerves • nervous condition
Pain	TOPICAL PAIN • CONTACT HEALER • POULTICE • headache
Reproductive System	*Female* regulates menstruation • diminished flow • vaginitis • douche • sore breasts • weaning
Skin, Tissue and Hair	ACNE • pimples • SKIN ERUPTIONS • SKIN IRRITATIONS

	• EMOLLIENT (softens and soothes skin when applied externally and mucous membranes when taken internally) • ANAL FISSURES • CHICKEN POX ITCH • ECZEMA • shingles • PSORIASIS (use gel form) • skin wrinkles • CELLULAR REGENERATION • promotes hair growth • SEBORRHEA
Urinary Tract	bladder infection • kidney infection

Key Properties:

CATHARTIC	*causes rapid bowel evacuation*
ACCELERATES HEALING	*cleanses out waste, fights infection, improves cell regeneration, soothes skin and mucous membranes*
BLOOD CLEANSING	*eliminates waste, balances acidity*
DIGESTIVE AID	*soothes, relieves gas, cleanses colon, expels worms*
Primarily affecting	*SKIN • STOMACH • COLON*

History	Aloe is known worldwide as a healing plant. It was considered to be a 'plant of immortality' in ancient Egypt, and it is reported to have been a secret beauty aid of Egyptian queens including Cleopatra and Nefertiti. The Egyptian secret of embalming is believed to include aloes in its process. Muhammadans, especially those in Egypt, regard the aloe as a religious symbol, and those who have made a pilgrimage to the shrine of the Prophet are entitled to hang the aloe over their doorway. They believe that this holy symbol protects a householder from evil influence. In Cairo, the Jews also adopted the practice of hanging up aloe. The word 'aloes' as used in the Bible (Psalms 45:8; Song of Solomon 4:14; Proverbs 7:17; and John 19:39) probably designates a plant totally distinct from aloes of today, namely the resinous wood of Aquilaria *agallocha*, a large tree growing in the Malayan Peninsula. Its wood constituted a drug which was valued for use as incense and is still esteemed in the East. The Greek historian Dioscorides, Roman philosopher Pliny in the first century, and 2nd century Greek philosopher Celsus wrote of aloes as effective treatments for burns, constipation, and kidney ailments.

An early record of aloe is found as an ancient cave painting in South Africa. In the 3rd century, Alexander the Great is said to have captured an island off Somalia for the sole purpose of possessing its luxurious crop of aloe.

Reference to aloe as one of the drugs recommended to Alfred the Great (King of England 871-899 AD) by the Patriarch of Jerusalem infers that its use was known in Britain as early as the 9th century. At that time, aloe was imported into Europe by way of the Red Sea and Alexandria.

In the early part of the 17th century, there was a direct trade in aloes between England and Socotra. In the records of the East India Company, there are notices of the drug being bought from the King of Socotra (the produce being a monopoly of the Sultan of the island at that time).

In 1935, aloe vera was reported as being used in the treatment of certain types of burns such as third-degree X-ray burns. (2) More recently, aloe vera has been acclaimed as a treatment for atomic radiation burns.

Today, aloe vera is most commonly known for its laxative, cleansing, and healing effects when taken internally. Applied topically, it is known for its abilities to moisturize, soothe, and regenerate skin cell tissues.

Attributes	Aloe vera is a widely used healing herb taken both internally and applied externally on the skin. It soothes irritations, builds up weakened bodies, helps tissues to heal faster, pulls poisons out of the body through the bowel and the skin, and acts as a bulk-forming laxative. The gel is mild tasting, while the juice scraped from the inside rind of the leaf is rather bitter.
Nutrients	**Key Components:** *(including, but not limited to)* *Vitamins* A • B9 (folic acid) • B12 • Choline • C • E • Calcium • Chromium • Copper • Iron • Magnesium • Manganese • Potassium • Selenium • Sodium • Zinc • 20 Amino Acids • 8 Enzymes (including Bradykinase, which helps reduce excessive inflammation when applied to the skin topically) • Sugars • Fatty Acids • Hormones (which help in wound healing and have anti-inflammatory action) • Anthraquinones (which are laxatives – including Aloin and Emodin)

Infectious Diseases	Aloe vera contains some 200 nutrients that have been found to be beneficial to man.

Aloe vera has antibacterial, antimicrobial and antifungal activities. Extracts have been shown to inhibit the growth of fungi that cause tinea (ringworm). (3) The inner-leaf gel from aloe vera has been shown to inhibit growth of the bacteria Streptococcus and Shigella. (4) |
| **External Uses**

Skin | Aloe vera gel is what is used topically on the skin for soothing, moisturizing, and healing. It is transdermal (passes through the skin barrier), penetrating quickly into the top three layers of skin, bringing nutrients and healing to the surrounding tissues.

Applied topically, aloe vera gel naturally balances the pH of skin. It seems the Egyptian queens knew what they were doing. The plant's enzymes soften the skin by accelerating the removal of dead cells, increasing moisture, stimulating the normal growth of living cells, fighting the effects of aging, and bringing health and beauty to the skin.

Aloe vera is added to many cosmetics and shampoos. Beware of products which also contain harmful additives, chemicals, or colorings, as these will penetrate the skin barrier along with the aloe vera gel. |
| *Burns* | If you know anything about aloe vera, you have heard of its healing properties associated with various types of burns. It is used to stop the burning sensation and to reduce the chance of infection and scarring. It is especially beneficial for first and second degree thermal and acid burns. Aloe vera gel helps prevent progressive skin damage caused by burns and frostbite.

A 2007 study review concludes that the cumulative evidence supports the use of aloe vera for the healing of first to second degree burns. (5) |
| *Caution* | Some aloe vera preparations contain lanolin, a product that softens and moisturizes the skin. However, lanolin will intensify a burn and should not be used in burn care. Read the label. Make sure the aloe vera product you use for burns does not contain lanolin. |

In addition, do not use aloe vera products on burns that have any type of toxic ingredients in them. It will absorb directly into the skin and inhibit the healing process.

Wounds

Aloe vera gel clearly promotes wound healing by penetrating and cleansing injured tissue, soothing and reducing inflammation, and opening the capillaries to increase blood flow to and from the injury. (6)(7)

The gel can be used for all manner of cuts, abrasions, rashes, skin irritations, and eruptions. It works to prevent and draw out infection, cleansing and healing wounds rapidly. Aloe vera stimulates circulation and the growth of new cells. A piece of white linen or cotton saturated in aloe vera water and applied to fresh wounds, as well as old ones, quickly closes them. It has also been used successfully by nursing mothers for easing sore breasts.

If ulcerous wounds progress to a running stage, sprinkle aloe vera powder thick enough to cover the open wound, secure with clean gauze, and repeat daily. The powder will absorb the morbid fluid matter, while encouraging healthy, new replacement tissue.

For radiation treatments given on the skin, aloe vera leaves prepared with castor oil or eucalyptus oil can moisturize, heal and prevent further complications.

Seborrhea

Seborrhea is a fairly common skin condition, leading to oily, red, and scaly eruptions in such areas as the eyebrows, eyelids, nose, ear, upper lip, chest, groin, and chin. A recent double-blind, placebo-controlled study indicates aloe vera may help relieve the symptoms of seborrheic dermatitis. In the study, 44 adults applied either an aloe vera ointment or a placebo cream to affected areas twice a day for 4-6 weeks. Of the aloe vera group, 62 percent (versus 25 percent for the placebo group) reported their symptoms improved significantly. Doctors also noted that those using aloe vera had fewer seborrheic areas, with reduced scaliness and itching. (8)

Herpes, Psoriasis

Topical application of aloe vera may be effective for genital herpes and psoriasis. (9)

Eyesight

You can use the pure gel as an eyedrop to improve circulation and eyesight.

ALOE — 17

Internal Uses

Digestion and Elimination

Both the gel and the inner and outer rind juice (or powdered form) are used internally.

Aloe vera increases digestion, absorption, and cleansing. It neutralizes body toxins, thus reducing arthritic pain caused by tissue toxicity. Aloe vera absorbs toxins and promotes the growth of friendly colon bacteria. Early studies suggest that internal use of aloe vera gel may reduce symptoms and inflammation in patients with ulcerative colitis. (10)

Aloe vera gel has laxative qualities, while the bitter 'latex' juice is a powerful purgative for acute or chronic constipation. The eliminative action of both forms is due to a stimulation of peristalsis (intestinal contractions that propel contents onward), particularly in the larger bowel. As its action is fairly limited to the colon, it is not recommended when the entire intestinal system requires cleansing.

Aloe vera juice may cause uncontrollable bowel spasms in its raw form. Taking ginger, slippery elm bark, fennel, and peppermint in tea or capsules will moderate the griping tendency. Aloes are one of the safest and best stimulating purgatives for persons of sedentary habits and sluggish constitutions. An ordinary small dose takes 15-18 hours to produce an effect. Its action on the large intestine makes it useful as a vermifuge (expelling worms).

The German pharmacopoeia recommends aloe vera for treating acute constipation, anal fissures, hemorrhoids, and other disorders in which defecation with a soft stool is desired. Also, for emptying the bowels before X-rays, and both before and after abdominal and rectal operations.

Aloe vera juice may be safely taken for several days. Be aware that prolonged use of purgative laxatives may tax the body and electrolyte mineral balance of the body. In my opinion, it is better to eliminate waste than to let it back up and damage the system. To compensate, replace minerals and electrolytes as needed, and discontinue laxative use if diarrhea occurs.

The FDA Regulates Aloin in over-the-counter (OTC) drugs: Aloin, naturally occurring in aloe plants, was a common ingredient in OTC laxative products in the United States prior to 2003. Because companies that manufactured them at the time did not provide necessary safety data, the FDA required that OTC aloe laxative products be reformulated or removed from the U.S. market. (1)

Processed aloe vera that contains aloin is used primarily as a laxative, whereas processed aloe vera juice that does not contain significant amounts of aloin is used as a digestive healer. Manufacturers commonly remove aloin in processing due to the FDA ruling.

Gingivitis and Plaque

In a double-blind clinical trial, the group using an aloe vera containing dentifrice demonstrated a statistically significant reduction of gingivitis and plaque. (11)

Diabetes

Aloe vera gel may improve blood sugar control in individuals with type 2 diabetes. The results of a single-blind, placebo-controlled trial showed significantly greater improvements in blood sugar levels among those given aloe vera over the two-week treatment period. (8)

Another single-blind, placebo-controlled trial evaluated the benefits of aloe vera in individuals who had failed to respond to their diabetes medications. Of the 36 individuals who completed the study, those taking aloe vera along with their medicine showed definite improvements in blood sugar levels over 42 days as compared to those taking their medicine and a placebo. (8)

Internal intake of aloe vera has been linked with improved blood glucose levels in diabetics. (12)(13) A dosage of one tablespoon of aloe vera juice twice daily has been used effectively in diabetic studies.

Psoriasis, Cankers and Blood Sugar

Human clinical trials also prove aloe vera effective for treating psoriasis, cankers, and lowering blood sugar. (14)

Heart

A study of 5,000 subjects found a positive effect of lowering risk factors in patients with heart disease. The study showed that by adding aloe vera gel and a bulking agent to the diet, there was a marked reduction in total lipids, overall serum cholesterol, serum triglycerides, fasting and post-meal blood sugar levels in diabetics, and an increase in HDL (high-density lipoproteins, the 'good' cholesterol). (15) Another study also showed lower blood lipids in hyperlipidaemic patients using aloe vera. (16)

Immune System

It is believed that by balancing the pH levels of the blood, aloe vera is able to boost the immune system.

	Researchers at Tokyo Women's Medical College in Japan have shown that certain proteins in aloe vera gel may stimulate the immune system to increase production of killer cells or naturally occurring lymphocytes that kill bacteria and tumor cells. (6) Studies in Japan and the Netherlands suggest that constituents in aloe vera gel can enhance the workings of the immune system by containing the killer cells' lethal chemicals, preventing them from damaging healthy, functional cells. (6)
Anti-Viral	A polysaccharide called acemannan from the aloe vera leaf rind has been found to impair the ability of viruses, including retroviruses like HIV (human immunodeficiency virus), to infect healthy T-cells. This effectively limits the HIV virus from going from one cell to the next, thus keeping the virus from moving through the body. The overall effect is to stabilize the body's natural life force and allow the immune system to get rid of the remaining invaders.
Women	Aloe vera facilitates and regularizes menstrual flow. It makes an excellent douche for vaginal discharge and irritation.
	Use with caution when pregnant. We recommend that you consult your health care practitioner. When given to nursing mothers, it can cause purging in the suckling infant. If this happens, discontinue use.
Herb Parts Used	The dried and fresh juice of the leaves, the whole leaves, gel from the water-storing tissue, and the roots are all used for medicinal purposes. The central, pulp, gel-like substance is believed to contain the wound-healing agents. The inside of the leaf is scraped and also harvested. This makes a yellow juice substance, sometimes called 'latex', which can be dried and powdered.
Preparations and Remedies	There are a wide variety of commercially processed aloe vera products. Read labels carefully to ensure you are getting what you want. In general, there are two unique (though related) aloe vera products found in the leaf. The gel (also made into a juice) and a juice scraped from the rind of the inside of the leaf surrounding the gel (referred to as aloe vera juice, aloe vera latex, or aloe aloin). Whole leaf aloe vera is also available, which seems to have a stronger effect on the immune system.

Aloe Vera Gel

The inner, jelly-like pulp of the leaf is called aloe vera gel. It is typically applied topically or made into a juice for internal healing applications.

The gel is extracted by various means commercially. Most involve pressing, but some methods entail solvent extraction, which can alter the properties of the gel. I do not recommend this method.

The gel is used in commercially made lotions, yogurt, beverages, and some desserts. Remember, aloe vera goes deep into the cells and takes toxins and chemicals that are added with it. Avoid aloe vera preparations with added preservatives and chemicals.

External Use

Apply gel as needed, several times a day on wounds and other skin conditions. Gel may be left on for up to two days without changing the application. If the whole leaf is being used, cut off the spines around the edges, fillet the leaf to expose the inner gel, and apply it directly to the site, leaving the outer leaf attached. You may also scrape the gel into a container and then apply it to the injury as you would a prepared gel purchased from a quality health store

Burns

1st degree burns - Reddened skin
Use cold water to stop further injury and to relieve the burning sensation. Open fresh aloe vera leaf or use a prepared aloe vera gel (no lanolin). You can also add a few drops of lavender essential oil to the gel before smoothing on the skin for its tissue-healing properties.

2nd degree burns - Reddened skin and blisters
Use cold water to relieve burning sensation. Then prepare a poultice made of aloe vera juice or gel and extra virgin olive oil, Vitamin E, or castor oil. Gently drop some oil on the skin before applying the poultice to prevent pulling when poultice is removed. Gently cover area with the poultice for further healing and regeneration of cell tissues.

3rd degree burns - Skin destroyed and charred
Seek medical care immediately! Do not apply water or remove clothing. Wrap the area in a cold, wet cloth and have the burned individual lie down and treat for shock as needed. If the skin is charred, use sterile, cold, moist cloths dipped in aloe vera juice or gel to relieve burning sensation and cleanse the area. When appropriate, apply a poultice as described for second degree

burns. Depending on the degree of burn and the percent of the body burned, additional medical assistance may be required.

Aloe Vera Juice (from the gel)

Externally:
A freshly broken leaf of the plant is the best source of aloe vera gel. The process of separating the gel and the inner-rind juice is not always complete, so aloe vera latex may be found in some aloe vera gels. This may or may not matter, depending on how it is being used.

Processed products are difficult to keep stable. Refrigeration may extend the quality of the product. Many commercial products add preservatives. Some are natural (Vitamin E oil, essential oils, etc.) and others are not.

It is a common practice for companies to add aloe vera gel, sap, or other aloe vera derivatives to their products (such as makeup, tissues, moisturizers, soaps, sunscreens, incense, razors, and shampoos). Read the label. Ingredient lists are arranged in descending order according to quantity. If aloe vera is listed in the middle or towards the end of the list, or if the product contains large amounts of filler, there is reason to suspect that the product is not of high medicinal value and may even harm skin and tissues.

I do not recommend using creams, lotions, sunscreens, soaps, shampoos, or any beauty products that have artificial ingredients added to aloe vera, as the natural aloe vera will bring the chemical toxins deep into the tissues.

Internally:
Used for consumption and relief of digestive issues. Take one to two teaspoons up to three times daily. Discontinue if diarrhea occurs. When it subsides, you can start again with a lesser amount.

Aloe Vera Juice/Powder

When collecting the yellow, bitter-tasting juice, the leaves (from the rind) are cut off close to the base of the stem and placed so that the juice is drained off into tubs. This juice is concentrated by evaporation or, more generally, by boiling until it becomes the consistency of thick honey. Once cooled, it is poured into containers and solidified. The color changes as it is exposed to air, becoming a dark brown resin.

ALOE — 22

Commercial aloin is a refined form of the resulting resin, which contains high concentrations of barbaloin (aloe vera's main laxative constituent). The resin is further processed into a powder or granule product and put into capsules or tablets for ingestion without the bitter taste.

Aloe vera latex is used for severe constipation and cleansing but should not be used in cases of bowel obstruction. It is highly effective and useful as a laxative when taken properly.

Pure aloe vera latex should be taken as recommended and may require the supervision of a qualified health professional. High doses or prolonged use may tax the body. (see **SAFETY** below)

Internally:
The recommended dose for acute constipation is 100-300 mg per day of the aloe vera resin/latex, before bed, in capsules or tablets. To reduce cramping, add orange peel or fennel seed. Follow the label's instruction for liquid gel latex.

Safety

Topical Aloe Vera Gel: No known adverse side effects.
Aloe Vera Gel Juice: Aloe vera gel juice taken internally may lower blood glucose levels. This should be taken into consideration when taking insulin and hypo- or hyper-glycemic therapies that also lower blood glucose levels.
Aloe Vera Latex: In large doses, aloe vera latex products may increase the action of other laxatives and should not be taken at the same time. With chronic use/abuse of purgative laxatives of any kind, a potassium deficiency may develop.
Avoid taking internally during pregnancy

Plant Profile

Natural Habitat:
Aloes are indigenous to East and South Africa but have been introduced into the West Indies (where they are extensively cultivated) and into tropical countries. One variety has been discovered in the remote districts of southwest Africa growing 30 to 60 feet in height, with stems as much as 10 feet in circumference.

After being introduced at the beginning of the 16th century, aloe vera products were produced on the island of Barbados, where it was then largely cultivated. It is still frequently, but improperly, called Barbados Aloes, for it is almost entirely grown commercially on the Dutch islands of Curacoa, Aruba, and Bonaire. Their dried juice product is usually opaque and varies in color from bright yellow or rich reddish brown to black.

It is also cultivated and found wild in northern Africa, the Near East, Asia, and in the southern Mediterranean region. The species has been widely cultivated throughout the world, having been introduced to China, India, Pakistan, and parts of southern Europe in the 17th century. Large scale agricultural production to supply the cosmetics industry with aloe vera gel is undertaken in Australia, Cuba, the Dominican Republic, China, Mexico, India, Jamaica, Kenya, South Africa, and the USA.

Plant Description

Aloe vera is a perennial (plant that lives for more than two years) which grows wild in temperate and tropical areas or may be grown as a houseplant in less favorable climates. The leaves grow from the center in a stemless rosette of spiny, tapered, succulent (thick and fleshy) green or gray-green leaves, with some varieties showing white flecks. The edges of the leaves are serrated with small white teeth.

The cuticle, which covers every part of the plant, is formed to absorb and retain moisture. A leaf separated from the parent plant can be laid in the sun for several weeks without becoming entirely shriveled. Even when dried by long heat exposure, it will become plump and fresh again in a few hours if placed in water.

Aloe vera grows as tall as two to three feet (or less if they are grown in a constricted space). Yellow or red bell-shaped flowers are borne atop a tall, erect stalk that can grow up to three feet tall in the summertime; however, they rarely flower in cool climates. The capsule-like fruits are triangular and contain many seeds.

Aloe veras are widely cultivated for their healing and commercial uses. While all aloe plants exhibit similar qualities, the aloe vera species is most commonly used medicinally and commercially. Its inner, mucus-like sap called 'gel' (resembling slightly-melted clear to lemon-colored gelatin) is rich in over 200 nutrients known to be beneficial to mankind and, due to the size and softness of the leaves, can easily produce a high quality, high-yield product.

Aloe vera juice (sometimes called aloe vera latex) is a bitter, yellow exudate found in the rind just beneath the outer skin of the leaves. Near the outer skin of the leaves is a row of fibrovascular bundles with enlarged cells filled with a yellow juice which exudes when the leaf is cut. Aloe veras require two or three year's growth before they yield their juice. The juice can be dried to produce aloe 'granules' (rich in aloin) and used as a laxative.

Growing Aloe Vera

Aloe veras grow naturally in arid climates and are best grown in tropical and warm zones with well-drained soil that is low in organic matter. The roots will rot if exposed to long periods of wet soil. If water and soil are too alkaline, growth may be slow. Aloe veras prefer full sun but can tolerate light shade. They do not tolerate temperatures below 41° F.

In climates with frost or snow, the species is best kept indoors or in heated glasshouses. Avoid over watering indoors and mix coarse sand with the potting soil to facilitate good drainage. Terracotta pots are practical as they are porous. Let potted plants completely dry prior to re-watering. During the winter, aloe veras may become dormant and require less moisture.

Planting

Aloe veras can be grown from seed or by division of the parent plant. New shoots must be 'pruned' or leaves turn bright green and grow horizontally rather than vertically. When new shoots are four inches tall, break them off from the parent and repot them in prepared soil. You may also cut off an overlong stalk and simply plant it in a pot. It will root readily. Water well and then leave for three weeks to form a network of water-seeking roots.

Harvesting

Cut leaves as needed. Aloe vera grows from the center. Cut the older, outside leaves that have more juice with a sharp knife at the base of the plant. Using the outer leaves will keep the plant in balance and promote new growth from the center. Leaves do not grow back once they are cut.

Storage

Whole leaf:
The gel is best used when it is fresh, but if needed, you may store cut leaves for a week or two by wrapping the whole leaf in cellophane at 50-70° F (the refrigerator is too cold).

Juice:
You may bottle the extracted gel or juice and keep it in the refrigerator for several days. To extract the juice, trim the thorny edges of the leaves and split the leaf across its width to extract the gooey gel. As the gel ceases to flow, scratch the exposed leaf and continue to do so until only the green leaf skin is left.

Barley

Latin Name: *Hordeum vulgare*

Also known as: Barley Grass, Pearl Barley, Pearled Barley, Pot Barley, Scotch Barley, Sprouted Barley, Sprouted Barley Malt

Scientific Classification

Traditional classification of barley divides similar forms of barley into separate species. For example, two-rowed barley with shattering spikes (wild barley) is Hordeum *spontaneum*; with non-shattering spikes, *H. distichum*; six-rowed barley with non-shattering spikes as *H. vulgare*, with shattering spikes as *H. agriocrithon*. These differences are minor. Form, structure, and function of the plants are similar, leading most recent classifications to treat these variations as a single species, *H. vulgare*.

Family: Poaceae / Gramineae – grass family
Genus: Hordeum – barley
Species: *H. vulgare* – common barley

H. distichum (and many more)

Influence on the Body	(PRINCIPAL ACTIONS are listed in CAPITAL LETTERS)
Addictions	Smoking
Blood and Circulatory System	ANEMIA • BLOOD PURIFIER • cholesterol • heart disease • high blood pressure
Body System	general ILLNESS • demulcent (softens and soothes inflammation of mucous membranes) • tonic (increases energy and strengthens the muscular and nervous system while improving digestion and assimilation, resulting in a general sense of well-being.
Cleansing	body odor • heavy metals • METAL POISONING • toxic conditions
Diabetes	Diabetes (blood sugar)
Digestive Tract	digestion • NUTRITIVE • ulcers • gastritis • constipation • POLYPS
Endocrine System	Pancreatitis
Infections and Immune System	allergies • hay fever • infections • FEVERS • virus attack • herpes • leprosy • CANCER • AIDS • immuno-stimulant
Inflammation	INFLAMMATION • ARTHRITIS • MUCOUS MEMBRANE

Liver	Hepatitis
Lungs and Respiratory System	bronchitis • asthma • tuberculosis
Muscles	lumbago (lower backache) • MUSCULAR DYSTROPHY
Nervous System	adapt genic (increases resistance to stress) • anxiety
Reproductive System	syphilis *Male:* impotence
Skin, Tissue and Hair	skin problems • emollient (softens and soothes skin when applied externally, and mucous membranes when taken internally) • acne • eczema • psoriasis • BOILS • LIVER SPOTS • ANTI-AGING
Urinary Tract	Kidney
Weight	EXCESSIVE APPETITE • obesity

Key Properties:

NUTRITIVE	*full of nutrients, builds blood, improves appetite, anti-aging, regulates blood sugar balance, provides bulk*
BLOOD CLEANSER	*cleanses system, lowers blood cholesterol*
Primarily affecting	BLOOD • COLON

History	Barley is one of the most ancient of cultivated grains. Barley seeds have been found in tombs in Asia Minor dating from about 3500 B.C. According to Deuteronomy 8:8, ancient Israel used barley as one of the "Seven Species" of crops that characterized the fertility of the Promised Land of Canaan, and it had a prominent role in Israelite sacrifices. (Numbers 5:15). Alongside wheat, barley was a staple cereal and known as a sacred grain in ancient Egypt, where it was used to make bread and beer. Greek athletes attributed much of their strength to their barley-rich training diets. Roman athletes continued this tradition. Gladiators were known as hordearii, which simply means 'eaters of barley.' In the grain form, barley is known for its soothing and strengthening properties. It is easy to assimilate into the digestive system. Barley water has been used for various medicinal purposes. An entire book on the benefits of gruel made from

barley was written by Hypocrites (460-377 BC).

In Islam, the Prophet Muhammad (570-630 AD) prescribed barley for seven diseases. These included grief, high cholesterol levels, heart disease, treatment of cancer, diabetes, hypertension, and the effects of aging. It was also said to soothe and calm the bowels.

In his 11th century work, *The Canon of Medicine*, Avicenna wrote of the healing effects of barley water, soup, and broth for fevers.

Europeans in the Middle Ages made bread with a combination of barley and rye because wheat was expensive and not always available. English herbalist and physician Nicholas Culpeper (1616 - 1654 AD) wrote of barley as giving 'great nourishment to persons troubled with fevers, agues, and heats in the stomach.'

The Spanish introduced barley to South America in the 16th century, while the English and Dutch settlers brought barley with them to the North American colonies in the 17th century. It was one of the first crops planted in the Virginia Colony in 1611.

Today, the largest commercial producers of barley are Canada, the United States, Germany, France, Spain, and the Russian Federation. Half of the United States' barley production is used as animal feed, with smaller amounts used for health food products and malting (principally for beer and whiskey manufacture).

Attributes

Whole Grain:
The whole grain cereal known as barley is a nutritious food source with significant contributions to health and healing. Although the grain is not considered an herb supplement, the health benefits are worth mentioning.

Barley Grass:
Young barley grass is what is typically referred to when discussing barley as an herb. It is used as a raw powder, freeze dried, evaporated powder or juiced product as health supplements.

Barley Grain

Barley is a wonderfully versatile cereal grain with a rich nut-like flavor and an appealing chewy, pasta-like consistency (due to its gluten content). Its appearance resembles wheat berries, although it is slightly lighter in color. Sprouted barley is naturally high in maltose, a sugar that serves as the basis for malt, syrup sweetener and (when fermented) as an ingredient in alcoholic and non-alcoholic beer and other alcoholic beverages.

Nutrition

Found in Whole Grain Cereal

Key Components: *(including, but not limited to)*

Vitamins B1 (thiamine) • B2 (riboflavin) • B3 (niacin or nicotinic acid) • B5 (pantothenic acid) • B6 (pyridoxine) • B9 (folic acid) • C • Calcium (most Americans do not get enough calcium in their diets) • Copper (a cofactor in essential enzymes affecting the substance and flexibility of blood vessels, bones and joints) • Iron • Magnesium • Manganese • Phosphorus (found in cell structures, bone matrix, DNA, and energy systems of the body) • Potassium • Selenium • Zinc • Dietary Fiber • Carbohydrates • Fats • Proteins • all eight Essential Amino Acids • Lignans

Digestion

For weak and fragile individuals, barley water and gruel has been used since ancient times to provide easily assimilated nourishment and for increasing strength and stamina.

Barley's fiber promotes regularity, overall intestinal protection, and relieves diarrhea, gastritis, and inflammatory bowel conditions. As a source of bulk, it decreases the transit time of fecal matter, lowering the risk of colon cancer and hemorrhoids.

Barley's dietary fiber provides food for the 'friendly' bacteria in the large intestine, and, as they grow in number, they crowd out pathogenic (disease-causing) bacteria from surviving in the intestinal tract. When these helpful bacteria break down barley's insoluble fiber, they produce a short-chain fatty acid called butyric acid, which helps maintain a healthy colon.

Cholesterol and Heart Disease

Numerous studies report a lowering of cholesterol and fatty lipids in the blood, measurably reducing the risk of high blood pressure and heart attack with the regular use of barley. (1)(2)(3)(4)(5)

Barley is one of the foods the FDA (U.S. Federal Drug Administration) permits to display a health claim stating consumption is linked to lower risk of heart disease and certain cancers. These include foods that have at least 51 percent whole grains by weight, low in fat, saturated fat, and cholesterol.

Blood Sugar

The dietary fiber in barley helps to prevent blood sugar levels from rising too high in people with diabetes. According to a recent study, eating whole grain barley can regulate blood sugar levels for up to 10 hours after consumption. (6)

Barley and other whole grains are a rich source of magnesium, a mineral that acts as a co-factor for more than 300 enzymes. These include enzymes affecting the body's use of glucose and insulin secretion. Research now suggests that regular consumption of whole grains reduces risk of type 2 diabetes. (7)(8)(9)

Asthma

Increasing consumption of whole grains and fish can reduce the risk of childhood asthma by about 50 percent, according to the International Study on Allergy and Asthma in Childhood. (10)

Cancer

Barley packs a two-sided attack against certain cancers. By providing fiber needed to minimize the amount of time cancer-causing substances spend in contact with colon cells, and by being a good source of selenium, which has been shown to significantly reduce the risk of colon cancer. (11)

Lignans found in barley are thought to protect against breast and other hormone-dependent cancers, as well as heart disease. Studies found that a diet rich in fiber from whole grains (such as barley) and fruit offered significant protection against breast cancer for pre-menopausal women. (12)(13)

Obesity

Studies have clearly shown that dietary fiber is an important tool in the prevention of obesity. Compared to an average American meal, a fiber-rich meal is processed more slowly, and nutrient absorption occurs over a longer period of time. Nutritionists conclude that fiber promotes satiety (feeling full) and satisfies the body's craving for nutrients by increasing the absorption of micronutrients. Long term observational studies consistently report lower weight in individuals consuming higher levels of fiber. (14)(15)(16)

Barley Grass

Young barley grass contains more concentrated nutrients than adult barley grass, having increased amounts of live enzymes, protein, vitamins, minerals, and chlorophyll. I have seen the biggest change and improvement in people's health when they add what I call 'greens' to their diet. By 'greens', I mean barley grass and alfalfa grass.

Taking 1 or more tablespoons of greens a day, mixed in juice or water, is like adding jet fuel to your engine. You feel it and your body responds by using the blast of added nutrients to help the body heal. I believe it to be, by far, the best daily supplement anyone can take. Try it for yourself. Take 1 tablespoon of greens for 30 days, and you will be a believer!

Nutrients in Barley Grass	Key Components: *(including, but not limited to)*
Vitamins	A (in the form of beta carotene, comparison tests have shown barley grass juice powder to have as much as 6 times more than that found in spinach) • B1 (thiamine - has 30 times more than cow's milk) • B2 (riboflavin) • B5 (pantothenic acid) • B6 (pyridoxine) • B9 (folic acid) • B12 (cobalamin, works to overcome fatigue and anemia) • C (has nearly 7 times more than an equal amount of oranges) • E
Minerals	• Calcium (11 times that found in cow's milk) • Copper • Iron (5 times the iron in spinach) • Magnesium • Manganese • Phosphorus • Potassium • Sodium • Zinc • trace minerals
Other Components	• Chlorophyll • Enzymes • Super Oxide Dismutase (SOD, a free radical scavenger, in greater amounts than most any other food source available. It is an excellent blood and immune builder) • eighteen Amino Acids (including all eight essential ones)
Chlorophyll	Barley grass has very high chlorophyll levels. Chlorophyll accounts for many of the health benefits derived from taking barley grass. It works synergistically with other nutrients in barley to renew cell growth, to cleanse the body of wastes, bacteria, toxins, heavy metals, and pollutants, to facilitate the oxygen exchange in blood, and to counter-balance acids and restore healthy pH levels (the measure of acidity and alkalinity) in the body.
Blood	An added benefit of green barley leaf proteins is that they are polypeptides (small proteins that can be directly absorbed by the blood), where they promote cell metabolism and neutralize substances that are bad for health.

The green pigment 'chlorophyll' is a protein found in most plants. Its molecular structure is similar to human red blood cell hemoglobin. So why don't we have green blood? The critical difference is the substitution of a magnesium molecule (in chlorophyll) in place of the iron (found in the heme group making up human hemoglobin). Chlorophyll in the blood has the same effect as iron, making it a natural blood builder and cleanser. This strengthens and may temporarily thicken the blood. As the body adjusts to the nutrients and cleanses the body of toxins and wastes, the blood ultimately thins to its natural level. |

BARLEY — 31

Cancer	According to Allan L. Goldstein, Ph.D., head of the biochemistry department at George Washington University's School of Medicine and Health Sciences in Washington, D.C., alpha-tocopherol succinate (a component of barley grass) seems to inhibit several types of cancer, including leukemia, brain tumors, and prostate cancer.
Cholesterol	Young barley grass and the juice powder helps reduce cholesterol.
Cleansing	Chlorophyll progressively cleans the blood, cells, tissues, and organs while providing nutrients for new cell life. It absorbs energy from the sun and has been called 'liquid sunshine.' In high enough amounts, chlorophyll is able to affect every cell and organ of the body (inside and out).
	Barley grass is a great cleanser. It detoxifies cells, normalizes metabolism, and neutralizes heavy metals such as lead and mercury.
Digestion	Barley grass and barley juice powder have been shown to be an anti-inflammatory agent, helping to heal stomach, duodenal ulcers and inflamed hemorrhoids.
Infections and Immune System	Barley grass boosts the immune system and reduces pancreas infections.
pH Balance	Barley grass contains buffer minerals: sodium, potassium, calcium, and magnesium, which help alkalinize the body and promote an ideal pH balance. Most processed foods (including red meat and coffee) are acidic. When we consume too many of them, the acidity/alkaline balance is upset.
Skin and Tissues	Barley grass promotes natural tissue repair and nourishes anti-aging mechanisms of the body. Chlorophyll accelerates the healing of damaged tissues by providing nutrients to the cells, increasing cell activity and growth, and cleansing out dead cell matter and wastes. It also stimulates wound healing on the skin and in the bowels while destroying toxins and disease-causing bacteria.
	In Japan, where barley grass extract is popular, it is reported to help the body heal from many illnesses. In one informal study, a Japanese dermatologist observed a group of seven patients with skin diseases ranging from melanosis (darkening of the skin) to

	eczema. The patients who took barley grass extract healed faster than those who did not take the extract. The patients taking barley grass extract also noticed improvements in appetite and bowel regularity. Antioxidants found in barley grass have been isolated and reported to have antioxidant activity equal or superior to that of Vitamin E. Research has further shown that when barley grass juice is added to injured cells, their DNA (deoxy-ribonucleic acid contains the genetic instructions for the development and function of living organisms) is rapidly repaired. This may contribute to preventing the changes that often lead to cancer and rapid aging.
Herb Parts Used	The whole grain cereal is considered a food, providing substantial health benefits, nutrients, and sustenance to the body. The young leaves and young grass made into powder are used for herbal supplementation.
Barley Grains	**Preparations and Remedies** Barley grain can be found in the market in various forms, including the following: *Hulled barley:* The outermost hull is removed. It is considered to be the whole-grain form of barley and is sometimes called dehulled or hull-less barley. *Pearl (or pearled) barley:* The grain is steam processed to remove the bran, then polished or 'pearled' to varying degrees. The total procedure takes off the outermost hull, the bran layer, and some of the inner layers. Most nutrients are in the outer bran layer. The amount of polishing determines the amount of nutrients lost in the end product. Pearl barley should always be washed before being boiled, as it is apt to accumulate dust. *Pot (or scotch) barley:* The grain is only slightly polished to remove the hull, leaving most of the grain intact. In many countries, pot barley is popular in soups, giving it its name. *Barley flakes:* Flattened and sliced, flakes are similar in shape to rolled oats.

Flakes can be made from hulled or pearl barley and varies in nutrient content for this reason.

Barley grits:
Barley that has been toasted and cracked. Grits are similar in appearance to bulgar. Barley grits can be made from hulled or pearl barley and varies in nutrient content for this reason.

Storage

Grain barley may be stored in tightly covered glass containers in a cool, dry place. Barley may also be stored in the refrigerator during periods of warmer weather.

Preparation Tips

Mix barley flour with wheat flour to make breads and muffins. Use cracked barley or barley flakes to make hot cereal.

Like all grains, rinse thoroughly before cooking barley, removing any dirt or debris that you may find. Add 1 part barley to 3-1/2 parts boiling water or broth. After the liquid has returned to a boil, turn down the heat, cover, and simmer. Pearled barley should be simmered for about 1 hour, while hulled barley should be cooked for about 90 minutes.

Combine cooked barley and healthy sautéed mushrooms for a pilaf. Toss chilled, cooked, hulled barley with chopped vegetables and dressing to make a tasty cold salad. Add barley to your favorite stews and soups to give them extra heartiness and flavor.

Poultices

A poultice made of barley meal, or flour boiled in vinegar and honey, eases inflammations where applied and has been used for swellings, leprosy, gout, and itching skin.

Decoction and Gruel

Barley Water (Decoction) and Gruel:
Barley prepared in the form of a watery decoction affords a mucilaginous drink much employed from the time of Hippocrates to the present. Pearl barley is preferred for the preparation of the decoction. It may be used for infants and convalescents, as it prevents large milk curd formation.

Pour four pints of boiling water over two ounces pearl barley. Boil away to two pints and strain. Use the infused liquid as barley water or mash the cooked barley for a nutritious gruel.

Keep the gruel closer to its liquid state for weaker stomachs (prone to vomiting), gradually adding more substance (cooked barley) as can be tolerated.

Optional: Lemon juice or raisins may be added to gruel for the last ten minutes of cooking time to suit taste.

Barley Grass

Vitamin and Nutrient Supplement:
Barley grass is generally cut, dried, and powered by evaporation at low temperatures (to protect the vital and sensitive nutrients found in barley grass) and used as a green drink powder in juice or water. It is also put into preparations or capsules for tasteless ingestion.

Eye Poultice:
Saturate white bread with the juice of freshly cut barley grass. Gently squeeze excess liquid from the bread and apply to the eyes while relaxing. This poultice will help clear eyes and relieve eye pain.

Barley Grass Juice Powder

Barley grass juice powder is made by separating the juice in the barley grass from the grass solids by rapid freeze-drying in an oxygen-free environment. This evaporates the water from the juice, leaving barley grass juice powder. The process of freeze-drying concentrates and preserves the food elements which are in the whole barley grass.

Safety

There are no known adverse side effects attributed to barley or barley grass.

Taking barley juice greens may temporarily alter blood thickness, as the body adjusts to available nutrients and blood cleansing actions. Dosage requirements for individuals taking blood thinning medications may be affected. Contact your health care professional to correctly monitor blood thickness and adjust medications if needed.

Plant Profile

Natural Habitat:
Barley originated and was cultivated for thousands of years in Ethiopia and Southeast Asia. It is now grown worldwide.
Barley is a highly adaptable crop. It is currently popular in temperate areas as a summer crop and in tropical areas as a winter crop. Its germination time is anywhere from one to three days. Barley has a short growing season and is relatively drought tolerant.

Barley can withstand more soil salinity than wheat, which might explain the increase of barley cultivation in Mesopotamia from the

2nd millennium BC onwards. Barley grows well in cool conditions but is not particularly winter hardy.

Plant Description

Barley is a cereal grain harvested from the annual (must be replanted yearly) grass Hordeum vulgare. The plant grows two to four feet high before harvesting. It has a long hollow stalk which bears an ear of grain at maturity. Each barley seed is enclosed in a strong hull which remains intact even during threshing. Barley is an important feed grain in many areas of the world.

Barley grass is the seedling of the barley plant. The young leaves are usually harvested about 200 days after germination, when the shoots are less than a foot tall. They have a tremendous ability to absorb nutrients from the soil and contain many vitamins, minerals, proteins, chlorophyll, and other nutrients that make it a valuable herb supplement.

Bilberry

Latin Name: *Vaccinium myrtillus*

Also known as: Blueberry (not the American variety of blueberry), European Blueberry, Myrtle Blueberry, Huckleberry, Whortleberry, Dyeberry, Blaeberry

Scientific Classification

In Europe, the bilberry is commonly called blueberry. It is related to the American blueberry, huckleberry, and cranberry, all different species of the Vaccinium genus. There are nearly 450 species of the genus Vaccinium.

Family: Ericaceae – heath family
Genus: Vaccinium – blueberry
Species: V. myrtillus – bilberry

Influence on the Body	(PRINCIPAL ACTIONS are listed in CAPITAL LETTERS)
Blood and Circulatory System	blood thinner • BLOOD VESSELS • scurvy (Vitamin C deficiency that can cause weakness and bleeding) • COLD HANDS and FEET • Raynaud's disease (pain and numbness in the outer extremities when cold) • atherosclerosis • edema • VARICOSE VEINS
Blood Sugar	DIABETES
Body System	Antioxidant
Digestive Tract	nutritive • DIARRHEA • DYSENTERY • HEMORRHOIDS
Eyes	eye problems • light sensitivity • NIGHT BLINDNESS • astringent (tightens and tones tissues)
Infections and Immune System	immune system • INFECTIONS • typhoid epidemics • antiseptic (prevents infection)
Inflammation	mouth and throat inflammation
Reproductive System	*Female:* anti-galactagogue (limits milk production)
Skin, Tissues and Hair	Ulcerative skin
Urinary Tract	kidney problems • URINARY PROBLEMS • BLADDER STONES • diuretic • water retention
Other Uses	BLUE DYE manufacture

Key Properties:

BLOOD CIRCULATION	improves blood circulation throughout the body, including the tiny end capillaries
EYE HEALTH	strengthens and supports eye health, particularly light and dark sensitivity
ASTRINGENT	increases the tone and firmness of tissues
DIURETIC	increases urine flow
Primarily affecting	EYES • BLOOD • KIDNEYS

History

The name bilberry is derived from 'blae', a northern Scottish old-country word meaning livid or bluish, and the Danish word 'bollebar' meaning dark berry.

Ancient Greek physicians used bilberries and Dioscorides (ca. 40-90 AD) spoke highly of them. The common use of bilberry fruits as an herbal medicine emerged in the Middle Ages. Saint Hildegard of Bingen (first woman to write an herbal, 1098-1179) recommended the plant for inducing menstruation flow.

Later, in the 1500s, German herbalists such as Hieronymus Bock recommended the berries for treatment of bladder stones, liver disorders, and in syrups for coughs and lung ailments. Use of bilberry fruits became widespread among herbalists and physicians over the following centuries. German physicians made berry preparations for various intestinal conditions, as well as typhoid fever, infections of the mouth, skin, and urinary tract, and for gout and rheumatism.

By the early 1900s, the dried berry tea was used as an astringent for diarrhea and dysentery, a diuretic and a cooling nutritive tonic. It was used to help stop bleeding and as an astringent-disinfectant mouthwash for inflammations of the mouth. Bilberries were at one time used to prevent scurvy (a Vitamin C deficiency) in Norway and other northern countries.

When stewed with a little sugar and lemon peel in an open tart, bilberries make a very enjoyable dish. Immense quantities were exported annually from Holland, Germany, and Scandinavia to be purchased largely by pastry cooks and restaurant owners.

At the time of World War II, it was noted that the British Royal Air

Force pilots who were consistently using bilberry jam on their bread, seemed to be far more successful at hitting their night mission targets. This initiated several studies to determine how bilberries affect the eyes.

Attributes

Bilberry contains high levels of anthocyanosides which are linked to health benefits for the heart, cardiovascular system, eyes and against cancer. (1)(2) Anthocyanosides strengthen blood vessel walls, reduce inflammation, and stabilize tissues containing collagen (tendons, ligaments, cartilage, etc).

Nutrition

Key Components: *(including, but not limited to)*

Vitamin C • Chromium • Tannins (with astringent qualities) • Anthocyanosides (derivatives of anthocyans – pigments responsible for the red, blue, or violet colors in flowers and fruits)

Eyes

In the mid-1900s, research was earnestly conducted on the health benefits of using bilberry for eye disorders. Bilberry was found to reduce eye irritation, fatigue, nearsightedness, and night blindness. These studies also noted bilberry's ability to extend the range and sharpness of vision, aid in the adaptation to darkness (by accelerating regeneration of the retina), and help limit the development of conditions such as glaucoma and cataracts.

Regular use of bilberry helps keep eyes clear, reduces the effect of aging on eyes, and improves night vision. Studies published in the late 1960s by Italian researchers showed that after taking a bilberry extract, both healthy individuals and patients with visual disorders had significant improvement in night vision, ability to more rapidly adapt to darkness, and faster restoration of vision following exposure to bright flashing lights.

Additional studies on air-traffic controllers, airplane pilots, and truck drivers showed that an extract of bilberry fruits helped to improve night vision and enhance adjustment to darkness.

In two clinical trials, Italian researchers found that 76 percent of patients with myopia (short or near sightedness) had a marked improvement in retinal sensibility. In these trials, patients were given 150 mg per day of a bilberry fruit extract for 15 days, along with Vitamin A.

Some diabetics develop diabetic retinopathy, a condition in which there is non-inflammatory degeneration of the retina. At least 3 double-blind, placebo-controlled studies conducted between 1982 and 1987 by Italian researchers showed improvements and a significant reduction or disappearance of hemorrhages in the retina. Patients in the study were given 320 to 480 mg per day of a high anthocyanoside-containing extract for 1-12 months.

A double-blind, placebo-controlled study on 40 healthy subjects found that a single dose of bilberry extract improved visual response for 2 hours.

Blood Vessel and Antioxidant Effects

Bilberry anthocyanosides serve to strengthen fragile capillaries and blood vessel walls, have antioxidant effects (protecting them from free radical damage), and stimulate the formation of new capillaries and healthy connective tissue.

More than 700 patients with various conditions related to poor microcirculation in cases of atherosclerosis, a tendency to bruise, hemorrhoids, and varicose veins participated in clinical studies that have shown bilberry extracts help reduce damage from free radicals and promote healthy circulation to the extremities. These studies involve extracts of the fruits standardized to contain 25-36 percent anthocyanosides.

Bilberry increases peripheral and connective tissue circulation, improves conditions such as Raynaud's disease (pain and spasms in the fingers and toes, when cold), and reduces edema. It also soothes inflammatory conditions such as arthritis.

European physicians have used bilberry's blood vessel-stabilizing properties as a treatment before surgery to reduce bleeding complications and bruising.

Modern laboratory studies on bilberry fruit extracts have confirmed a slight relaxation effect on smooth vascular muscles and documented its possible role in reducing factors associated with chronic inflammatory diseases.

In a placebo-controlled study that followed 60 people with varicose veins for 30 days, the use of bilberry extract resulted in a significant decrease in subjective symptoms such as a feeling of heaviness, pain in the legs and ankles, and sensations of burning, pricking, or numbness of the skin. Similar results were seen in a 30-day double-blind trial involving 47 individuals. (3)

Astringent

The dried berries of bilberry, in the form of a syrup, may be used for their astringent qualities (ability to tighten and tone tissues) in the treatment of dysentery and diarrhea.

Mucous Membranes	The German Commission E has produced a positive monograph on bilberry fruits, which are allowed in that country for the treatment of acute diarrhea and mild inflammations of the mucous membranes of the mouth and throat.
Women	Bilberry is a beneficial herb to use during pregnancy. It can be a strong but gentle astringent and will fortify veins, support capillaries, aid kidney function, and reduce bloating (as a mild diuretic). Bilberry is an anti-galactagogue (substance that limits milk secretions) when a woman finishes nursing.
Industrial Use	Bilberry is used as a home and industrial leather dye of brown and yellow colors. It is combined with other chemicals to produce violet, red, green, and blue for wool, cotton, and linen materials.
Herb Parts Used	The berries of the plant are used medicinally. Bilberry leaves, when used, are to be applied topically.
Preparations and Remedies	The small purple fruits may be eaten like blueberries, made into a syrup or extract, dried to make a tea, or dried and powdered to put in formulas, capsules, tablets, or extracts
Infusions	*Bilberry Tea:* Add one teaspoon dried berries in a cup of water and take once daily. Infants and children may drink bilberry tea for diarrhea.
Bilberry Jam	Owing to its rich, sweet tasting juice, bilberries do not require a large quantity of sugar when making into jam; add only half a pound of sugar to a pound of berries, if the preserve is to be eaten right away. Their small seeds make them ideal for jam. In a preserving pan, combine 3 pounds clean fruit with 1 ½ pounds raw sugar and 1 cup of water. Heat to a boil. Boil rapidly for 40 minutes. You may use apple juice made from windfalls and peelings instead of the water. It improves the taste. To make apple juice, cover the apples with water, stew down, and strain the juice through thick muslin. If the jam is to be kept long, it must be bottled hot in screw-top jars
Safety	Bilberry fruit is a food, and as such, is quite safe. No health hazards or side effects are known with proper dosages. Digestive complaints due to high tannin content are possible. Bilberry does not appear to interfere with blood clotting.

High doses of 'bilberry leaf' or 'leaf' extract are considered by many to be unsafe to ingest due to possible toxic side effects. If you choose to use preparations with bilberry leaf, do so only in designated doses as recommended on the bottle, or under the care of a health care practitioner.

Plant Profile	*Natural Habitat:* Bilberry is native to northern Europe and Asia and is now common to North America. V. myrtillus thrives in cool, damp, acid soils in vast areas which include woods, sandy or rocky soils, and is a scrub shrub of high mountains. It grows abundantly in Northwest England and Western Mongolia, then jumps the Pacific to Western North America, ranging from British Columbia, southward to Utah, Arizona, and New Mexico. The bilberry fruits and leaves of commerce are wild collected in European countries, particularly in Bosnia, Herzegovina, Bulgaria, Croatia, Romania, Macedonia, Serbia, Montenegro, and Kosovo, with significant amounts increasingly being wild collected under organic certification in the Russian Federation, Bulgaria, Romania, Sweden, Poland, Ukraine, and Finland.
Description	The species V. myrtillus, consists of low-growing shrubs that bear fruit. Bilberry is a small, woody shrub, rarely growing over a foot high, bearing greenish-pink, bell-shaped flowers in late spring and early summer, followed by bluish-black, round fruits (though one variety bears white fruit). Both the dried and fresh fruit should have a sweet and slightly astringent, acidic taste. The leathery leaves (similar to the shape of myrtle leaves, hence its species name) are at first rosy, then yellowish-green, and in autumn, turn red and are very ornamental. The easiest way to distinguish the bilberry plant from American blueberries is that it produces single or paired berries on the bush, while blueberries grow in clusters. The fruit of the bilberry plant is similar in taste to blueberries, but in size, they are somewhat smaller. Bilberries are darker in color, softer, and juicier than blueberries. While the bilberry's fruit pulp is red or purple (heavily staining the fingers and lips when eating the raw fruit), the blueberry's inner fruit is light green. In the wild regions of Europe, the plant flowers in May and the fruits ripen and are harvested from July through September.

Black Cohosh

Latin Name: *Cimicifuga racemosa or Actaea racemosa*

Also known as: Black Snakeroot, Snakeroot, Rattlesnake Root, Blacksnake Root, Rattleweed, Rattleroot, Squaw Root, Bugbane, Bugwort, Richweed, Macrotys

Scientific Classification

Family:	Ranunculaceae – buttercup family
Genus/Species:	Cimicifuga *racemosa* – in earlier classifications *Actaea *racemosa* (recently re-classified) – baneberry. *Actaea is part of the baneberry genus, and plants within it usually produce berries. However, black cohosh bears its seeds in a follicle, which is more consistent with the Cimicifuga genus

Influence on the Body	**(PRINCIPAL ACTIONS are listed in CAPITAL LETTERS)**
Addictions	smoking • delirium tremens (from alcohol poisoning)
Autoimmune Disorders	RHEUMATISM
Blood and Circulatory System	angina • heart palpitations • cardiac stimulant • circulation • DROPSY (edema) • HIGH BLOOD PRESSURE • BLOOD CLEANSER
Body System	astringent (tightens and tones tissues)
Blood Sugar	Diabetes
Digestive Tract	digestive disorders • bowels • DIARRHEA • expels worms
Endocrine System	Thyroid
First Aid	SORES • INSECT BITES • BEE STINGS
Infections and Immune System	coughs • FEVERS • typhoid fever • MEASLES • smallpox • scarlet fever • cholera • MALARIA • WHOOPING COUGH
Inflammation	anti-inflammatory (of all kinds) • RHEUMATISM • arthritis
Liver	liver • gallstones
Lungs and Respiratory System	EXPECTORANT • sore throat • CHRONIC BRONCHITIS • LUNGS • ASTHMA • TUBERCULOSIS
Muscles	lumbago (lower backache) • relaxes muscles

Nervous System	chorea (nervous disease causing involuntary muscle movements) • convulsions • SPASMS • EPILEPSY • ST. VITUS DANCE • sciatica • paralysis • SPINAL MENINGITIS • HYSTERIA • nervous disorders • NEURALGIA • NERVINE (improves nerve function)
Pain	pain • headaches
Poison	POISON ANTIDOTE • POISONOUS BITES • SNAKE BITES
Reproductive System	syphilis *Female:* ESTROGEN • ESTROGEN DEFICIENCY • HORMONE BALANCER • DYSMENORRHEA • MENSTRUAL PROBLEMS • MENSTRUAL CRAMPS • EMMENAGOGUE (promotes menstrual flow) • female aphrodisiac • uterine problems • CHILDBIRTH • CHILDBIRTH PAIN • HOT FLASHES • MENOPAUSE
Skin, Tissues and Hair	skin disorders • diaphoretic (increases perspiration)
Sleep	insomnia • sedative
Urinary Tract	kidney ailments • diuretic (increases urine flow)

Key Properties:

FEMALE HERB	*used especially for menopause and hormone replacement, regulates menstrual flow*
EXPECTORANT	*loosens and removes phlegm in the respiratory tract*
NERVINE	*strengthens nerve function, relieves spasms, calms nerves and acts as a sedative* *Anti-Inflammatory • ANTI-VENOMOUS*
Primarily affecting	*UTERUS • NERVES • LUNGS • HEART*
History	The bruised root was used by Native Americans as an antidote for snake bites, applying it to the wound and taking the juice (in small amounts) internally. They also found it helped relieve arthritis and fatigue. Native American women knew of black cohosh's ability to relieve pain during menstrual periods and used it extensively during childbirth. The Delaware (living in the area we now call Oklahoma), steeped black cohosh tea (in combination with other herbs) for a female tonic. The Iroquois (of New York area) used a strong root tea as a foot bath, soaking the feet and bathing sore, stiff areas of the body to treat rheumatism.

The Cherokee (Southeastern states area) are said to have treated rheumatism and various female conditions with a root preparation. They also valued black cohosh as a tonic and diuretic.

Early American Colonists used black cohosh for yellow fever, malaria, fevers, bronchitis, dropsy (swelling of ankles and legs due to heart insufficiency), uterine problems, and nervous disorders. European colonists rapidly adopted the herb for similar uses.

In the late 19th century, black cohosh was the principal ingredient in the wildly popular herb compound of Lydia E. Pinkham. The label on the bottle read, 'Vegetable Herbal Compound', but everybody knew it as 'A baby in every bottle' (meaning it helped heal infertility).

The importance of black cohosh as a medicinal plant was recognized in the first works on American herbs, dating back to 1801. It was widely prescribed by physicians in 19th century America, where it had a great reputation as an anti-inflammatory for arthritis and rheumatism and played important roles in normalizing suppressed, painful, or difficult menses and relieving pain after childbirth. It was also used for nervous disorders. The root was an official drug of the United States Pharmacopoeia from 1820 to 1926.

Migrating across the Atlantic, black cohosh became a popular European treatment for women's problems, arthritis, and high blood pressure. Black cohosh also has a long history of use in Asia.

Attributes	Key Components: *(including, but not limited to)*
Nutrition	Vitamins A • B5 (pantothenic acid) • Calcium • Iron • Magnesium • Phosphorous • Potassium • other Trace Minerals • Phytoestrogens • Phytosterin • Isoferulic Acid • Salicylic Acid (a precursor to aspirin) • Starches • Sugars • Tannins • Fatty Acids • Gum • Resin (in the root) • Wax • Volatile Material (when fresh, but lost with maturity)
Women	Black cohosh is widely known for supporting women's health and relieving unpleasant symptoms associated with hormone imbalance, particularly during menopause. It was widely thought to contain phytoestrogens (plant-derived estrogens) and other

BLACK COHOSH — 45

compounds that help balance the female system. The latest studies show that black cohosh might not contain any phytoestrogens but helps balance the body in other ways.

In my opinion, this just shows the remarkable nature of herbs. Whether black cohosh has phytoestrogens or not really doesn't matter. What matters is that our body knows what to do when we feed it with the right nutrients. Herbs like black cohosh have historically proven themselves over and over again for hundreds and, sometimes, even thousands of years. For me, supportive studies are just a bonus.

Black cohosh can stimulate blood flow to the pelvic area and restore menstruation when it is sluggish. Used with ginger, it can help relieve menstrual cramps. Black cohosh helps initiate uterine contractions, curbs hemorrhaging, and allays the nervousness and afterpains of delivery.

The German Commission E Report allows black cohosh products to be labeled for premenstrual discomfort, dysmenorrhea (painful or difficult menstruation), or climacteric (menopausal), neurovegetative ailments. (1)

Reported active properties of black cohosh include an estrogen-like action (binding to estrogen receptors) and the suppression of luteinizing hormones of the pituitary gland (reducing the occurrence of hot flashes). (2)

Researchers found that after 6-8 weeks of treatment, 80 percent of patients had beneficial effects in a 629 patient German clinical study. There was dramatic relief from, and reduction of, hot flashes, sweating, headache, vertigo, palpitation, and tinnitus in over 49 percent of the volunteers. Over 39 percent reported significant reductions of these symptoms, along with diminished nervousness, irritability, and depression. (3)

A 1987 German double blind study produced significant reduction of menopausal symptoms and depression. (4)

In a 1988 German clinical study, the authors concluded that in cases where conventional hormone therapy is contraindicated, black cohosh extract is the therapy of choice. (5) (It makes me wonder why the authors of the study wouldn't recommend a natural choice first).

Hormone Replacement Therapy (HRT) Study (1994-2002)

A significant interest in using black cohosh and other 'female' herbs for the relief of menopausal discomfort developed at the premature termination of a monumental Hormone Replacement Therapy (HRT) study involving more than 16,000 women. In 1994, a long-term study led by the National Institutes of Health called the Women's Health Initiative (WHI) was initiated with the hope of establishing proof that Premarin and Provera (estrogen replacement medications) would not only relieve menopause symptoms but continuous HRT could be used to protect aging women from heart attacks, strokes, osteoporosis, and cancer.

However, on July 9, 2002, the WHI came to an abrupt halt. The HRT study had proven unequivocally that the drugs were unsafe and, in fact, were significant factors causing increased risk of breast and uterine cancers, heart attacks, strokes, brain tumors, and dementia in the women they were following.

Women who take synthetic estrogen have been able to switch to black cohosh immediately with no side effects or drug withdrawal symptoms. Black cohosh does not exhibit the same cancer-causing agents as traditional HRT. Black cohosh works even better when mixed with other hormone-balancing herbs.

A more recent (2005) trial involving 304 postmenopausal women showed that black cohosh extract was significantly more effective than the placebo was in decreasing menopausal symptoms, particularly hot flashes. Liver enzyme levels watched during the study (liver enzymes increase when liver is damaged) did not show clinically relevant changes in the primarily important hepatic enzymes (GGT, AST, ALT) in comparison to placebo. (6)

Heart

Black cohosh slightly lowers the heart rate, while it increases the force of its beat and equalizes circulation. The herb reduces arterial action and is a mild cardiac tonic, especially useful for fatty hearts. Its action on the central nervous system, heart, and circulation resembles the action of digitalis (a medicinal heart stimulant, originally extracted from the herb foxglove). It contracts the heart muscle and helps relieve chest pains.

Nervous System

Black cohosh is used as a tonic for the central nervous system in both men and women and is regarded as a nervine (strengthens nerve function). It works directly on the nervous system, relieves nervous tension, soothes local pain, and alleviates headaches.

	This versatile herb is also an excellent and safe sedative.

The medulla oblongata (the lower half of the brainstem) deals with autonomic functions such as breathing and blood pressure. Black cohosh is reported to help heal medulla oblongata damage caused by hallucinogenic drugs.

The herb relieves or prevents spasms and is used for epilepsy. It helps reduce tinnitus (ringing in the ears) and has been used effectively for spinal meningitis. |
Inflammation	Black cohosh can be used in a poultice to help ease all kinds of inflammation and can diminish the effects of inflammation due to bee sting allergies.
Lungs and Mucous Membranes	Black cohosh has a stimulating effect on secretions of the spleen, liver, kidneys, and lymphatic system. It is a viable expectorant for acute, chronic, pulmonary and bronchial conditions. Because it breaks up mucus and phlegm deposits, it is found in many sinus combinations.
Muscles	Black cohosh has a strong effect on the muscular system. It relaxes and soothes inflammation and is a remedy of the greatest importance in muscular rheumatism.
Anti-venomous	The plant's genus name, Cimicifuga, from the Latin 'cimex' (bug) and 'fugare' (to drive away), is so named because certain species tend to drive away bugs and other insects. It can also be used as an antidote for the venom of serpents.
Herb Parts Used	Preparations of black cohosh are made from its roots and rhizomes (underground stems).
Preparations and Remedies *Powdered*	Black cohosh is used fresh, or in dried form, and made into infusions (teas), capsules, pills, and tinctures (liquid extracts). *Black cohosh is even more effective when taken with other female herbs (such as blue cohosh, dong quai, red raspberry leaf, bayberry bark, squawvine and damiana). Black cohosh taken alone may take up to four to six weeks to produce its full benefits.*

Tea	*Simmer one teaspoon of the cut and sifted herb for every cup of water for 5-15 minutes. Drink one cup twice daily.*
Safety	No health hazards are known when used in proper amounts. If taken in larger amounts than needed, black cohosh may cause a headache at the base of the skull. If headaches or nausea occur while taking this herb, take smaller doses or discontinue use. Black cohosh is not to be taken during early pregnancy. It may be taken in the final weeks of pregnancy, but only to ease or induce labor.
Plant Profile	*Natural Habitat:* The plant is native to eastern North America from the extreme south of Ontario, Canada down into the United States to central Georgia and west to Missouri and Arkansas. Black cohosh grows in a variety of woodland situations and is often found in small woodland openings. It is now cultivated in Europe and Asia as well.
Description	Black cohosh flourishes in the deep shade of moist hillsides. It has striking, bushy foliage with tall stems which bloom May through September (depending on the climate). Black cohosh is a tall perennial herb (it grows back without replanting) with a large, knotty root. The flowers bloom on a tall stem, which grows 2-1/2 to 8 feet tall in racemes up to 20 inches long. They have no petals or sepals; only a tight cluster of 55-110 white stamens, each about a half-inch long surrounding the white stigma. When flowering, black cohosh exhibits a strong, distinctively sweet smell that repels some insects, earning its name 'bugbane.' Its fruit is a dry follicle about a half-inch long that contains several seeds.

Blessed Thistle

Latin Name: *Cnicus benedictus*

Also known as: St. Benedict Thistle, Spotted Thistle, Bitter Thistle, Cardin, Blessed Cardus, Holy Thistle

Scientific Classification

Blessed Thistle is classified in other genus and species combinations. The same plant (or closely related) with various names.

Family: Asteraceae – aster, daisy and sunflower family
Compositae – in earlier classifications.

Genus Cnicus

Species C. benedictus – The sole species in the genus Cnicus is this thistle-like plant

Genus /Species: Other classifications commonly used:
Carduus *sanctus*, Carduus *benedictus*
Carbenia *benedicta*
Centaurea *benedicta*

Influence on the Body	(PRINCIPAL ACTIONS are listed in CAPITAL LETTERS)
Blood and Circulatory System	strengthens HEART • ANGINA (chest pains) • dropsy (edema due to heart insufficiency) • BLOOD PURIFIER • BLOOD CIRCULATION • circulation to the BRAIN
Body System	STIMULANT TONIC (increases energy and strength throughout the body) • diaphoretic (promotes perspiration, increasing elimination through the skin)
Cancer	CANCER
Digestive Tract	stimulates appetite • DIGESTIVE DISORDERS • carminative (brings warmth, circulation, relieves intestinal gas discomfort, and promotes peristalsis) • GAS • CONSTIPATION • emetic (causes vomiting in large doses) • anthelmintic (kills parasites and worms) • expels worms
Infections and Immune System	reduces FEVER • spleen
Inflammation	Arthritis

Liver	LIVER CONDITIONS • jaundice • GALLBLADDER • cholagogue (promotes the flow of bile)
Lungs and Respiratory System	strengthens LUNGS • respiratory infection
Nervous System	nervine (improves nerve function) • STRENGTHENS MEMORY • inability to concentrate • DEPRESSION • senility • HEADACHES • migraine headaches • HYSTERIA
Reproductive System	*Female:* HORMONE BALANCER • FEMALE HORMONES • FEMALE DISORDERS • MENSTRUAL CRAMPS • painful MENSTRUATION • EMMENAGOGUE (promotes menstrual flow) • birth control • leucorrhea (vaginal discharge due to infection) • vaginal discharge • PREGNANCY • enriches BREAST MILK • LACTATION • NURSING
Urinary Tract	kidneys • urinary disorders • diuretic (increases urine flow)

Key Properties:

EMMENAGOGUE	*promotes menstrual flow, safe during pregnancy in small Amounts*
GALACTAGOGUE	*enhances lactation of nursing mothers*
STOMACH TONIC ALTERATIVE	*purifies the blood*
TONIC • nervine	*strengthens nerve function*
Emetic	*causes vomiting in large doses*
Primarily affecting	*STOMACH • HEART • BLOOD • BRAIN • MAMMARY GLANDS • UTERUS*

History	Early herbalists believed that blessed thistle was a cure-all. They noted that the plant could prevent and stop headaches, provoke sweat, help memory, strengthen the heart and stomach, and treat external problems such as festering sores, boils, and itching rashes. Blessed thistle has been utilized for many years for digestive problems and for liver and gallbladder diseases. In 17th century England, the herbalist Culpepper listed blessed thistle for use in headaches, female complaints, and fevers. European monks once grew blessed thistle as a cure for smallpox, which is when it is believed to have received its name.

BLESSED THISTLE — 51

	The Native American Quinault tribe used the whole plant to create a birth-control medicinal, and 19th century herbalists recommended blessed thistle tea made from the plant tops as a treatment for fevers and respiratory ailments.

In herbal medicine today, blessed thistle is used as a 'female' herb (helping to nourish and balance female hormones), yet it is effective in balancing men's hormones as well. It aids in digestion and has health benefits derived from purifying blood and improving circulation. |
| **Attributes** | The 'bitter' principle was named 'cnicin' by Nativelle in 1839. He proposed that the reason bitter foods increased the appetite was due to the stimulation of the bitter taste buds on the tongue resulting in increased secretion of saliva and digestive juices. In turn, these secretions help protect the tissues found in the digestive tract, enhance bile flow and improve pancreatic functions.

Key Components: (including, but not limited to)

Cnicin (a 'bitter') • Other 'Bitter' components • Tannins |
| *Blood Circulation* | Blessed thistle is believed to have great power in improving blood circulation. It is such an excellent blood purifier that drinking a cup of blessed thistle tea twice a day can alleviate chronic headaches over time and gradually detoxify the spleen, liver, kidneys, and bowels. Blessed thistle is good for all urinary, pulmonary and liver disorders. Better circulation also strengthens the heart, lungs, and brain functions. Blessed thistle acts as a brain food by bringing oxygen and nourishment to the cells and stimulating memory. |
| *Women* | Helping to balance female hormones, blessed thistle has been effective in relieving cramps, painful menstruation and menopausal headaches. When given to girls before the onset of puberty, it can help to prevent future cramping and menstrual problems.

Blessed thistle is used in formulas for pregnancy, not as the main herb, but as a supportive herb. Blessed thistle is wonderful for enriching and increasing milk production in nursing mothers (even more so when taken in combination with red raspberry). |
| *Digestion* | Blessed thistle has a long history of use as a digestive aid and general tonic. It improves the appetite, reduces gas in the |

BLESSED THISTLE — 52

	intestines, relieves constipation, and helps to heal digestive liver problems. The leaves, dried and powdered, are good for expelling worms.
Infections and Immune System	Laboratory studies show that blessed thistle and its components (including cnicin) act against several types of bacteria and help to reduce and control fevers.
Inflammation	There is some evidence that blessed thistle also has anti-inflammatory properties.
Cancer	Along with other herbs, it has been taken internally to help the body heal cancer.
Perspiration	Blessed thistle can cause profuse perspiration when taken in a hot infusion. Perspiration cools down the body and helps it get rid of unwanted toxins through the skin.
Herb Parts Used	The leaves, stems, seeds, and flowers are used medicinally
Preparations and Remedies	The leaves and flowers may be eaten fresh like watercress, though the taste is very bitter. Fresh or dried parts of the blessed thistle plant may be made into an infusion tea (taken hot or cold), fluid extract, or dried and powdered to put into capsules singly or in combination with other herbs.
Infusions	Taken as a cold infusion, blessed thistle is a tonic. When taken warm, it can induce perspiration and help normalize menstrual flow. *Lactation Tea:* To enhance the quality and quantity of mother's milk, make a blessed thistle tea mixed with equal parts of red raspberry leaves, marshmallow root, goat's rue, and fenugreek. Steep for several hours, strain, and then keep in the refrigerator to drink throughout the day. Take three or more cups per day according to need. *Ginger Tea:* (see GINGER preparations)
Powdered Form	The herb may be ground up and encapsulated. Take four to twenty capsules per day.
Safety	During pregnancy, blessed thistle should be taken in small amounts and in combination with other pregnancy herbs. It is not to be taken alone or in large amounts during pregnancy.

Taken in large doses, blessed thistle may induce vomiting. It is better to take smaller quantities several times throughout the day.

Plant Profile	*Natural Habitat:* Although native to southern Europe and the eastern Mediterranean region, blessed thistle is now cultivated in many areas of the world, including parts of North America. The herb prefers dry, sunny places in arable, stony, and waste ground areas, and is easily grown in ordinary garden soil.
Description	Blessed thistle is an annual plant (it germinates, flowers, sets seed, and dies within one year), growing up to two feet tall. It has leathery, hairy leaves up to a foot long and three inches broad with small spines on the margins. The plant produces numerous yellow flowers (about one inch in diameter) arranged in a head at the tip of a branch or stem. The flower is surrounded by long, yellowish-red spines and almost hidden by upper leaves. Blessed thistle is sometimes considered to be a noxious weed. The herb has a feeble, unpleasant odor and an intensely bitter taste more disagreeable when fresh than in the dried plant. The leaves and tops are at peak medicinal quality when the plant flowers appear, usually between May and August. For best potency, the harvested plant should be thoroughly and speedily dried in a well-ventilated, moisture-free dark area.

Brigham Tea

Latin Name: *Ephedra viridis*

Also known as: Ephedra, American Ephedra, Mormon Tea, Miner's Tea, Desert Tea, Squaw Tea, Joint Fir, Yellow River, General of Respiration

Scientific Classification

There are approximately 40 species of ephedra,
each with similar and unique characteristics of varying potency.

Family: Ephedraceae – Mormon-tea family

Genus Ephedra – Joint fir

Species E. viridis – Mormon tea
E. nevadensis – also known as Mormon tea

Not to be confused with:
E. sinica – Chinese ephedra, also called Ma Huang,
E. sinica is currently FDA regulated because of reported health risks associated with the abuse of products that contained the isolated, extracted, and synthesized alkaloid 'ephedrine' (naturally found in abundance in this herb, and in lesser amounts in Brigham Tea).

Influence on the Body	(PRINCIPAL ACTIONS are listed in CAPITAL LETTERS)
Blood and Circulatory System	vasoconstrictor (narrows blood-vessel openings, restricting the flow of blood through them)
Infections and Immune System	allergies • malarial fevers • myasthenia gravis (disease characterized by the wasting of muscles, particularly those associated with swallowing) • hay fever
Lungs and Respiratory Tract	EXPECTORANT • BRONCHIAL ASTHMA • emphysema (painful condition in which air spaces in the lungs are enlarged)
Nervous System	epilepsy • depression • NERVINE STIMULANT
Weight	weight loss • increased metabolism

Key Properties:

STIMULANT — increases internal heat, dispels internal chill, and strengthens metabolism and circulation

BRONCHIAL DILATION EXPECTORANT — loosens and removes phlegm in the respiratory tract

BRIGHAM TEA — 55

Astringent	*tightens tissues and decreases swelling*
Diuretic	*increases urine flow*
Primarily affecting	CIRCULATION • LUNGS • HEART

History	Ephedra viridis (Brigham Tea) is a relative to the powerful, medicinal, Chinese plant Ephedra sinica. Both Ephedra plants have similar active components. Though Brigham Tea has considerably less quantities of the active component 'ephedrine', it makes an effective substitute for Ma Huang and, along with the other elements it contains, is an excellent herb in its own right.
Ma Huang (E. sinica)	Ma Huang is highly regarded in Chinese herbalogy, where it has been used effectively and safely for over 5,000 years to treat colds, coughs, fevers (including malaria), headaches, and skin eruptions.
	The Divine Husbandman's Classic of Materia Medica, 220 BC, is the first known record concerning the medicinal uses of herbs. Written by the Chinese, it records the use of Ma Huang as being a part of Chinese medicine.
	In recent years, scientists have extracted the stimulant alkaloid 'ephedrine' from the herb Ma Huang and chemically produced it as 'epinephrine' (synthetic adrenalin). When chemically produced in this way, the resulting drug can be dangerous to some individuals when taken in excess or combined with synthetic caffeine. This result became apparent when weight-loss products that contained these synthesized compounds in a laboratory were promoted and became popular in the United States and European countries.
	Major health threats became associated with synthetic ephedrine use, including hypertension (high blood pressure), tachycardia, CNS (central nervous system) excitation, arrhythmia, myocardial infarction (heart attack), stroke, and death.
FDA Ruling	On February 11, 2004, the U.S. Food and Drug Administration (FDA) issued a final ruling that prohibited the sale of dietary supplements with ephedrine alkaloids (ephedra) because they believed such supplements presented an unreasonable risk of illness or injury.

Brigham Tea
(E. viridis)

The shame of this whole thing is that the FDA grouped natural Ma Huang in with the laboratory-created chemical called ephedrine and made both illegal in the USA.

In five thousand years of whole plant use, not one negative side effect has been reported. When the whole plant is used, all of the chemical constituents are present, including those that balance out the active constituents. When one alkaloid is singled out and extracted, it becomes a powerful pharmaceutical that is unsafe for individuals with high blood pressure or heart problems.

There are several American ephedra species that contain little or no ephedrine and are *not* banned by the FDA. Brigham Tea contains less ephedrine than its Asian cousin, Ma Huang.

The Native American Navajo tribe are said to have brewed the tops of the Brigham Tea plant for cough medicine. Other tribes roasted the seeds and ate them whole or ground them into a meal. The Hopi used the plant to treat syphilis. The Paiute and Shoshones steeped tea made from the twigs to normalize kidney and bladder disorders. The Kawaiisu (from what is now California) used the tea for backaches. Today, it is still valued by many tribes as a tonic beverage and blood purifier.

The friendly Native Americans taught the pioneers how to use Brigham Tea. The herb grew abundantly in the Uinta Basin (Utah and surrounding areas), and the coarse green shrub became nicknamed 'Brigham Tea' or sometimes 'Mormon tea' because Brigham Young, a prophet of the Mormon pioneers, drank it often and recommended it for the health and vitality of his parishioners.

As long as I can remember, my Mother and Grandmother drank Brigham Tea. They always fed it to us children when we were sick and told us it was 'good for us.' My Mom always talked about it being a blood purifier. She taught me how to wildcraft it and how to store it in a brown paper bag so it didn't mold. We would gather large boxes of it so that it would last us all year long. Mom would fill her coffeemaker with the whole herb, run hot water on it, and let it steep for 30 minutes. Then she would add honey and drink it hot or put it in the refrigerator for a nice cool drink later. Mom reused the same herb until the water ran clear, then threw the used herb into the compost pile. Thanks, Mom, for teaching me about this wholesome herb!

Attributes	The 'bitter' principle was named 'cnicin' by Nativelle in 1839. He proposed that the reason bitter foods increased the appetite was due to the stimulation of the bitter taste buds on the tongue resulting in increased secretion of saliva and digestive juices. In turn, these secretions help protect the tissues found in the digestive tract, enhance bile flow, and improve pancreatic functions.
	Key Components: (including, but not limited to) • Phosphorus • Ephedrine • Pseudo ephedrine • Resin • Tannins
Opens Bronchioles and Blood Vessels	*Ephedrine*: The ephedrine component found in Brigham Tea accounts for much of its therapeutic action. To a lesser degree, ephedrine acts similarly to adrenalin. Brigham Tea has a milder action on the body than does adrenalin, but it lasts longer in the blood.
	Brigham Tea stimulates the heart muscles, thereby constricting blood vessels, increasing circulation, and normalizing blood pressure. This forces more blood to the extremities (head, arms, hands, legs, and feet), provides a stimulant action on the brain and nerve centers, and reduces fatigue and weariness.
	It is recommended by some that this herb should be avoided by those who are hypertensive and have a history of increased blood pressure.
Respiration and Chest Congestion	Brigham Tea stimulates and increases the depth of respiration. Ephedrine is a bronchial-dilator (relaxes and opens the bronchioles) and has been a life-saving herb in extreme cases of chronic asthma.
	Ephedrine reinforces heart action and dilates the bronchi, especially during spasms, which is why it is used for bronchial asthma. It can relax and relieve muscle spasms in the bronchial tubes.
	Ephedra acts as a decongestant and expectorant (loosens and removes phlegm) for relieving respiratory congestion. It has also been useful for acute sinusitis and hay fever.
Central Nervous System	Ephedrine stimulates the central nervous system and is an energy tonic that strengthens and restores body vitality. It acts to stimulate the body and calm the mind, making it excellent for increasing mental energy during a long test or meditation. It has

also been used effectively as a treatment for depression and narcolepsy (a chronic sleep disorder). Brigham Tea can cause sleeplessness if taken before bedtime.

Weight

Brigham Tea's ability to increase metabolism and 'warm' the body gives it some weight-loss benefits. The safest way to enjoy the benefits of Brigham Tea is to prepare it using the whole herb.

Diuretic

Pseudoephedrine:
Pseudoephedrine has a similar but weaker adrenalin effect than that of ephedrine, yet it has a stronger diuretic effect (increases urine flow). Brigham Tea also has astringent properties that can reduce swelling.

Allergic Reactions and Poisons

Brigham Tea can reduce the allergic response in a wide range of conditions, including bee stings. It has been used as a treatment for snake bites.

Herb Parts Used

The whole plant has been used medicinally

Preparations and Remedies

All parts of the plant may be used to make teas, infusions, decoctions, and tinctures; or the herb can be dried, powdered, and put into capsules.

Infusions

Brigham Tea:
It is most commonly used as a pleasant beverage. Steep for five to fifteen minutes. The plant is greenish gray but produces a beautiful light pink liquid when made into a tea.

Safety

Ephedra can increase nervousness and restlessness in some people and is contraindicated in certain cases of heart problems and high blood pressure.

It should be noted that plants of the Ephedra family have been used medicinally for thousands of years. There have been no reported undesirable side effects when the entire herb is used in its natural state.

Plant Profile

Natural Habitat:
Mormon tea ephedra (Brigham Tea) is native to the American Southwest. It is found in arid areas of the Northern Hemisphere, especially in the southwest deserts. Ma Huang ephedra (E. sinica) is indigenous to China, South Siberia, and Japan.

Description

The vivid green foliage of the Brigham Tea plant presents a striking contrast to an often gray desert environment. This perennial shrub is broom like, with jointed green stems and branches that grow two to four feet long. Two or three scale-like leaves grow at the joints in the stems and branches. Male and female cones appear on separate plants. The male cones have yellow pollen sacs.

The plant prefers full sun and very fast draining soil. It remains hardy to 10° F. To plant, scarify lightly and sow seeds in warm, fast-draining mix. Individuate the plants and grow out in pots for a year or two before transplanting to landscape soil.

It is best to harvest Brigham Tea in the fall to winter, after the new growth has subsided. The coloring of the plant will change to an olive greenish gray. Harvesting Brigham Tea too early in the season causes an odd tasting tea, somewhat like when you have eaten an unripe banana.

Burdock

Latin Name: *Arctium lappa*

Also known as: Turkey Burrseed, Hurr-bur, Hareburr, Hardock, Great Burr, Thorny Burr, Cockle Buttons, Beggars Buttons, Fox's Cloth, Lappa, Philanthropium, Sticky Bob, Gobo (in Japan)

Scientific Classification

Family: Asteraceae – aster, daisy and sunflower family
Compositae – in earlier classifications

Genus: Arctium – burdock

Species: A. *lappa* – greater burdock
A. *minus* – lesser burdock

Influence on the Body	(PRINCIPAL ACTIONS are listed in CAPITAL LETTERS)
Autoimmune Disorders	lupus • RHEUMATISM
Blood and Circulatory System	BLOOD CLEANSER • BLOOD PURIFIER • blood poisoning • scurvy • DEPURATIVE (cleanses blood by promoting eliminative functions)
Blood Sugar	HYPERGLYCEMIA • HYPOGLYCEMIA
Body System	demulcent (softens and soothes inflammation of mucous membranes) • degenerative conditions • endurance • energy • fatigue • TONIC (increases energy and strengthens the muscular and nervous system while improving digestion and assimilation resulting in a general sense of well-being) • INTERNAL ABSCESSES
Cancer	CANCER • TUMORS of glands and spleen
Digestive Tract	bitter (stimulates digestive juices and improves appetite) • stomach disorders • ulcers • carminative (relieves intestinal gas discomfort, and promotes peristalsis) • CONSTIPATION • LAXATIVE • HEMORRHOIDS
Eyes	Styes
First Aid	wounds • burns
Infections and Immune System	ALLERGIES • hay fever • LYMPHATIC CONGESTION • LYMPHATIC SYSTEM • lymph glands • CHRONIC INFECTIONS • COLDS • bactericide (kills bacteria) • coughs

	• FEVERS • MEASLES • CHICKEN POX (treat both internally and externally) • LEPROSY
Inflammation	inflammation • RHEUMATISM • ARTHRITIS • BURSITIS • GOUT
Liver	LIVER PROBLEMS • gallbladder • gallstones • cholagogue (promotes the flow of bile)
Lungs and Respiratory System	bronchitis • lungs • pneumonia • tuberculosis
Mouth and Throat	CANKER SORES • TONSILLITIS • sore throats
Nervous System	nervous conditions • SCIATICA NERVE
Poisons	poisons • antidote (neutralizes poison)
Reproductive System	SYPHILIS • venereal diseases • gonorrhea Female: prolapsed uterus
Skin, Tissues and Hair	BRUISES • SORES • ACNE (blood cleansing) • PIMPLES • BOILS • carbuncles (boil) • SKIN DISORDERS • skin eruptions • IMPETIGO (highly contagious skin disease) • ECZEMA • PSORIASIS • rosacea (symptomatic red nose) • RASHES • HERPES • ITCHING • POISON IVY • POISON OAK • BURNS/ SCALDS • FLUID RETENTION • SWELLING •dandruff • hair growth • hair loss • baldness
Urinary Tract	BLADDER INFECTIONS • BLADDER PAIN • KIDNEY PROBLEMS • cystitis • diuretic (increases urine flow) • lithotriptic (dissolves urinary stones)
Weight	Obesity

Key Properties:

ALTERATIVE	*(root and seeds)* *purifies the BLOOD; specific for the LIVER and SKIN*
DIAPHORETIC	*(root)* *increases perspiration*
DIURETIC	*(root and seeds)*
Demulcent	*(root)* *softens and soothes; specific for the DIGESTIVE TRACT & SKIN*
TONIC **Nutritive**	*(leaves)*

BURDOCK — 62

Primarily affecting *BLOOD • KIDNEYS • STOMACH • LIVER • SKIN*

History	Burdock has the historical reputation of being an 'alterative,' meaning herbalists have considered it as a good source of nutrients to help build up and cleanse the body. In the early 1900s, plants like dandelion and burdock were called 'blood purifiers.' Menominee and Micmac Native American used burdock for skin sores while the Cherokees used it for a broader base of ailments. In ancient China and India, herbalists used burdock in the treatment of respiratory infections, abscesses, and joint pain. Chinese physicians also used it for measles and skin sores as well. During the Middle Ages, Europeans began using burdock to treat cancerous tumors, skin conditions, venereal disease, and bladder and kidney problems. Interestingly, in the early 1940s, the hooked burr of the burdock thistle inspired Swiss inventor George de Mestral to create the popular fastener 'Velcro.'
Attributes *Nutrients*	**Key Components: (including, but not limited to)** • Phosphorus • Ephedrine • Pseudo-ephedrine • Resin • Tannins Vitamins A • B1 (thiamine) • B3 (niacin) • B5 (pantothenic acid) • B6 (pyridoxine) • B9 (folic acid) • B12 (cobalamin) • Biotin • Choline • Inositol • PABA (Para-Amino Benzoic Acid) • C • Bioflavonoids • E • Calcium • Copper • Iron (a good source) • Potassium • Sulfur • Zinc • other Trace Minerals Burdock is an excellent choice for treating iron deficiencies. Inulin (27-45 percent) • Amino Acids • Bitter • Volatile oils Inulin is a low-calorie starch important in the metabolism of carbohydrates. It promotes the growth of healthy intestinal bacteria and increases calcium (and possibly magnesium) absorption. (1)(2)(3) Nutritionally, inulin is considered a form of soluble fiber (called gobo dietary fiber, or GDF, in Japanese cuisine) and is sometimes categorized as a prebiotic (helps good bacteria grow and flourish). Unlike other sugars and starches, inulin has a

BURDOCK — 63

minimal impact on blood sugar levels, has a rather low glycemic index (measure of the effect food has on blood sugar levels), and does not raise triglyceride levels. Because of its inulin component, burdock is generally considered to be suitable for diabetics and potentially helpful in managing blood sugar related diseases.

General	Burdock has been used for centuries as a blood purifier for clearing the bloodstream of toxins and moving them out of the body, a diuretic for helping rid the body of excess water by increasing urine output, and a topical remedy for skin problems such as acne, eczema, rosacea, and psoriasis.
Blood	Burdock is an excellent restorative cleanser and detoxifier. It rapidly eliminates long-term impurities from the blood without causing nausea or irritation. Continued cleansing of the blood will then detoxify the cells, tissues, and organs (specifically the liver, kidneys, bowels, and skin).
Poisoning	Burdock has the ability to neutralize most poisons, relieving both the kidney and lymphatic systems.
Soothing Skin and Mucous Membranes	Burdock root is a first-class blood and lymph purifier, cleansing the lymphatic vessels, serous membranes, and mucous membranes. Burdock works well for clearing up skin problems, acne, etc. It is especially indicated in chronic cutaneous lesions like eczema and psoriasis.
Immune System	Burdock relieves congestion of the lymphatic system and promotes perspiration. This is especially helpful in cases of fever.
Liver	The root helps ease liver congestion and fat digestion. It is a strong, liver-purifying, hormone-balancing herb with particular value for skin, arthritic, and glandular problems.
Inflammation	Use the root or the seeds for rheumatism and mild to advanced cases of arthritis. Burdock is excellent for gout. It helps to reduce swelling and breaks down the calcification deposits of joints and knuckles. Burdock also soothes, cleanses, and relieves inflammation and congestion of bronchial tissue.
Urinary Tract	Burdock naturally increases the flow of urine which can relieve pain in the bladder and help to fight kidney and bladder infections. This reduces any water retention in tissues and joints. It is also useful for weight loss.

Endocrine System

Burdock works on the pituitary gland by helping it to release protein in proper amounts, thus maintaining a healthy hormonal balance.

Women and Infants

Burdock is an herb that women can use during pregnancy. It helps balance all systems, reduces water retention, and helps prevent jaundice in the baby.

In Europe, it has been used as a remedy in cases where there was a prolapsed and displaced uterus.

Skin

Burdock tea makes a good wash for acne, burns, and sores. Hot fomentations (towel soaked in infusion or decoction and placed on affected area) help heal swellings. Used as a poultice, burdock has been found to be an effective remedy when applied to sores and bug bites.

Burdock is one of the best herbs for taking care of chronic skin problems. Used internally and externally for skin problems, burdock and red clover (or yellow dock and sarsaparilla) are traditionally taken as a tea to treat eczema.

The seeds help restore smoothness to the skin. They have limited tonic qualities and work as a relaxant and demulcent on mucous membranes.

Burns

The leaves are used externally for burns, skin problems, and wounds. Burn care workers report that burdock eases dressing changes, appears to impede bacterial growth on the wound site, and provides a great moisture barrier. (4)

Cancer

Burdock has been used by some for cancer, as it is such an excellent alterative (cleans toxins and purifies blood). It has manifested great effectiveness when used as a poultice on skin cancers and is one of the four ingredients in the reportedly successful Essiac Tea formula.

Essiac strengthens the immune system, allowing the body to take care of itself and heal. It is also an excellent cancer preventative.

Renée Caisse

In 1922, Renée Caisse, a Canadian nurse, received an herbal recipe from an elderly female patient in an Ontario hospital where Renée was the head nurse. The recipe Renée received had been given to the older woman years before by an Ojibwa Medicine Man.

Renée began using the formula on critically ill volunteers, calling the recipe 'Essiac' (Caisse spelled backwards is Essiac). The majority of those whom she treated came on referral with letters from their physicians certifying they had incurable or terminal forms of cancer and they had been given up by the medical profession as untreatable.

In cases where there was severe damage to life support organs, her patients died, but they lived longer than the medical profession had predicted and, more significantly, they lived, in large part, free of pain. Still others, listed as hopeless and terminal, but without severe damage to vital organs, were healed and lived 35-45 more years.

Some of the positive results noted were: Cessation of pain, increased appetite (emaciated patients gained weight), improved sleep, feeling of well-being, energy, a noted decrease in depression, anxiety, and fear, a prolongation of life, and a decrease of nodular masses.

Renée paid a price for her success. She was censored by her government, and her clinical data and records were destroyed at her death. Her story survived through friends and patients she served. (5)

I have had a lot of experience with Renee's formula. The first time I read about it was in an article that was given to my mother by Mr. Marshal. The article was an interview with Dr. Gary Glum. He had written a book about Renée Caisse entitled *'Calling of an Angel.'* Dr. Glum's article gave me hope. The drinking of Essiac was a turning point in my health and healing. I also watched hundreds of others take Essiac while I worked as an Herbalist at alternative treatment clinics. I never saw anyone respond as positively and as dramatically with any other of the many variations of this formula than I did with the original four-herb formula that was disclosed in a court battle in the 1980s.

If you use Essiac, please make it exactly as directed. It is well worth the effort. I am so grateful to Mr. Marshall, Dr. Gary Glum, and Renée Caisse for their sacrifice and dedication to helping others heal. See Renée Caisse's Essiac formula below.

Hair Growth

In Russia, burdock oil is used as a hair tonic to strengthen and encourage the growth of new hair. This can be done if the hair follicles are just dormant and not completely destroyed. It usually

	takes from six to eight months for a noticeable change.
Herb Substitution	Burdock is an effective replacement for chaparral.
Herb Parts Used	Roots, seeds, and sometimes, the leaves are used.
Preparations and Remedies	Young roots are best for eating. They are long, thin, very crisp, and have a sweet, mild, pungent flavor. Slice one or two crisp, juicy, fresh roots and add to a soup or stew. Any harshness in the taste can be reduced by soaking julienned/shredded roots in water for five to ten minutes.
Fresh	Burdock root (fresh when possible) is the best for healing arthritis and any joint problems (a twisted ankle, pulled shoulder, etc.). Skin the root, cut into pieces, and blend with water. Strain and drink a quart or more of the liquid per day. The raw root is excellent when grated and marinated. Served hot, it will fortify the system against disease, strengthen all body systems, and accelerate recovery. The stalk is nutritive when cut before the flower opens and, stripped of the bitter rind, it can be boiled or used raw in salads. Its delicate flavor is similar to asparagus.
Powdered or Cut	The herb may be used in capsules, extracts, infusions, and in topical preparations. The seeds made into an extract are good for skin and kidney diseases.
Tea or Wash	Use as a wash to rinse the affected area or make a fomentation by soaking a towel in the infusion or decoction and placing it as needed. Apply on large sores, skin diseases, inflammation, swelling, rashes, boils, and hemorrhoids. Drink as a tea for an added benefit. Bruised leaves or tea have been used successfully for poison ivy or poison oak and for fevers (applied to the forehead or to the soles of the feet). The tea also makes a wash for acne, burns, and sores.
Poultices	Apply a poultice of the root over painful joints. Steamed roots can be mashed and applied to the affected area as hot as can be

tolerated. Fresh leaves may be lightly steamed and applied hot. Burdock poultices can draw out splinters, poisons, and pus. They improve blood flow to injured or infected areas, help fight infection, reduce tumors and gouty swellings, relieve bruises and inflammation, and speed the healing process.

For burns, shred the bruised leaves fine and fold into a stiffly beaten egg white; it will take out the heat, relieve the pain, and hasten healing.

The seeds may be ground up or bruised, soaked overnight in the liquid of choice to macerate (soften), then briefly blended the following day before applying topically. Burdock seeds are wonderful for soothing, healing, and softening the skin.

Ointment

Itch Ointment:
1 pound Burdock root, freshly grated
(4 oz of dried herb may be used if fresh is not available)
8 oz Extra Virgin Olive Oil
1 oz Beeswax

Simmer ingredients slowly for two hours. Strain through coarse cloth or fine wire sieve, stir until solidified, and place into jars. Apply to affected parts morning and night. Also drink the root decoction internally for an increased benefit.

Infusions

Burdock tea of the leaves can be used as a stomach tonic and for indigestion. **When using for debilitating illness, it is crucial to follow directions exactly!**

Burdock Root Decoction (strong tea):
4 oz Burdock root, cut or powdered
3 pints Distilled Water
8 oz Glycerin (for longer preservation)

Simmer the herb root in distilled water for 30 minutes. Strain, sweeten with honey, allow to cool, bottle, and keep in a cool place. Take 2-4 ounces 3-4 times a day internally for fevers and skin problems such as boils, styes, carbuncles, and canker sores.

For Longer Preservation:
Prepare as described (without honey), then return the liquid to the pan, heat, and reduce by simmering to one pint. Strain, allow to

cool, add glycerin, and shake well. Keep in a cool place and sweeten at time of use.

Stronger Decoction:
4 oz Burdock root, cut
2 quarts Distilled Water
1/4 pint Glycerin

Bring herb and water to a boil. Remove from heat and soak the herb for 8 hours or overnight. Bring to a boil again and reduce by simmering to 1 quart. Strain then return the liquid to a clean pan and reduce by simmering to 3/4 pint. Add glycerin, mix well, and allow to cool. Bottle and store in a cool place.

Take 1-3 teaspoons in water each dose. The decoction is 3 times as strong as the infusion. Large amounts may purge the bowels, so regulate the dosage accordingly.

System Cleanse Tea: (see CHAPARRAL PREPARATIONS)

Essiac Tea by Renée Caisse
6-1/2 cups Burdock (A. *lappa*) root, cut form
16 oz. Sheep Sorrel leaf, powdered
1 oz. Rhubarb root (Turkey), powdered
4 oz. Slippery Elm bark, powdered

Rinse clean large pot and lid with hydrogen peroxide to sterilize. Pour 2 gallons of distilled water into sterilized pot. Bring water to a rolling boil with lid on (approximately 30 minutes). Stir in 1 cup Essiac Tea herbs. Replace lid and continue to boil for 10 more minutes. Turn off stove. Scrape down sides of pot and stir with sterilized spatula or spoon. Replace lid and let pot remain closed for 12 hours.

Turn stove to full heat for 20 minutes. While Essiac Tea is heating, rinse bottles, lids, funnel, strainer, and other pot or bowl with hydrogen peroxide. Turn off stove after the 20 minutes and strain liquid into another pot. Use funnel to pour hot liquid into amber bottles immediately, taking care to tighten caps. Allow bottles to cool and tighten caps again. Refrigerate in light-proof bottles.

Suggested use: 2 ounces liquid 2-3 times a day on an empty stomach (2 hours after you have eaten or 15 minutes before you

	eat). Essiac may be warmed on the stove or taken cold. For babies, use 1 ounce of the liquid 2 times a day.
Safety	No health hazards or adverse side effects are known with proper dosages. Plant burrs may cause contact irritation.

Burdock is beneficial during pregnancy. The intensely bitter seed extract is a concentrated preparation and should not be used during the first two trimesters of pregnancy.

Used alone, the herb will sometimes cause expulsion of toxins through the skin and may result in the formation of temporary pustules. When combined with a diuretic (such as dandelion or juniper berry), toxins move out more effectively through the urine, rather than the skin. |
| **Plant Profile** | *Natural Habitat:*
A. lappa comes from southern Europe but is cultivated in northern Asia and North America, primarily in the north part of the United States. *A. minus* is the American source of the root and is found in most areas of the continental United States. |
| *Description* | Burdock prefers cool climates and grows as a weed along roadsides and rich waste places. Burdock is any one of a group of biennial thistles in the genus Arctium. The plants grow three to nine feet tall and have large (up to 18 inches), dark green leaves. Its leaves are coarse and ovate, with the lower ones being heart-shaped; the underside of the leaves are woolly to hairy. The leafstalks are generally hollow. Crimson to purple flowers bloom in July and August, after which they dry out and the base becomes the troublesome, half-inch burr that easily catches onto clothes and animal fur. |
| *Growing Burdock* | *Planting*:
Burdock seeds are direct sown in the spring to midsummer. The plant prefers full sunlight and freshly worked soil rich in humus.

Alternate planting method:
For easy harvesting of the root, burdock may be grown in a bale of hay. Take an old bale of wet hay and connect four 1x4 boards, like an empty-bottomed flat, to fit on top of the hay bale. Fill the bottomless flat with garden soil and plant burdock seeds. Seeds |

Harvesting

will germinate and send their roots down into the hay. When harvesting, remove the boards and pull apart the hay to reveal perfectly formed and tender burdock roots.

The root is dug up during or after the first growing season and used fresh or dried (older roots are too fibrous). Seeds are harvested at maturity in the fall of the second growing season and dried. Immature flower stalks may be harvested for eating in late spring before flowers appear. After the stem matures, the taste becomes quite bitter. The root and seeds have a mucilaginous (slimy), somewhat sweet, and slightly bitter taste. The leaves and adult stems are bitter.

Catnip

Latin Name: *Nepeta cataria*

Also known as: Catswort, Catmint, Catnep, Catrup, Field Balm

Scientific Classification

There are about 250 species of the Nepeta genus.

Family: Lamiaceae – mint family
Genus Nepeta – catnip
Species N. *cataria* – catnip

Influence on the Body	(PRINCIPAL ACTIONS are listed in CAPITAL LETTERS)
Addictions	ADDICTIONS • drug withdrawal • nicotine withdrawal
Blood and Circulatory System	anemia • improves circulation
Blood Sugar	Hypoglycemia
Body System	fatigue • stress • tension • stimulant (increases internal heat, dispels internal chill, and strengthens metabolism and circulation)
Digestive Tract	aperitive (improves the appetite) • aromatic (has volatile oils, which aid digestion and relieve gas) • bitter (stimulates digestive juices and improves appetite) • DIGESTION • indigestion • nausea • ACID STOMACH • STOMACHIC • upset stomach • vomiting • DIARRHEA • constipation • ENEMA • COLIC • relieves GAS • hemorrhoids • expels worms
Infections and Immune System	COLDS • coughs • ADULT AND CHILD FEVERS • REFRIGERANT (produces coolness and reduces fever) • FLU • CHILDHOOD DISEASES • MEASLES • MUMPS • CHICKEN POX (prevention) • smallpox
Inflammation	Inflammation
Liver	Liver
Lungs and Respiratory System	bronchitis • hiccups • lung congestion • CROUP
Muscles	ACHES • muscular cramps
Nervous System	NERVOUSNESS • nervous headaches • dizziness • shock

	• restlessness • sedative (calms and exerts soothing or tranquilizing effect) • RELAXANT (relaxes nerves and muscles, relieves tension) • INSOMNIA • SLEEPLESSNESS • SPASMS • CONVULSIONS • epilepsy • hysteria • insanity • mental illness
Pain	PAIN RELIEVER • toothache
Reproductive System	Female: stimulates menstruation • menstrual cramps • infertility • amenorrhea (menstrual failure) • MORNING SICKNESS • uterine problems • MISCARRIAGE (helps prevent)
Skin, Tissues and Hair	skin problems • external sores • ACNE
Urinary Tract	bladder • water retention • kidney stones
Other Uses	CAT STIMULANT • insect repellant (MOSQUITOES & cockroaches)

	Key Properties:
DIGESTIVE AID	*relieves gas and intestinal spasms, improves appetite and increases peristalsis*
	Specific for <u>CHILDHOOD DISEASES</u>
RELAXANT	*relaxes nerves and muscles; relieves tension*
DIAPHORETIC	*increases perspiration*
Nervine	*improves nerve function*
Primarily affecting	*NERVES • INTESTINES*

History	Catnip is in the mint family. In Elizabethan England, it was called cat mint and was the most popular tea before black tea was introduced. Catnip tea has a very pleasant smell and taste and is calming to the nerves. Europeans also used catnip tea for bronchitis and diarrhea.
	Culpepper (1616-1654) mentions catnip as a topical aid for hemorrhoids. North American Natives used catnip for its sedative effect on the nervous system and for treating colic in infants.
Attributes	**<u>Key Components:</u>** (including, but not limited to)
Nutrients	Vitamins A • B1 (thiamine) • B2 (riboflavin) • B3 (niacin)

CATNIP — 73

• B5 (pantothenic acid) • B6 (pyridoxine) • B9 (folic acid)
• B12 (cobalamin) • Biotin • Choline • Inositol • PABA (Para-Amino Benzoic Acid) • C • Iron (good source) • Magnesium • Manganese • Phosphorous • Sodium • Sulfur
Volatile oils (chiefly Nepetalactone - for distinctive smell)
• Bitters • Tannins

Digestion

Catnip relieves gas and generally soothes and relaxes the bowels. The tea has a diuretic effect which reduces swollen tissues (including puffy eyes) and increases gallbladder activity.

Catnip enemas cleanse the colon, reduce spasms, and increase urination. It is often used as a warm enema because of its relaxing action. Use the tea enema in large amounts to expel worms, release gas, and to treat fevers and nervous headaches.

Children

Catnip is a gentle antispasmodic that relieves indigestion and gas in babies and young children with colic, stomach pains, and fevers. It is also helpful for babies who are teething.

A catnip and fennel extract combination are an excellent liquid form that babies and children can take easily. It is famous for settling the stomach and soothing nerves.

Catnip works quickly to overcome convulsions in children. It also helps to control restlessness and colic by calming the nerves.

Blood and Circulation

It has been documented that catnip normalizes blood pressure. It improves circulation and helps to reduce fatigue from muscle exhaustion.

Nerves

Catnip relieves pain, prevents spasms, and calms the nerves. The herb elevates the mood and promotes a feeling of well-being.

Warm catnip tea is also used as a sedative for treating insomnia, dispelling headaches, and sweating out fevers.

Immune System

Catnip reduces excess mucus in the body and is often used for colds and flus, especially in children. It produces 'perspiration inducing sleep' without increasing body temperature. The sweat-releasing effects, in this sense, help the body to evacuate poisons and lower body temperature. Catnip enemas reduce fevers quickly in both adults and children.

Addictions

It is said that putting several drops of catnip extract on the back of the tongue will decrease the desire for cigarettes.

Insect Repellant	Using nepetalactone from catnip to repel mosquitoes was reported to be ten times more effective than using the same amount of DEET (an ingredient in commercial insect repellents).

Evidence that catnip repels flies and cockroaches was observed in preliminary studies. |
Cats	It must be mentioned that catnip is a favorite of cats, many of which develop an almost unnatural affection for it. The bruised, fresh herb may be given to cats to make them happy or to silence nighttime yowling. Catnip affects about two-thirds of cats in this way.
Herb Parts Used	Leaves and flowers are harvested during the early flowering stage, without the stem, and used fresh or dried as an herb.
Preparations and Remedies	***Never boil catnip. Much of the therapeutic value is in the volatile oil and will be lost.***
Fresh	Chew the fresh leaves for a toothache.

Catnip and Fennel Extract:
For colic, gas, and indigestion |
| *Powdered Formula* | *Liver Formula:* (see MILK THISTLE preparations). |
| *Infusions* | *Catnip Tea:*
Make tea with 1 tablespoon herb to 1 cup water. Steep 5-15 minutes. Drink 1-8 ounces of the tea as needed. Catnip tea may be used for headaches caused by digestive disturbances. It makes a mild, aromatic tea for colds, flu, fevers, and fussiness in children. Warm catnip tea is often effective in bringing on a delayed menstrual period. Take the infusion cold to treat suppressed urination. |
| *Enemas* | *Catnip Enema:*
This enema is particularly useful in bringing down fevers, eliminating mucus, relaxing the colon, easing cramping, dislodging congestion in the colon, releasing gas, expelling worms, increasing urination, treating nervous headaches, hiccups, menstrual cramps, and relieving the aches of flu.

4 tablespoons Catnip herb
1 quart Distilled Water

Pour boiling water over catnip in a one quart jar, cover, and let |

steep for ten minutes. Strain and cool until lukewarm. Pour into enema bag with rectal tip and proceed with enema.

Catnip and Garlic Enemas:
A very effective enema combination is equal parts catnip and garlic together in the same bag. Garlic fights infection, pulls mucus, kills germs, bacteria, virus, and parasites, and increases peristaltic action of the colon. Catnip helps ease cramping of the colon, brings down fevers, pulls mucus, helps stop pain, and relaxes and soothes the whole system. These two herbs are a powerful enema combination.

Make catnip tea as described above for catnip enema. Add garlic solution (below) in equal parts in the enema bag.

Garlic Solution:
Blend ten to twelve garlic cloves in one cup of hot water. Strain and add enough water to fill an enema bag.

As an alternative to fresh garlic:
Eight garlic capsules or one teaspoon herbal garlic powder (not the kind found in grocery stores) may be used, but fresh garlic is always preferred. For babies, use one small garlic clove to one pint of water. See additional information in the Garlic chapter.

The enema solution should feel neutral when drops are put on the wrist. Fill the bag according to the child's size. Use one-quarter bag (about one pint) for babies, one bag for small children, and one to two bags for older children.

How to Give an Enema to Babies and Children

Have child lie on their left side if possible. Lubricate the end of the enema tube. Insert it a few inches into the rectum past the sphincter muscle. Do not force. Allow water to flow until there is a cramp or the need to expel. Children should not take the whole bag at once. Their colon is too small. The solution should never be forced. Children need only take the amount that is comfortable. Allow them to expel when they feel the need.

It is helpful to gently massage the colon during an enema. Somewhat following the path of the large intestine, start on the right side of the child's abdomen, massage over to the middle section above the navel, then to the left side, and finally, work down towards the rectum.

Babies may be laid on a towel in the tub. Allow water to enter very slowly. When the baby feels the urge, it will expel.

Safety	No health hazards or adverse side effects are known.
	Catnip has historically been used as a uterine stimulant during childbirth, so it is generally recommended that it not be used during pregnancy.
Plant Profile	*Natural Habitat:* Indigenous to Europe, catnip originated in the Mediterranean area. It is now commonly found in England, North America, and Canada. Catnip is considered to be a common, ditch-bank weed.
Description	Catnip is an aromatic, herbaceous plant that cats love. It resembles mint in appearance and grows two to five feet tall. The tall, erect stalks have very fine whitish hairs and branching stems. The flowers are small and white with purple dots and grow in large tufts at the tops of the branches. The leaves are heart shaped (one to two and a half inches long) with finely scalloped margins, a green upper surface, a grayish-green underside, and whitish hairs.
	Catnip's odor is distinctive and faintly mint like. The herb has a pungent, bitter taste. The plant readily spreads and reseeds itself once it is established.

Cayenne or Capsicum

Latin Name: *Capsicum annum*

Also known as: Red Pepper, Bird Pepper, African Bird Pepper, Pipo

Scientific Classification

The capsicum genus has many herbs in it,
cayenne, chili pepper, bell pepper, pimento, paprika, tabasco pepper, etc.

Family: Solanaceae – potato family
Genus Capsicum – pepper
Species C. annuum – cayenne pepper

Influence on the Body	(PRINCIPAL ACTIONS are listed in CAPITAL LETTERS)
Addictions	HANGOVER
Autoimmune Disorders	RHEUMATISM
Blood and Circulatory System	HEART • HEART ATTACKS • PALPITATION • BLOOD PRESSURE EQUALIZER • HIGH BLOOD PRESSURE • HYPOTENSION • LOW BLOOD PRESSURE • CARDIOVASCULAR TONIC • CIRCULATORY DISORDERS • blood thinner • blood cleanser • arteriosclerosis • external and internal BLEEDING • HEMORRHAGE • NOSEBLEEDS • VARICOSE VEINS • VEIN ELASTICITY • PHLEBITIS (inflammation of veins)
Blood Sugar	DIABETES
Body System	ENERGY • GENERAL TONIC (increases energy and strengthens the muscular and nervous system, while improving digestion and assimilation, resulting in a general sense of well-being) • fatigue • lethargy • preparation for SURGERY • CATALYST (enhances function) • astringent (increases the tone and firmness of tissues, lessens mucous discharge from the nose, intestines, vagina and draining sores) • increases PERSPIRATION • promotes SWEATING • diaphoretic (promotes perspiration, increasing elimination through the skin)
Cancer	TUMORS
Digestive Tract	APPETITE STIMULANT • aromatic (has a spicy taste, contains volatile oils which aid digestion and relieve gas) • digestive disorders • STOMACH ULCERS • ULCERS

	• CARMINATIVE (brings warmth, circulation, relieves intestinal gas discomfort, and promotes peristalsis) • gas • COLON • COLON INDIGESTION
Endocrine System	Pancreas
Eyes and Nose	eyes • sinus problems
First Aid	bruises • burns • sunburn • cuts • WOUNDS (stops bleeding) • vulnerary (promotes healing of wounds by protecting against infection and stimulating cellular growth) • SHOCK • prevents FROSTBITE • insect bites and stings • sprains
Infections and Immune System	CHILLS • COLDS • coughs • hay fever • antipyretic (reduces fever) • INFECTION • antiseptic • antibacterial • spleen • contagious diseases • lock jaw (tetanus) • diphtheria • malaria
Inflammation	inflammation • ARTHRITIS • RHEUMATISM
Liver	jaundice • liver
Lungs and Respiratory System	ASTHMA • BRONCHITIS • GENERAL CONGESTION • fluid in the LUNGS • mucus • pleurisy
Mouth and Throat	offensive breath • pyorrhea (a gum disease) • LARYNGITIS • SORE THROAT • TONSILLITIS
Nervous System	cluster headaches • CONVULSIONS • palsy • spasms • Parkinson's disease • STROKES • paralysis • SENILITY
Pain	chronic pain • external backache • cramps
Reproductive System	*Male:* male tonic *Female:* menorrhagia (excessive bleeding during menstruation)
Skin, Tissues and Hair	shingles • skin problems • diaphoretic (promotes perspiration, increasing elimination through the skin) • rubefacient (increases blood flow to the skin causing local reddening)
Urinary Tract	Kidneys
Other Uses	CATALYST in herb formula combinations (enhances the function of other herbs)

Key Properties:

HEART and CIRCULATION DIGESTIVE AID	*relieves gas, increases gastric secretions and appetite, repairs ulcers*

CAYENNE OR CAPSICUM

STIMULANT	*increases internal heat, dispels chill, strengthens metabolism and circulation*
Analgesic	*relieves pain • <u>mucous decongestant</u> • <u>antispasmodic</u> • <u>antiseptic</u>*
Primarily affecting	HEART • CIRCULATION • STOMACH • NERVES

History	References to cayenne have been found on plaques in Egyptian tombs. It was cultivated for hundreds of years in Africa, India, and tropical areas, including the tropical Americas. Healers from India have used cayenne as an Ayurvedic (Indian traditional medicine) herb for many centuries. The North American Cherokee natives used cayenne for its stimulating properties, while the Navajos used it as a means of weaning children. The hot, pungent taste of the cayenne pepper was introduced to Europe by Columbus on his return trip from the Americas. John Lindley (1799-1865) wrote in his Flora Medica (1838) about capsicum annuum being employed as a gargle, administered internally, and for treating gout, gas, and paralysis. In 1943, the Dispensary of the United States of America reported, 'Capsicum is a powerful local stimulant, producing, when swallowed, a sense of heat in the stomach and a general glow over the body without narcotic effect.' Cayenne and related peppers have a long history of use as digestive aids in many parts of the world, but the herb's recent popularity has come through conventional medicine. Capsaicin, the 'heat' component in peppers, has been approved by the FDA (U.S. Federal Drug Administration) for treatment of pain that often lingers after an attack of shingles. There is also evidence that capsaicin creams may be helpful for relieving various types of arthritis. My Mom taught us how to use cayenne from a young age. If she was cold, she would mix a teaspoon of cayenne (40,000 HU) in a cup of water and drink it down. She would also put cayenne between two pairs of socks before my brothers would go hiking in the snow of the Sierra Nevadas. The first time I really experienced the majesty of cayenne was when a young friend of my son was playing at our home and cut his hand on the top of a can. I ran it under water and put pressure

on it, but it still wouldn't stop bleeding. I remembered the cayenne and poured it on his hand. It stopped bleeding immediately and alleviated any discomfort he was experiencing.

More recently, I mixed cayenne into a natural cream for my aging mother's 'burning' feet. After just three applications, her discomfort stopped. She had been suffering for over six months with this condition. I also make up an easy and effective cough syrup (recipe to follow). I am grateful each time I remember the wisdom with which I was raised. I hope you will pass on this wisdom to the next generation and beyond.

Attributes	**Key Components:** (including, but not limited to)
Nutrients	Vitamins A (partially responsible for its red color) • Carotenes • Lutein (yellow carotenoid pigment) • B1 (thiamine) • B2 (riboflavin) • B3 (niacin) • B5 (pantothenic acid) • B6 (pyridoxine) • B9 (folic acid) • B12 (cobalamin) • Biotin • Choline • Inositol • PABA (Para-Amino Benzoic Acid) • C • Bioflavonoids • E • K • Calcium • Iron • Magnesium • Phosphorous • Potassium • Sulfur • Phytosterols • Capsaicin (effective for blocking the transmission of the pain impulse to the brain)
Heat Units (HU)	The 'heat' of the herbs in the pepper family is measured by a Heat Unit (HU) rating system, which is equivalent to BTU (British Thermal Units). In other words, the rating of how 'hot' the herbs are. Cayenne is the hot capsicum pepper, generally rated from 40,000 HU on up to the hottest at around 300,000 HU. Most cayenne is in the range of 40,000 to 100,000 HU. The hotter the heat unit does not necessarily mean the herb is more effective. I recommend 90,000 HU cayenne. It seems to be tolerated by most people and is very effective.
Stimulant	Cayenne stimulates circulation and the nervous system. The effect is almost immediate and the benefits linger. Circulation is equalized everywhere. The heart is given immediate support and nutrition. It beats more firmly and steady, and the blood vessels dilate. Nutrients from foods will reach and penetrate damaged muscle and nerve tissues more efficiently when cayenne is eaten in strong doses with meals. Profuse perspiration cleanses the pores of the skin and the effect on the nervous system is electrifying.

Stimulation is the key to healing. When the body and its organs are properly stimulated, they heal, cleanse and return to normal function. If taken regularly, cayenne will reach and rejuvenate every part of the body. It has been used specifically in the treatment of the spleen, pancreas, kidneys, and ulcers of the stomach.

Heart and Circulatory System

Capsicum gives the cardiovascular system a little lift by stimulating the heart and enhancing circulation without raising blood pressure (it actually adjusts itself to normal). Pulse rate does not get faster, but each beat of the heart is given more power. Cayenne influences the heart immediately, then gradually extends its effects; feeding, restoring the elasticity, and healing ulcers in the cell structures of the walls of arteries, veins and capillaries.

Cayenne is used for strengthening the heart muscle. In emergency situations (such as heart failure), cayenne can be administered to stimulate the heart muscle, restore active circulation, and normalize blood pressure. Capsicum is excellent for equalizing blood circulation, which works to prevent strokes and heart attacks, and will bring one quickly out of shock. It is reported that capsicum significantly lowers serum cholesterol and triglycerides and improves the ratio of HDL (high-density lipoprotein - good cholesterol) and LDL (low- density lipoprotein - bad cholesterol) elements, reducing the risk of heart disease.

Bleeding

Cayenne is useful in arresting hemorrhages, both externally and internally. Even when the bone is exposed in a deep injury, cayenne pepper can be poured onto the wound to stop bleeding, cleanse and accelerate healing.

Red Skin

As blood flow increases to the skin, it may cause local reddening and feel warm. When people see this, they may think that the skin is irritated, but cayenne is a counter-irritant (there is no itching involved). Cayenne brings the blood to the surface (causing redness) to take away toxic poisons and begin the healing process. The warm, burning sensation heals, rather than damages, the tissues.

Warms the Body

Sprinkle a small amount of cayenne into shoes to keep the feet warm on a cold day (too much cayenne will over heat and produce a burning sensation). Sprinkle a small amount of powder into socks to prevent frostbite.

Promotes Perspiration

Interestingly, many people who live in hot tropical areas consume goodly amounts of hot peppers every day to cool down. Perspiration is the natural cooling mechanism of the body. Capsicum promotes perspiration and increases elimination through the skin.

Weight

By increasing circulation, cayenne raises the metabolic rate of the body, especially when combined with other substances that increase metabolism. Cayenne also stimulates the liver, increases the number of liver enzymes responsible for fat metabolism, and decreases the fat deposits in the liver caused by a high fat diet.

Digestion

Like many spices, cayenne pepper increases the flow of digestive secretions from salivary, gastric, and intestinal glands. This stimulates the appetite, improves digestion, relieves gas discomfort and distension, and promotes peristalsis in the intestines. Cayenne enhances the body's ability to digest food in the stomach, assimilate nutrients in the intestines, and expel wastes through the colon.

Capsicum supports the cleansing and removal of ulcerous tissue from the stomach and the acceleration of tissue regeneration and healing.

Catalyst for Herb Formulas

Capsicum is used as a catalyst in many herb combinations. It aids in the absorption and effectiveness of most any herb formula. The nutrients are assimilated far faster into the body and moved to where they are needed more efficiently.

Arthritis

Those suffering from osteoarthritis and rheumatoid arthritis have received relief by using a rub-on cream made with capsaicin, an ingredient of capsicum. It is possible to make a liniment with cayenne extract or the powdered herb to relieve inflammation. Rub the extract over arthritic joints and wrap with a cotton flannel cloth overnight, or make a poultice with the powdered herb. Although the 'heat' of the herb may be severe, there is usually no reddening or blistering of the skin. Capsaicin primarily affects sensory nerves, having very little action upon blood vessels.

Toothaches	Capsicum is useful for relieving toothaches. Rub the powder on the affected area.
Poultice	Combining capsicum and plantain and applying them externally in a poultice can draw out foreign items embedded in the skin.
Infections and Immune System	Cayenne is excellent for disease prevention and the quick improvement of conditions caused by the flu or a cold. In the case of diarrhea caused by exotic bacteria, cayenne (especially taken in capsule form) will often elicit a rapid return to normal gastrointestinal function.
Alcohol Addiction	Capsicum is said to be able to help people end their addiction to alcohol, possibly by reducing the dilated blood vessels and thus relieving chronic congestion.
Cancer	The herb may be taken as part of a daily diet to ward off disease in general and, specifically, to act as a cancer preventative.
Herb Parts Used	Whole red peppers, with or without the seeds, used fresh or dried.
Preparations and Remedies	***When heated, cayenne loses most of its healing qualities and becomes an irritant.***
Fresh	The fresh chilies are the most nutritious, with the most Vitamin C. They also contain a beneficial essential oil that aids digestion. Be cautious and wear rubber gloves when preparing fresh peppers and their seeds, as their oil can burn the skin. Cayenne may be added to soups and salads. Home-made Hot Sauce: Cover the fresh or dried peppers with vinegar in a macerating jar (a non-porous container with a lid); soak overnight. Blend and continue to macerate for a week. (Maceration is the process of breaking down the fruit of a plant to a soft, mushy consistency, releasing some of its moisture, flavor and properties into a liquid of choice.) Next, express the pulp out and add salt to taste. This makes a thin hot sauce that may be used freely according to preference and tolerance.

Powder

The cayenne pepper of grocery stores is largely a mixture of paprika and true pepper. Paprika (Hungarian pepper) has scarcely more than one-sixth the pungency of real cayenne pepper.

Color does not entirely determine the quality of powdered peppers. The red color of cayenne does fade when exposed to light, however, some types of red peppers are naturally lighter in color, yet still very potent and powerful. The value of any specimen may be fairly estimated by the intensity of its odor (which is peculiar, somewhat aromatic, and extremely irritant) and by its acrid, burning taste.

First Aid

A teaspoon of cayenne in a cup of water can help stop a heart attack, bring someone out of shock, help a headache vanish, and assist in warming a body in hypothermia. Cayenne can help stop bleeding when applied to a wound or taken internally. Cayenne is a disinfectant and will actually reduce pain when applied to a cut.

Cayenne is used in nearly all external applications where speed is important, or when quick relief (as in arthritis, rheumatism, bursitis, and sore muscles) is desired. Cayenne may be added to all natural creams or lotions and used for external discomfort or circulation problems.

Sprinkle powdered cayenne on bleeding cuts, wounds, or abrasions and it almost immediately stops the bleeding. Cayenne powder or liquid extract may be rubbed directly on toothaches or swellings for relief.

Liquid Extract

The liquid extract is valuable to have on hand for emergencies. Use it moderately, as it is many times stronger than the tea. Place the powder or extract on or under the tongue for crisis situations such as shock, hemorrhage, or heart attack.

Tea/Infusion

Cayenne is seldom used in a decoction because some value is lost when it is simmered for any length of time.

Cayenne Tea:
A tea may be made by pouring hot water over the cayenne and letting it steep.

Valerian Tea: (see VALERIAN preparations)

Washes

Pregnancy Decoction: (see WILD YAM preparations)

Eye Wash: (see GOLDENSEAL preparations)

Fomentations

Cayenne is effective as a fomentation (towel soaked in warm infusion and placed on affected area) for rheumatism, inflammation, pleurisy, sores and wounds. It soothes discomfort and promotes healing and circulation.

Soothing Fomentation: (see LOBELIA preparations)

Breathe Easy Fomentation: (see MULLEIN preparations)

Poultices

Cayenne added to any poultice will promote circulation.

Healing Poultice:
1 part comfrey leaves
1 part plantain
1/16 part cayenne
Optional: add two parts slippery elm for binding a wound and soothing inflammation.

Mix powdered herbs with warm water and make a paste. Spread on the affected area and cover with a natural fiber cloth. Apply heat if desired.

Slippery Elm Poultice: (see SLIPPERY ELM preparations)

Poultice for Boils and Abscesses: (see ECHINACEA preparations)

Liniment Rub

Cayenne Liniment Rub:
1 cup raw apple cider vinegar
1-1/2 teaspoon cayenne
Pour hot vinegar over cayenne. Cover and let steep for a few hours. Use immediately or continue to macerate (soak to soften and release constituents) for up to two weeks for greater strength. Store liniment rub in a light-proof bottle and apply externally when needed for sprains, swellings, inflammation, and deep-seated internal congestion.

	Alternative: Once the liniment is cool, add 1/4 teaspoon wintergreen essential oil (about 25 drops). Shake capped bottle vigorously each time before using to disperse the oil.
Spray	Cayenne Spray: Distilled Water Cayenne to tolerance Glycerin (optional) for greater adherence Mix water with cayenne. Filter out any grittiness by running the mixture through an unbleached coffee strainer. Put in spray bottle. The spray is slightly numbing. Use for the discomfort of arthritis, painful joints, sore muscles, neuropathy, and numbness or burning in the extremities.
Ointments	Easy Cayenne Cream or Ointment: Add cayenne powder or extract (to tolerance) to a simple, organic cream or ointment (without synthetic ingredients). Cayenne ointment is extremely valuable due to its powerful ability to bring out toxic poisons and as a counter-irritant, easing arthritic and sore muscle discomfort. It may be used safely without burning or blistering.
Internal Uses	**When used as a catalyst in herb formulas, cayenne is generally used as a one-eighth part compared to other herbs used in the formulation, unless otherwise stated.**
Capsules	Taking cayenne powder in capsules carries the herb deep into the gastrointestinal tract and eliminates the feeling of 'heat' in the mouth. At the first sign of a cold, take two capsules of capsicum every hour with a large glass of water. By eating nothing else, an oncoming illness can be warded off within a few hours. It is not recommended to take more than eight capsules in a twenty-four hour period. Colon discomfort and purging may result.
Tonic	Daily Tonic: (four days a week) Taking 1/4 teaspoon powder in water or juice, up to 3 times a day, will benefit the heart and circulation in the body.

Bleeding	For Internal Bleeding: Take a teaspoonful of cayenne in a glass of extra-warm water and drink it down. By the count of ten, in most cases, the bleeding will stop.
Cough Syrups	2 tablespoons freshly squeezed lemon juice (or raw apple cider vinegar) 2 tablespoons honey ¼ tsp or more cayenne (depending on tolerance) Mix and keep in the fridge. Shake well before using. For sore, scratchy throat or cough, take one teaspoon cough syrup as needed. Garlic Syrup: (see GARLIC preparations) Ginger Cough Syrup: (see GINGER preparations) Slippery Elm Cough Syrup: (see SLIPPERY ELM preparations)
Enemas	Garlic Enema: (see GARLIC preparations)
Safety	Cayenne should not be used internally for hemorrhage during childbirth. It can stop bleeding temporally, but as the circulation increases, bleeding could resume after a short period of time. A skilled midwife may choose to use cayenne directly in the uterus, as she deems necessary. Handle fresh cayenne with great respect and keep out of eyes and away from mucous membranes. Contact with cayenne herb or extract will not permanently damage the eyes or mucous membranes, but it can cause serious discomfort. If cayenne gets into the eyes or mucous membranes, flush the area freely with cold milk until the burning abates. If skin contact with cayenne becomes uncomfortable, first rinse with plain rubbing alcohol and then wash with soap and water. Wear a filter mask when grinding dried cayenne. Grinders used to process cayenne must be cleaned with alcohol, then soap and water, otherwise, potent oils and resins will affect subsequent products.

Cayenne sometimes gives a burning sensation to the throat and stomach, but it does not damage them. In fact, studies show that cayenne helps heal ulcers. For the first few days of taking cayenne, it may feel hot going in and hot going out. The body eventually becomes accustomed to the sensation. With continuous use, it feels more like a warm glow.

Plant Profile

Natural Habitat:
Indigenous to Mexico and Central America, cayenne is now cultivated in all warmer regions of the globe. While the species can tolerate most climates, they are especially productive in warm and dry climates.

Description

The varieties of capsicum fruits vary greatly in size, color and 'heat' of taste. The hottest is the yellowish red fruit of Sierra Leone, West Africa. These African birdseye cayenne have small (1/3 to 1/2 inch long), pungent, bright pods. Once consumed, the 'heat' is retained longer in the body than any other variety. The African varieties grow on shrub-size plants with small and pungent fruit, while the American varieties are herb-size plants with larger, heart-shaped fruit.

The red pepper 'cayenne' is a perennial shrub in its native South America and other warm parts of the world. In northern gardens, it is an annual, dying out each year.

The plant grows 20-60 inches. The leaves are covered with short, soft hairs. Single white flowers, purple-tinged and ornamental, bear thin, long pods that are very shiny and thick-skinned. The pods are initially green and eventually turn red or yellow.

Cayenne is readily recognized by its characteristic 'heat', due to the high concentration of the compound known as capsaicin (from the Greek word 'to bite'). Capsicum has been aptly described as the plant that bites back.

Growing Cayenne Pepper

Planting:
Don't set plants out too early. Peppers are heat-lovers and prefer warm climates. In cooler areas, grow the plant in a greenhouse or amid sheltered borders out of doors, in full sun. The plant flowers in midsummer. Protect the blossoms from sun and wind damage by planting them with taller plants.

Harvesting — When fruits are uniformly red, cut them from the plant, leaving a stem of at least ½ inch long. Dry them immediately on screens, or string together using a needle and heavy thread. The entire plant may also be pulled out of the ground to dry.

Storage — Do not put cayenne in a paper sack. Paper takes the precious oils out of it. Do not refrigerate. Store peppers whole or ground in tightly sealed containers. Keep cayenne powder at room temperature. Cayenne fades in the light and should always be kept in dark containers. When kept sealed in proper conditions, it will keep its potency for six months to a year. Cayenne will last longer if made into a fluid extract.

Chamomile

Latin Name: *Matricaria rectita (German)*
or *Chamaemelum nobile (Roman)*

Also known as: Ground Apple, Wild Chamomile, Camomile, German Chamomile, Roman (or English) Chamomile, Manzanilla (in Latin America)

Scientific Classification

Chamomile is a common name for several daisy-like plants. German chamomile and Roman chamomile are the two major herb types used for health purposes.

Family:	Asteraceae – aster, daisy and sunflower family
	Compositae – in earlier classifications
Genus	Matricaria – mayweed
Species	*Matricaria recutita* – German chamomile
Genus	Chamaemelum – dogfennel
Species	*Chamaemelum nobile* – Roman chamomile
	Anthemis nobilis – in earlier classifications

Influence on the Body	(PRINCIPAL ACTIONS are listed in CAPITAL LETTERS)
Addictions	ALCOHOLISM • DRUG ADDICTION • SMOKING (calms nerves) • DRUG WITHDRAWAL
Blood and Circulatory System	blood disorders • blood purifier • POOR CIRCULATION
Body System	• dropsy (edema due to poor heart function) • hemorrhage tonic (increases energy and strength throughout the body) • stimulant (increases internal heat, dispels internal chill, and strengthens metabolism and circulation) • ABSCESSES • air pollution
Cancer	Tumors
Digestive Tract	APPETITE STIMULANT • aromatic (has a spicy taste, contains volatile oils which aid digestion and relieve gas) • bitter (stimulates digestive juices and improves appetite) • heartburn • DIGESTION • INDIGESTION • nausea • stomach upset • stomach cramps • COLIC • carminative (brings warmth, circulation, relieves intestinal gas discomfort, and promotes peristalsis) • ulcerations • peptic ulcers • colitis • constipation • diarrhea • diverticulitis • expels GAS • hemorrhoids • expels worms • parasites

Ears	earaches • dizziness
Eyes	sore eyes • eye wash
First Aid	wounds • open sores • bruises • sprains
Infections and Immune System	childhood diseases • colds • antibiotic • antifungal • coughs • reduces FEVERS • flus • measles • spleen • typhoid
Inflammation	anti-inflammatory
Liver	gallstones • jaundice • stimulates liver • sluggish liver
Lungs and Respiratory System	bronchial tubes • BRONCHITIS • mucous discharge • expectorant (loosens and removes phlegm in the respiratory tract) • lungs • asthma
Mouth and Throat	teething • TOOTHACHE • sore throat • throat gargle
Muscles	MUSCLE PAIN • leg cramps
Nervous System	NERVINE (improves nerve function) • anxiety • NERVOUS DISORDERS • INSOMNIA • calmative (gently calms nerves) • sedative (calming, exerts soothing or tranquilizing effect) • SLEEP • headaches • migraine headaches • relieves pain • anodyne (relieves pain and reduces nerve excitability) • spasms • HYSTERIA
Pain	pain reliever
Reproductive System	*Female:* menstrual regulator • painful MENSTRUATION • emmenagogue (promotes menstrual flow) • menstrual cramps • BREAST CYSTS • UTERUS
Skin, Tissues and Hair	gangrenous sores • callouses • CORNS • dandruff
Urinary Tract	bladder problems • kidneys • diuretic (increases urine flow) • bedwetting

Key Properties:

NERVES	*calms and heals nerves, mildly sedative and anti-spasmodic*
DIGESTIVE AID	*increases appetite and relieves gas*
analgesic	*relieves pain*
boosts immunity	*promotes menstrual flow*
emmenagogue	

CHAMOMILE — 92

Primarily affecting *NERVES • STOMACH • UTERUS*

History	Early Egyptian physicians used chamomile for fevers. The Greeks called it 'ground apple' (kamai for 'on the ground' and melon for 'apple'), due to the apple-like scent of its flower and the way it grows as low ground cover. The Greeks and Romans used the herb for headaches.
	Anglo-Saxons believed it was one of the nine sacred herbs given to humans by the god Woden. Nicholas Culpepper, an English herbalist, claimed that chamomile had the ability to take away weariness and ease pain wherever it was applied. English author Beatrix Potter had Peter Rabbit's mother give him chamomile tea after his frightful adventure.
	Chamomile has been used for centuries to quiet an upset stomach, promote urination, relieve colic, and induce sleep. The Cherokee Indians used it in cases of colic, bowel complaints, and vomiting.
	In 1921, a German manufacturer introduced a topical form of chamomile which became a popular treatment for a wide variety of skin disorders. Germany's Commission E report authorizes the use of various topical chamomile preparations for diseases of the skin and mouth. It has authorized taking chamomile internally for pain and inflammation in the stomach and intestines and using inhaled chamomile-vapor for asthma and other lung problems.
	In Europe today, chamomile is used to treat inflammations and irritations of the skin and mucous membranes, soothe aches, and heal cuts, sores, and bruises.
Attributes	Chamomile calms and soothes irritating conditions, is anti-inflammatory, and is anti-spasmodic. It is used for digestive problems, headaches, stress, irritability, nervousness, allergies, and swollen or inflamed tissues.
Nutrients	**Key Components:** (including, but not limited to)
	Vitamins A • Calcium • Iron • Magnesium • Manganese • Potassium • Zinc • Bitter
Nerves	Although chamomile is a stimulant, its abilities to equalize circulation and strengthen, quiet, and heal nerve endings result in soothing the nervous system and relaxing the body. In Europe,

chamomile is commonly used as a sleep-inducing herb. It quickly helps one to settle down for quality sleep and is often used for preventing migraine headaches.

Digestion

The tea tones and heals the complete digestive tract. It improves appetite and aids digestion by increasing blood circulation in the intestinal tract, reducing gas and muscle spasms and helping to expel worms and parasites.

Those who have sinus troubles often have bowel problems as well. Using chamomile tea as a digestive aid can help get bowels moving properly and relieve other congestions in the body.

Muscle Spasm

Drinking chamomile tea is associated with an increase in urinary levels of glycine, an amino acid that has been shown to relieve muscle spasms. This may explain why the tea appears to be helpful in easing menstrual, gastro-intestinal, and leg muscle cramps.

Glycine is also known to act as a nerve relaxant. Scientists believe the tea seems to act as a mild sedative for this reason.

Children

Chamomile is popular as a children's remedy for earaches, convulsions, teething, calming and relaxing nerves, stomach disorders, and controlling bedwetting. At first, it may seem that drinking tea before going to bed would not be advisable to control bedwetting, but it is very effective. It seems to help children relax while going to sleep, thereby allowing them to feel the urge to urinate.

The medical professions in France and Spain recognize chamomile as a valuable tonic for the young with such problems as colic, upset stomachs, and sleep difficulties. It is reportedly useful as a remedy for nightmares (especially in children).

Fever

Chamomile is used as a relaxing diaphoretic (to induce perspiration), making it excellent for fevers and colds.

External Use

As a poultice, chamomile reduces swelling without drawing the poison to a head. It can often prevent or remove gangrene. Chamomile is excellent for bruises and sprains by crushing the herb, moistening with vinegar, and applying topically.

It also eases pain, itch, and irritation of the skin. One double-blind study of 161 individuals found chamomile cream equally effective as 25 percent hydrocortisone cream for the treatment of eczema.

Anti-bacterial	Researchers found that drinking chamomile tea was associated with a significant increase in urinary levels of hippurate (a breakdown product of certain plant-based compounds known as phenolics) associated with increased antibacterial activity. This could help explain why the tea is able to boost the immune system and fight infections associated with colds.
Anti-inflammatory	Studies have found that chamazulene, a component of the essential oil of German chamomile, has both anti-inflammatory and antiseptic activities. Chamazulene is also found in Roman chamomile, but in lesser concentrations. Its anti-inflammatory activity stems from its ability to inhibit inflammatory prostaglandin (hormone-like substance) production.
	Chamomile is contained in many skin creams and, because it is virtually anti-toxic, helps to prevent skin infections. A chamomile extract also proved effective in promoting wound healing. (1)(2)(3)
	The essential oil of chamomile can be applied directly to the skin, but it is best diluted in a carrier oil or lotion. Traditionally, chamomile extracts are used topically to treat diaper rash and orally to treat mouth infections.
Women	As a uterine agent, chamomile (when taken cold) relieves congestion and stimulates menstrual flow. It has been effectively used for menstrual cramps as well. Chamomile (manzanilla) is found in almost all Latin American homes for use before, during, and after childbirth.
Hair	Chamomile will add luster and golden tint highlights when used as a hair rinse. It has also been used to overcome dandruff.
Addictions	Chamomile has been used very successfully as a toxin cleanser for long-time drug users.
Herb Substitute	For those who find yarrow bitter, chamomile often makes an excellent substitute.
Other Uses	Industrial manufacture of essential oils of the chamomile flowers:
	Roman chamomile essential oil is used in perfume, shampoo powder, hair rinse, and flavoring for tobacco.
	German chamomile essential oil is used in the perfumery process

	for blending compounds, often in combination with oils of patchouli, lavender, and oak moss. It is also used as a solvent for platinum chloride in the process of coating glass and porcelain with platinum.
Herb Parts Used	The entire flower.
Preparations and Remedies	Chamomile is prepared as bulk dried flowers, tea, capsules, tincture, cream salve, or as a bath product. When given warm, chamomile will favor perspiration and soften the skin. The cold infusion acts as a tonic and is more suitable for stomach disorders, typhoid fever, and fevers in general.
Tea/Infusion	Chamomile tea or tincture are valuable for insomnia and nervousness. As a digestive aid, it improves appetite, relieves spasms and inflammatory conditions of the gastrointestinal tract, and helps heal peptic ulcers. The tea and tincture are used for menstrual cramps and kidney, bladder, and spleen problems. When making the tea, hold in the essential oils by using a cover. Steep (do not boil) fresh or dried flowers for 10 to 30 minutes in hot water. **Boiling chamomile flowers will allow volatile oils (possessing much of the therapeutic value) to escape.** *Yarrow Tea:* (see YARROW preparations)
Eye Wash	Use chamomile tea as a wash for open sores of the skin or irritated eyes. Chamomile tea bags may be steeped in a small amount of hot water, allowed to cool, and placed on closed eyes as well.
Compress/Fomentation	Apply as a compress, fomentation (towel soaked in infusion and placed on affected area), or cream for sore muscles, swellings, and painful joints.
Poultice	When used externally as a poultice, chamomile has a drawing and cooling effect.
Enemas	*Garlic Enema:* (see GARLIC preparations)
Relaxing Herb Bath	Three methods: 1. Put four to eight ounces chamomile (dry or fresh) in a thin muslin cloth bag and put in bath water. 2. Make a gallon of tea and add to the bath. 3. For soaking applications, use one teaspoonful (5 ml) of the

	tincture in a basin of Himalayan or Real Salt water and soak as needed.
Hair Rinse	Make one quart of a strong chamomile tea and use as a rinse at lukewarm temperature after shampooing. It improves color and texture of the hair and fights dandruff.
Essential Oil	Chamomile essential oil is especially helpful when applied to areas of rheumatic joint pain.
Safety	Bulk dried flowers are widely available. Herbal chamomile is sometimes confused with a similar-looking plant which does not have the same medicinal qualities, is bad-tasting, and is highly allergenic. Even when dried, chamomile flowers should be white and yellow-colored (not brown or dingy), and there should be a fresh, characteristic, fruity smell (rather than a musty odor).
	Chamomile is an herb that is beneficial to use during pregnancy. It relaxes the body for sound sleep and helps with digestive and bowel problems.
	Rare allergic reactions occur in persons sensitive to ragweed (another member of the aster family) or the many varieties of chrysanthemum.
	Chamomile is listed on the Federal Drug Administration's GRAS (generally recognized as safe) list.
Plant Profile	*Natural Habitat:* German chamomile is indigenous to Europe and northwest Asia and naturalized elsewhere in places such as North America. Major suppliers of German chamomile include Argentina, Egypt, the Czech Republic, Slovakia, Germany, Hungary, and Poland. Roman (or English) chamomile is native to England and western Europe to Northern Ireland and now grows other places including North America.
Description	The uses of both German and Roman chamomile parallel each other. It is generally considered that both have similar effects on the body, although German chamomile may be slightly stronger. Most research has been done on German chamomile, which is more commonly used everywhere except in England (where Roman chamomile is more often used).

Chamomile flowers from late spring to late summer and has an attractive, apple-like fragrance. Teas made with the herb are aromatic and flavorful. The herb itself has a slightly bitter taste. Both German and Roman chamomile have the same characteristic, thready, lacy leaves, and small, daisy-like blossoms, but the plants have different growth habits.

German chamomile is an annual (must be grown from seed each year) and grows much taller (one to two feet high) than its Roman cousin. The many terminal flower heads are about a half an inch in diameter. The flowers have a yellow center surrounded by ten to twenty white ray petals.

The Roman (or English) species is a low-growing perennial (lives for more than two years, growing back from a persistent rootstock in the spring) which spreads gracefully over the earth, reaching only six to twelve inches in height. It is often grown in herb gardens as a low, mat-like ground cover and can be mowed similar to a lawn. It thrives in dry, light, sandy soil in full sunlight. The flower heads are about an inch across and sparse when compared to German chamomile. A solitary flower head sits atop each stalk. The yellow center is encircled with white, daisy-like petals (though sometimes absent).

Chamomile contributes to the health of the soil and keeps away pests. It has been called 'the plant's physician.'

Growing Chamomile

Planting:
Both German and Roman chamomile varieties are best sown in early spring for flowering by early summer. Direct-seed sow (on the surface and pressed in) German chamomile seeds six inches apart and provide full sun, regular water, and good drainage.
It is better to grow Roman chamomile seeds first in pots and then transplant. As a perennial, the plant self-propagates each year, and plant starts can be made by root division or layering runners. Space new plantings six inches apart.

Harvesting

Harvest the entire full-bloom flower in the morning, just after the dew has evaporated on a warm, dry day. Use the herb fresh or spread flowers out to dry on screens or paper

Storage

Store in tightly sealed containers when dry. Flowers may be frozen for up to six months to retain freshness.

Chaparral

Latin Name: *Larrea tridentata, L. divaricata*

Also known as: Chaparro, Creosote Bush, Greasewood, Stinkweed, Gobernadora

Scientific Classification

Chaparral refers to over one hundred different botanical plant types. It is closely related to the South American Larrea divaricata and was formerly treated as the same species.

Family: Zygophyllaceae – creosote bush family
Genus Larrea - creosote bush
Species L. tridentata - creosote bush
Species L. divaricata - South American variety

Influence on the Body	(PRINCIPAL ACTIONS are listed in CAPITAL LETTERS)
Blood and Circulatory System	blood cleanser • blood poisoning • BLOOD PURIFIER • ALTERATIVE (purifies the blood, cleanses, and induces efficient removal of waste products) • circulation • lowers blood pressure
Body System	potent ANTIOXIDANT • tonic (increases energy and strength throughout the body)
Cancer	CANCER • LEUKEMIA • TUMORS
Digestive Tract	bitter (stimulates digestive juices and improves appetite) • stomach disorders • lower bowels • hemorrhoids • intestinal parasites • expels WORMS
Eyes	strengthens eyes • cataracts • glaucoma
First Aid	cuts • wounds • bruises • snake bites
Infections and Immune System	allergies • hay fever • colds • flus • viral diseases • antibiotic • anti bacterial • antiseptic • anti fungal • candida yeast • chicken pox • herpes • HIV • tetanus
Inflammation	bursitis • anti-inflammatory • ARTHRITIS • osteoarthritis • RHEUMATISM
Lungs and Respiratory System	respiratory system • EXPECTORANT • lungs • asthma • tuberculosis

Muscles	leg cramps
Nervous System	insomnia • anodyne (relieves pain and lessens the excitability of nerves)
Pain	pain • aches • chronic backache
Reproductive System	venereal diseases Male: prostate problems Female: hormone • menopause balancing • prolapsed uterus
Skin, Tissues and Hair	bruises • sores • swelling • boils • SKIN DISEASES • skin problems (blotches) • acne • eczema • psoriasis • warts • athlete's foot • fibrositis (overgrowth of fibrous tissues due to injury) • promotes hair growth • dandruff
Urinary Tract	diuretic • kidney infection • kidney stones • bladder problems
Weight	weight reduction • obesity

Key Properties:

ALTERATIVE - BLOOD PURIFIER	cleanses toxins from blood and eliminative organs
ANTI CARCINOGENIC	*Anti cancerous*
ANTIOXIDANT	
IMMUNE STIMULATOR	
ANTI MICROBIAL	*Inhibits bacterial, viral, and fungal infections*
Primarily affecting	BLOOD and liver • DIGESTIVE TRACT • URINARY TRACT • LUNGS • IMMUNE SYSTEM
History	The word 'chaparral' comes from the Spanish language, meaning 'a low-growing shrub.' Native Americans of the southwest called chaparral the 'Mother of All Plants.' It plays a prominent role in the creation stories of the Pima tribe. They believe the creator planted the bush shortly after creating the world. Papago, Pima, and Maricopa tribes of the southwestern states area boiled the leaves and branches for bruises and rheumatism. The dry-heated leaves and branches were applied as a poultice for chest and other pains of the body. The tips of young chaparral branches were sharpened, placed in the fire until hot, and inserted into tooth cavities to relieve discomfort.

The Kawaiisu, Paiute, and Shoshone tribes used the creosote bush for ailments relating to sepsis (bacteria infection) and digestive elimination. Resin from the leaves was rubbed on burns, scratches, sores, and wounds. They used chaparral tea to treat colds, bronchitis, chicken pox, snake bite, and arthritis.

White settlers were taught by friendly Native Americans and adopted the plant, using it for bruises, rashes, dandruff, and wounds. They used it internally for diarrhea, stomach upset, menstrual problems, venereal diseases, and cancers of the liver, kidney, and stomach. In Mexico, chaparral has been used for centuries as an anti-cancer remedy.

My Mom drank chaparral tea, and my Grandma drank it. Grandma even had a pan she used just for her chaparral tea. The oily creosote formed a thick, oily residue on the inside of the pan that could never be completely cleaned out. (Please note when making chaparral tea over and over, it may ruin the pan you are using.)

Grandma drank chaparral tea every day of her life after she went into menopause in her early 50s. She said it helped with her menopausal symptoms and kept her pretty healthy. She lived to be 98 years old. Near the end, when others were caring for her, she wasn't able to make the tea regularly. Once she stopped taking it, she seemed to deteriorate much faster.

Attributes

Nutrients

Key Components: (including, but not limited to)

Ascorbic Acid (increased levels in the adrenal glands after ingestion) • Aluminum • Barium • Chlorine • Potassium • Silicon • Sodium • Sulfur • Tin • other essential Trace Minerals
Bitter • Protein • Nordihydro-guaiaretic acid (NDGA)

The protein content of chaparral is similar to alfalfa in quantity and has been used as cattle feed. NDGA is used commercially as a preservative in lard and animal shortenings and approved for human consumption by the U.S. Department of Agriculture. NDGA is a powerful antioxidant (especially for fats and oils), and is thought to be largely responsible for chaparral's anti-cancer, anti-tumor, and medicinal properties.

Circulation

Chaparral increases circulation through vasodilation (opening of blood vessels), promotes sweating, and improves elimination of toxins from the liver and skin. It has the ability to cleanse deep into muscles and tissues. The lymph and respiratory systems are cleansed of toxins as well, rejuvenating the entire body and easing the symptoms of colds, flu, and bronchitis.

Blood Toxicity

Those who suffer with arthritis, rheumatism, sinusitis, and bursitis may find their condition significantly improved after blood purification with chaparral.

Toxins can accumulate in people who work with photography or industrial chemicals on a regular basis. Toxic headaches or breathing problems often result. Once the blood is cleansed, these complaints are alleviated.

Chaparral is excellent for getting rid of the chemical build up from processed foods. It has been used to eliminate the residue of LSD drugs from the body, helping to prevent recurrent symptoms. Of course, one must stop continued chemical and/or drug exposure to obtain total relief of symptoms.

Heavy users of drugs, including caffeine, alcohol, and chemotherapy may experience headaches and nausea when taking chaparral. This is a result of getting toxins moving in the blood and through the system for elimination. Adjust the use of blood purifying herbs (including chaparral) to tolerance as you cleanse.

Inflammation

The oil from chaparral's resin has been shown to reduce inflammation of the intestinal and respiratory tracts and is reportedly a strong pain killer.

Eliminative Organs

Chaparral cleanses the lower bowel and tones peristaltic muscles (intestinal muscles that contract to move contents onward). Take chaparral with fluids, as it is a strong cleansing herb for the kidneys and a potent healer of the urethral tract, blood, liver, and lymphatic system. Chaparral tones the system and helps rebuild tissues.

Expectorant

Chaparral was listed in the United States Pharmacopoeia from 1842 through 1942 as an expectorant (substance used to clear mucus from the respiratory system) and as a bronchial antiseptic.

Immunity Stimulant and Anti Microbe

Chaparral is an excellent antiseptic, antibacterial, and antifungal herb. Chaparral infusions are used to alleviate athlete's foot and for external sores and wounds. Chaparral is so powerful, parasites will leave the system and dangerous microbes will either leave or perish.

Strong smelling and nasty tasting chaparral is the supreme blood cleanser and immune stimulator. It removes heavy metals and all forms of putrefaction and decay. Decoctions or strong teas have been taken historically for cancer, HIV, and all serious diseases (see Safety section below).

Candida

People with large abdomens usually have a dramatic overgrowth of yeast in their body. Chaparral is one of the primary herbs to get rid of candida yeast. It is famous for eliminating candida from the body as a vaginal wash and as a topical wash on the skin. The tea is also effective when taken internally. Chaparral works particularly well against candida when dried and powdered and taken in a capsule along with the herbs pau d'arco, olive leaf, and myrrh.

Anti-Aging

As a strong antioxidant, the plant is known to act against free radicals, thereby helping to prevent degenerative diseases associated with aging.

Cancer

Chaparral contains elements which have definite anti-cancer potential to help decrease tumors and combat leukemia. Many universities have tested chaparral and found it to be an aid in dissolving tumors and fighting cancer. Some suggest chaparral's ingredient NDGA is an anti-tumor agent as well as a powerful antioxidant. Others attribute its anti-carcinogenic properties to its ability to purify the blood and tissues of toxins.

For more than 100 years, chaparral has been used as a treatment for cancer. The medical literature from the National Cancer Institute contains several case reports of tumor reduction in people who used chaparral. One case published in the Cancer Chemotherapy Reports tells of a man diagnosed by University of Utah physicians as having malignant melanoma, a serious skin cancer. The doctors urged surgery, but the man refused, saying he intended to treat himself with chaparral tea. The Utah medical team was aghast but, eight months later, the man returned. To their credit, it was noted he had 'marked regression' of his cancer at that time.

FDA Warning	On December 10, 1992, the FDA (Federal Drug Administration) issued a press release warning of the potential link between the use of chaparral and liver toxicity. Many manufacturers and distributors voluntarily suspended sale of the herb shortly after this time. It has been our experience chaparral is a potent blood cleanser that may increase the workload of the liver while eliminating toxins and pollutants of all sorts from the body. I highly recommend individuals with weakened livers first support and strengthen the liver with appropriate herbs before cleansing toxins from the body. Chaparral has a 2,000 year recorded history of effective medicinal use. It is a wonderful and powerfully safe herb when used properly and without abuse.
Herb Parts Used	Leaves and twigs
Preparations and Remedies	The powdered or cut form of chaparral is used in capsules, in tablets, and for infusions.
Infusions	Chaparral Tea: Pour one cup of boiling water over one teaspoon of chaparral leaf and leave to stand for ten minutes. This is excellent to relieve bad reactions to some food or to speed recovery after alcohol over-indulgence. Use the infusion as a wash for bruises, cuts, and minor wounds or as a vaginal douche for women. Make a hot fomentation (towel soaked in liquid and placed on affected area) of the infusion for old sores and inflammation.
Soak	Athlete's Foot Soak: This fungal infection can be alleviated by soaking the feet in a double strength chaparral tea (two teaspoons herb to one cup of hot water) several times a day until healed. A paste of chaparral and slippery elm powders mixed with aloe vera gel will further improve the condition.
Decoctions	Native American Decoction:

Place one tablespoon of creosote bush leaves and small twigs into a glass screw-top jar. Pour one pint of boiling water over this, cover, and let stand overnight. Do not refrigerate. Do not remove surface sediment. Drink a quarter of the liquid a half hour before each meal and at bedtime.

Approximately 40 percent of the active ingredient is utilized (taken in the above amounts) with a total daily intake around 200-250 milligrams. Herbalists combine other herbs with creosote bush as the case requires.

Nine Day Chaparral Cleanse:
Make a quart of this tea every day, using the same herb for up to three days in a row before discarding. Fill one fourth of a quart jar with dried chaparral (the fresh herbs may also be used if you have them). Continue filling the jar with boiling water. Throughout the day, drink the entire quart of tea. Repeat for a total of nine days.

This cleanse is incredibly potent. It will help purify the blood, cells, tissues, and skin of toxins and help rid the body of candida. You should be aware this is a very intense cleanse and often brings out emotional issues associated with diseases that may have been hiding in the tissues. I recommend you take the time to seclude yourself and do this cleanse on your own when possible.

Alternative:
A milder type of cleanse may be done by taking just a tablespoon of the tea two or three times a day for a longer period of time.

System Cleanse Tea:
1 part Buckthorn bark, cut
1 part Burdock root, cut
1 part Chaparral, cut
1 part Licorice root, cut
1 part Red Clover blossoms, cut or whole
1 part Dandelion root, cut
1 part Barberry root, cut
1 part Cascara Sagrada bark, cut

Add 1 cup of the above combined herbs to 2 quarts of distilled water. Use only a stainless steel or glass pot. Never use aluminum! Bring to a light simmer. Turn the stove down and

	continue to simmer for 20 minutes. Strain out the wet herb and return it to the same pan. Add 2 more quarts of distilled water to the pot and repeat the process of heating. Refrigerate. Discard the used herb when done. Suggested use: Take 1/2 to 1 cup of the prepared System Cleanse Tea 2-3 times a day for six weeks. Take a two-week break and repeat usage for six weeks. Then take another two-week break and repeat for a final six weeks. Normal bowel movements occur at least 2-3 times a day. The body must be able to eliminate unhealthy cells and dead matter from the body. If constipated, increase the amount of times System Cleanse Tea is taken each day. If bowels become too loose, decrease the amount of each dose and/or how often it is taken. This formula helps cleanse every system of the body, beginning with digestion. It generally takes three days to clean out the digestive tract, then it starts on the other body systems, blood, lymph, cells, lungs, etc. It takes about two weeks to be an effective parasite cleanse. CAUTION: Using System Cleanse Tea may cause some weakness if the body is already fragile or if the individual has had chemotherapy treatments. System Cleanse Tea has powerful herbs that draw chemicals and poisons from tissues in order to eliminate them. Sometimes, it is too much for a frail body to take all at once. Use this tea wisely. Ease off if needed, nourish and strengthen the body, then try again when ready. It is an excellent idea to build the body with kidney and liver herbs (milk thistle, dandelion, etc.) for at least a month before going on an extensive cleanse.
Safety	Do not use with compromised kidney or liver conditions until these organs are stabilized and functional. It is recommended appropriate herbs be taken to support the liver during a deep cleanse such as milk thistle and dandelion.
Plant Profile	*Natural Habitat:*

Description

The chaparral bush grows in low altitudes (sometimes up to 3000 feet above sea level) and is commonly found in desert regions of the southwestern United States and Mexico. It covers thousands of square miles from California, Utah, Arizona, and New Mexico west to Texas and south to Mexico.

Chaparral is a very long-lived perennial (the plant grows back each year from a persistent rootstock). As it grows, its oldest branches die and its crown splits into separate crowns, making 'clones' of the original plant. This normally happens when the plant is 30 to 90 years old. Eventually, the old crown dies and the new clones continue growing and splitting. One chaparral plant near Lucerne Valley, California has been named 'King Clone' and has been carbon dated to be over 11,700 years old.

Chaparral is a common desert shrub that grows 12 or 15 feet high. The bush is considered to be a dominant plant of the desert flora. It appears to take up most of the available water where it grows, leaving other plants to wither and die when water is scarce.

Stems and leaves are dark green or, if in a drought season, pale or yellowish green. Its small leaves exude a waxy resin that smells like creosote (an oil which is used to treat wood) and is the source of its popular names: stinkweed, grease-wood, and creosote bush (though the plant does not contain actual creosote components).

Bright-yellow flowers (of about one inch in diameter when fully grown) appear in early spring, and small, white, hairy fruits follow shortly thereafter.

Harvesting

The best time to gather seeds for replanting is when they are well developed in the springtime or in the fall (do not hesitate to gather at other times as well). The fresh leaves and twigs are harvested as the viable herb. When drying, take care to preserve the valuable volatile oils.

Chaste Tree

Latin Name: *Vitex Agnus-Castus*

Also known as: Chasteberry, Vitex, Monk's Pepper

Scientific Classification

Vitex is a genus of about 270 species of shrubs and trees. Two other species demonstrate similar medicinal activity: V. negundo and V. trifolia.

Order:	Lamiales
Family:	Verbenaceae – verbena family
Genus	Vitex – chastetree
Species	V. agnus-castus – lilac chastetree

Influence on the Body	(PRINCIPAL ACTIONS are listed in CAPITAL LETTERS)
Nervous System	depression • anxiety • migraine
Reproductive System	*Male:* impotence *Female:* PMS • mastodynia (cyclic breast pain) • bloating • MENSTRUAL CYCLE irregularities • female infertility • inadequate milk secretion • promotes lactation • MENOPAUSE difficulties
Skin, Tissues and Hair	Acne

Key Properties:

HORMONE BALANCING GALACTAGOGUE	*enhances lactation of nursing mothers*
Primarily affecting	PITUITARY • REPRODUCTIVE SYSTEM
History	In Greek mythology, the goddess Hera (champion of marriage and family) was said to have been born under the chaste tree. Young women celebrating the festival of Demeter (goddess of fertility) wore chasteberry blossoms to show they were remaining pure in honor of the goddess. The plant became a symbol of chastity through the ages and for a time was thought to counter sexual desire. A drink prepared from the plant's seeds was used by the Romans to diminish libido, and monks in the Middle Ages used the fruit for similar purposes (yielding the common name 'monk's pepper'). Despite the

common use, there is no scientific evidence that chasteberry diminishes libido.

Chaste tree has been used more effectively to treat female gynecological disorders. Hippocrates (460-377 BC) wrote of its use by women to stop afterbirth hemorrhaging and, three centuries later, the Roman physician Pliny wrote of its ability to normalize menstruation and increase lactation.

In the 1950s, the German pharmaceutical firm 'Madaus Company' first produced a standardized extract of the herb. Chaste tree became a standard European treatment for the cyclical breast tenderness that is often associated with PMS and other symptoms of monthly irregularity. Chaste tree continues to be one of the principal herbs to help normalize the balance of female hormones and support women's gynecological health.

Attributes	**Key Components: (including, but not limited to)**
	Flavonoids (contribute to the effectiveness of the herb)
	Chaste tree has relaxant and pain-relieving properties, but it is best known for its hormone-balancing effects. It is commonly used for lactation support and to overcome pre-menstrual syndrome (PMS) and menstrual irregularities.
Lactation	Herbalists have recommended chaste tree as an effective galactagogue (increases the flow of breast milk) for nearly 2,000 years.
Menstrual Irregularity	Scientists have not found any hormone-like components in chaste tree. It appears to act on the pituitary gland to lower abnormal release of prolactin. High levels of the hormone prolactin in non-pregnant women may cause cyclic breast tenderness and other PMS symptoms and, ultimately, result in an imbalance and irregularity in the female hormone cycle. Chasteberry is often used for irregular or absent menstrual flow.
	In a study of 52 women with irregular menstruation, 'significant improvements' were shown after three months of using chasteberry as a supplement.
PMS	German health authorities allow chaste tree preparations for pressure and swelling in the breasts, heavy or too-frequent

Other	periods, acyclic bleeding, infertility, suppressed menses, and PMS (premenstrual syndrome). In two studies enrolling about 3,000 women, doctors rated chasteberry as being 90 percent effective in showing significant or complete improvement in symptoms such as breast pain, fluid retention, headache, and fatigue. Another study of 175 women found marked reduction of PMS symptoms including breast tenderness, edema, tension, headache, constipation, and depression. It was found useful in 80 percent of the women, and results were rated by practitioners as being excellent in over 24 percent of the cases. Chaste tree has been shown to be effective for helping women ease off birth control pills. In Germany, chaste tree has had good results in reducing certain kinds of teenage acne (it was less effective for those having a strong family history of severe acne with continuous break out).
Herb Parts Used	Ripe fruits gathered in the autumn
Preparations and Remedies	Chasteberry is effectively used in liquid tincture form, powdered, capsules, and tablets. Teas are seldom used.
Fresh	The berries may be taken fresh one after another, held in the mouth, slowly crunched, and then consumed.
Powdered	The berries must be crushed or milled to a coarse powder before adding the menstruum (liquid of choice), then macerated (soaked to soften and release constituents).
Safety	Widespread use in Germany has not led to any reports of significant adverse effects. Because it lowers prolactin levels, chaste tree berries are not recommended by many during pregnancy.
Plant Profile	*Natural Habitat:* Chaste tree is commonly found along riverbanks and nearby foothills in central Asia and around the Mediterranean Sea. It is naturalized in much of the southeastern United States. The fruits

Description

are grown commercially in Europe. It thrives in most types of soil, is drought tolerant, and may be grown from seed or cuttings.

Chaste tree is a large shrub or small tree (growing 3-18 feet) that is cultivated as an ornamental and medicinal plant.

Its abundant lavender (occasionally purple, mauve, or pink) flowers cluster on spikes in the height of the summer. The plant has dull-green, palm-like leaves that are lighter on the underside. There are up to nine leaflets radiating from each leaf stalk. The flowers and leaves exude an exotic, pepper-like aroma and flavor.

After its flowers have bloomed, a dark reddish-black, peppercorn-like fruit grows to less than a quarter of an inch long. It can be harvested in the autumn at full maturity and dried for herbal use.

Comfrey

Latin Name: *Symphytum officinale*

Also known as: Knitbone, Bruisewort, Woundwort, Slippery Root, Boneset, Gum Plant, Nipbone, Knitback, Salsify, Wallwort, Blackwort, Black Root

Scientific Classification

Family:	Boraginaceae – borage family
Genus	Symphytum – comfrey
Species	S. officinale – common comfrey

Influence on the Body	(PRINCIPAL ACTIONS are listed in CAPITAL LETTERS)
Blood and Circulatory System	BLOOD CLEANSER • ANEMIA • hemorrhage • styptic (contracts blood vessels)
Body System	tonic (increases energy and strength) • fatigue • energy • astringent (tightens and tones) • MUCOUS MEMBRANES • mucilage (soft and slippery sugar molecules that protect mucous membranes and inflamed tissues) • demulcent (softens and soothes inflammation of mucous membranes)
Bones and Teeth	BROKEN BONES • FRACTURES
Cancer	cancer • tumors
Digestive Tract	nutritive (supplies nutrients and aids in building and toning the body) • bitter (stimulates digestive juices and improves appetite) • DIGESTION • digestive problems • stomach • ulcers • ULCERATED BOWELS • diarrhea • dysentery • laxative • colon • colitis • hemorrhoids
Endocrine System	Pancreas
Eyes	EYES (painful or injured)
First Aid	BRUISES • SORES • gangrenous sores • SPRAINS • pulled tendons • SWELLINGS • BURNS • WOUNDS • CUTS • CELL PROLIFERANT (enhances the formation of new tissue) • INSECT BITES • BEE STINGS • GANGRENE
Infections and Immune System	ALLERGIES • HAY FEVER • COUGHS • colds • fevers • INFECTIONS • YEAST INFECTION • HERPES • ATHLETE'S FOOT

Inflammation	INFLAMMATIONS • ARTHRITIS • rheumatism • GOUT • BURSITIS
Liver	Gallbladder
Lungs and Respiratory System	respiratory problems • dissolves and expels mucus • expectorant (loosens and removes phlegm in the respiratory tract) • sinusitis • BRONCHITIS • CONGESTION • moistens LUNGS • asthma • pneumonia • pleurisy • EMPHYSEMA • tuberculosis
Mouth and Throat	COLD SORES • MOUTHWASH • bleeding gum disease • pyorrhea • throat • hoarseness • gargle • tonsillitis
Muscles	leg cramps
Pain	PAIN • headache
Reproductive System	*Female:* sore breasts • female disorders • menstruation • leukorrhea • vaginal discharge • VAGINAL DOUCHE
Skin, Tissues and Hair	SKIN • ACNE • BOILS • eczema • psoriasis • diaper rash • ITCHING • dandruff
Urinary Tract	kidneys • kidney stones • BLADDER PROBLEMS • bloody urine

Key Properties:

VULNERARY	promotes cell regeneration in damaged bones and tissues by stimulating cellular growth and warding off infection
DEMULCENT	soothes inflammation of mucous membranes
EXPECTORANT	loosens and removes phlegm in the respiratory tract
alterative	purifies the blood, cleanses, and induces efficient removal of waste products
astringent	increases the tone and firmness of tissues, reduces mucous discharge from nose, intestines, vagina, and draining sores
nutritive	supplies substantial amounts of nutrients and aids in building and toning the body
Primarily affecting	BONES • TISSUES • MUCOUS MEMBRANES • LUNGS

History	Comfrey was a well-known healer for both people and animals as early as 400 BC. It was noted for its ability to promote tissue repair.

Comfrey's genus name 'symptium' is the Greek word meaning to unite, and 'comfrey' is a corruption of 'con firma', alluding to the uniting of bones. Dioscorides, a Greek physician, used the plant to heal wounds and mend broken bones. The Greeks and Romans made poultices out of comfrey leaves and roots to treat external wounds, and they drank comfrey tea for stomach disorders, internal bleeding, diarrhea, bronchial problems, and other ailments.

Through the ages, comfrey continued to be a popular treatment for a wide variety of ailments. It was considered a gentle remedy for diarrhea and dysentery, an effective treatment for bronchitis, whooping cough, and tuberculosis, and used in cases of internal bleeding, ulcers, and hemorrhoids. Ointments and other preparations of the roots and leaves were applied to bruises, sprains, strains, broken bones, torn ligaments, severe cuts, boils and burns, arthritis, gangrene, and almost any kind of inflamed swelling.

Native Americans discovered the healing qualities of comfrey and used it with other herbs.

Farmers have long fed comfrey to their livestock for various ailments or as a spring tonic after a long winter of standing in barnyard mire beneath overcast skies. Farmers have also fed comfrey to their families as a nearly unparalleled source of protein, potassium, calcium, and Vitamins A, B12, and C. The general rule was 'if anything is broken, use comfrey.'

Our family's use of comfrey is quite extensive. My Mom bought a small comfrey plant 45 years ago from a local health food store. She was told it could help my little brother, Phil, with his weakened lung condition that kept landing him in the hospital. Mom would cut the leaves from the plant and put them in the blender with some pineapple juice. He immediately started to heal. From that point on, he never had to go back into the hospital for lung problems. Eventually, he stopped taking comfrey altogether, as it seemed his lungs had healed.

Fast forward to 1990. Phil was in the Desert Storm War. He started having severe respiratory problems, and the Army was considering a medical discharge for him. Our Mom sent him a package of dried comfrey leaves from her garden and, in no time,

Phil's lungs began repairing. He just recently retired from the Army.

My Dad planted comfrey in our backyard, and Mom always fed comfrey to us kids, especially when we were sick or had a broken bone. When it died down in the winter, he roto-tilled it into the ground in preparation for next year's garden. In the spring, my parents were surprised to be greeted by hundreds of comfrey plants all over the yard. A day hardly goes by that my Mom and Dad don't eat comfrey in some form, whether dried and put into a tea or processed fresh in a blender with juice as a 'green smoothie.' Wherever they have moved, they have taken it with them.

Since 2001, comfrey preparations made only for topical use have been approved for sale in the United States.

Attributes	Key Components: (including, but not limited to)
Nutrition	Vitamins A (carotene) • B12 (cobalamin, high concentrations) • C • E • Calcium • Copper • Iron • Magnesium • Phosphorus • Potassium • Sulfur • Zinc Mucilage (helps in healing) • Chlorophyll • Bitter • Allantoin (stimulates cell growth, also found in aloe vera) • Proteins • Alkaloids (thought by some to be toxic to liver when taken internally in large amounts. It is found in the root and young leaves, see **Safety** section.)
Cell Regeneration	Comfrey contains allantoin (a cell proliferant) which stimulates new cell growth and rapid healing of tissues and bone. It reduces or eliminates scar tissue and accelerates the healing of sprains, wounds, and broken or fractured bones. Comfrey is well known as the 'bone knitter.' The extract of comfrey poured into a cleaned wound can close it (often avoiding stitches).
Wound Healing	As a 'contact healer', comfrey relieves pain and starts to repair and heal on contact. It soothes inflammations on skin, in joints and pulled muscles, and in mucous membranes of the digestive tract and lungs. Swelling is checked, and bleeding and hemorrhaging are arrested by comfrey's astringent and capillary constricting properties. Comfrey will join cleanly, even when

bones have been badly set or will not heal.

Comfrey is applied as a poultice to cuts and abrasions, sore breasts, burns, sprains, and bites. A hot poultice of the fresh, bruised leaves helps ease the pain of gout, bursitis, and joint inflammations (often within an hour). Nothing compares with comfrey's healing effects on traumatic eye injuries.

When comfrey extract is applied topically to mosquito bites, the itching stops and the swelling goes down. The extract is easily applied to help heal acne, sores, and athlete's foot.

Women

Use poultices on sore, full (with infection), or caked breasts to quickly relieve tenderness, as the tissues are soothed and healed.

Comfrey teas and extracts have been used as a douche for yeast infections.

Anti-Bacterial

In a study on the effectiveness of comfrey to hinder streptococcus agalactiae and staphylococcal bacteria, Daniel O. Noorlander demonstrated when comfrey extract was introduced topically to the bacteria, the walls of the bacteria cells weakened and then burst, destroying the bacteria within 20-30 minutes.

Internal Preparations Banned (2001)

Comfrey-containing herbal products for internal consumption were banned in the United States in 2001. Topical preparations are still available. (see discussion in Safety section)

Comfrey has been used historically for the following internal applications:

Comfrey was used to normalize the calcium-phosphorus balance, promoting healthy skin and strong bones. It was used to feed the pituitary with its natural hormones and help regulate blood sugar levels by supporting the pancreas.

Mucous Membranes

Comfrey has an abundance of mucilage, which gives it the ability to calm inflammation and soothe mucous membranes of the digestive and respiratory tracts.

Digestive Tract

Comfrey was used to promote the secretion of pepsin (to aid digestion) and soothe inflammatory disorders of the gastrointestinal tract (including ulcers and dysentery). It was used as a mild laxative to expel wastes.

Respiratory System	Comfrey was used as a healer of the respiratory system, acting as a general stimulant to the mucous membranes and helping to increase expectoration. It was considered to be a powerful remedy for coughs, throat and bronchial tubes, and was used to stop the hemorrhaging of weakened lungs.
Herb Parts Used	Leaves and root harvested anytime during the growth cycle (but preferably not when in full flower) used fresh or dried.
Preparations and Remedies	As a poultice, bruise the fresh leaves and apply to burns, wounds, bites, sprains, swellings, sore breasts, and gangrene. The tea and decoction may also be used as a fomentation.
Infusions	*Comfrey Tea:* Steep leaves for 30 minutes *Comfrey Root Decoction:* Simmer the dried, cut root for 30 minutes. Remove from heat and allow to sit for at least 8 hours. Reheat uncovered, simmering to concentrate until desired strength is achieved (approximately 10-15 minutes). *Mullein Decoction:* (see MULLEIN preparations)
Syrup	*Cough Syrup:* (see SLIPPERY ELM preparations)
Wash	*Comfrey Tea Wash:* The tea used as a wash is especially helpful for skin ailments that cover large areas, such as a sunburn or widespread topical staph infection. Slowly pour the infusion over the injury, allowing excess liquid to drip into a basin or bathtub. Let the infusion remain on the site for a few minutes without washing it off or drying with a towel. *Soothing Eye Compress:* (see EYEBRIGHT preparations)
Fomentations	Comfrey leaves subdue every kind of inflammatory swelling when used as a fomentation (towel soaked in infusion or decoction and placed on affected area).
Poultices	Plantain works synergistically with comfrey in poultice and fomentation applications. Plantain absorbs toxins and poisons and is particularly helpful in cases of itching, skin irritation, rash,

and discomfort. Comfrey has been used to ease the pain of gout and inflamed joints.

There are several ways to prepare an effective comfrey poultice. Here are a few:

1. Bruise the fresh leaves and apply directly to burns, wounds, bites, sprains, swellings, sore breasts, and gangrene.

2. An easy poultice may be made by spooning dried comfrey leaves or powder into a large 'empty' tea bag and sealing the open edge. (Open-ended tea bags are made to be filled and ironed shut). Moisten the closed comfrey 'tea bag' in hot water and lay on the injury when cooled enough to touch. The tea bag may be reheated in hot water several times and reapplied.

3. Put fresh leaves and/or root in a blender (or food processor) with a small amount of water, and then grind into a paste for direct application.

4. If you have dried, powdered comfrey, just mix it with a little water so that it makes a thick, slimy paste before applying.

5. Brew a decoction (strong tea) by first boiling 2 cups of water, then chopping up a cup of fresh comfrey leaves and/or root (or a half-cup of dried plant material). Use fresh plants when they are available. Reduce the heat to a simmer, and then cook slowly for about 20 minutes.

Allow decoction to cool before applying it to the skin. Use a towel with plastic wrap or adhesive tape to hold the poultice in place. Leave in place for up to several hours or even overnight. Re-apply a fresh poultice the following day if needed.

Flaxseed Poultice: (see FLAXSEED preparations)
Comfrey/Plantain Poultice: (see CAYENNE preparations)
Boils and Abscess Poultice: (see ECHINACEA preparations)

Salves

Drawing Salve:
The drawing qualities of this salve make it useful to pull out the last bit of infection from scabbed-over wounds to soothe and accelerate healing. As with any salve, it is best to let wounds drain and close on their own before sealing them off with the salve.

1 oz. Plantain leaves, crushed or powdered
1 oz. Comfrey root, powdered

4 oz. Extra Virgin Olive Oil
1/4 oz. Beeswax

Note: It is possible to make more than one batch at a time.
Heat oil in a crock pot on the warm setting. Temperature should not reach higher than 80-100° F. Stir in herbs and maintain this temperature (with a lid on) for 1-3 days, stirring occasionally.

When the mixture is ready (partially determined by the loss of herb color and smell), line a colander with two layers of unbleached broadcloth or muslin. Place the colander inside a collector bowl and pour in the contents of the crock pot. Strain and squeeze out all possible oil into the collector bowl (you may want to use gloves while squeezing). Return the used herbs (left inside the cloth) to the soil or discard them.

Return the herb-infused oil to the wiped down, clean crock-pot. Cut in the beeswax and slowly heat until melted (beeswax liquefies at 148.4° F). Once melted, turn off the heat. To determine if enough beeswax has been added, spoon a small amount onto a plate to cool. The room-temperature consistency should be gel-like, without liquefying. In warmer climates, it is necessary to add additional beeswax to set up properly. When satisfied, pour mixture into clean ointment jars (1-2 ounce jars are a convenient size for single or family use). This salve lasts up to 3 years in the refrigerator or for several months when stored at room temperature.

Lobelia Salve: (see LOBELIA preparations)

Safety

In the late 1970s, researchers raised concerns about a toxic alkaloid found in the root and young leaves of comfrey, which may cause liver damage when taken in large amounts (more than the liver can process and eliminate at one time).

In 2001, the FDA (Federal Drug Administration) banned comfrey from all commercially produced herbal supplements to be taken internally.

Bear in mind that the FDA decided to ban the plant only after injecting unnaturally large amounts of the plant's extracted alkaloids into animal test subjects, which then died of liver failure or got cancer (just as they would have done had the alkaloids been extracted from a carrot and then concentrated and injected into the animal's blood streams). 'Scientists that did the original experiments did tell the news media later that when the product (comfrey) was given to the rats in its whole and natural state, that this did not happen.' Jack Ritchason N.D.

Plant Profile

Natural Habitat:
Comfrey is native to Europe, growing in damp, grassy places, and is widespread throughout the British Isles and Asia on riverbanks and ditches. It is naturalized in much of North America.

Description

This large perennial herb (plant grows back from a persistent rootstock in the spring after dying down in the winter) grows from two to four feet. The stalk is hollow and hairy with large, dark green, hairy leaves that reach ten to twelve inches long near the base and grow smaller the higher they are on the stalk.

The joints of the stalk divide into many branches. At the ends of the branches, comfrey bears white, cream, purple, or pink clusters of drooping, bell-shaped flowers in May through summer, after which come small black seeds in August.

The slick quality of its rhizome (principal root which is black with a juicy white flesh within) gives rise to its nickname of slippery root. It contains a large amount of mucilage (soft and slippery material), and is rich in easily assimilated organic calcium with a bland and faintly astringent taste. Comfrey's other name, knit-bone, comes from its use in healing bones and tissues.

Growing Comfrey

Planting:
Comfrey can be grown in the spring by direct seed planting, cuttings at any stage of the life cycle, or root division in the fall. Sow seeds just under the surface and tamp in securely. Keep warm and moist until germination, which takes approximately ten days. Seedlings may be grown in pots for about three months, and then transplanted to the garden about three feet apart.

Comfrey prefers a full to part sun position (shaded plants will be smaller and have fewer blossoms), with rich, moist but well-drained soil, and has a cold hardiness to 15° F. Sandy soil is fine, as long as the plants are watered consistently during the growing season (fleshy herbs like comfrey need a great deal of water). Divide the plants every few years to prevent crowding. Cutting the flowers will encourage more leaf growth.

Comfrey is generally trouble free once established, although weaker or stressed plants may suffer from rust or mildew. These fungal diseases rarely reduce plant growth seriously, thus they do not generally require control. Infected plants should not be used for propagation purposes.

The plant dies down over the winter but makes a strong recovery in the spring. Comfrey can be quite invasive in the garden, overrunning other plants once it takes hold. To avoid this, cut them back when they make flowers and mulch the crowns with their own stems, leaves, and flowers. This will keep the seed from maturing and dropping and will quickly improve the soil and make large and healthy plants. Comfrey can form an attractive backdrop to other plants when they are confined to distant parts of the garden.

Removing Comfrey

It is difficult to remove comfrey once it is established, as it has deep roots, and any fragments left in the soil will regrow. The best way to eradicate comfrey is to carefully dig it out, removing as much of the root as possible. This is best done in hot, dry, summer weather when dry conditions help to kill any remaining root stumps.

Harvesting and Storage

Mature comfrey plants may be harvested up to four or five times a year once they are about two feet high. It is said that the *best* time to cut comfrey is shortly before flowering, for this is when the leaves are at their peak potency. Pinch off leaves or cut the entire plant down to about two inches above the ground. Dry and store in airtight containers. Leaves may be frozen for up to six months.

The roots should be unearthed in the spring or fall. Split the roots down the middle and dry them in moderate temperatures on screens or in an oven. Store roots in airtight containers.

Dandelion

Latin Name: *Taraxacum officinale*

Also known as: Lion's Tooth, Priest's Crown, Puffball, Blowball, Cankerwort, Wild Endive

Scientific Classification

There are more than 50 species in the Taraxacum genus, all taprooted biennials or perennials that contain a milky latex

Family:	Asteraceae – aster, daisy and sunflower family
	Compositae – in earlier classifications
Genus	Taraxacum – dandelion
Species	T. officinale – common dandelion

Influence on the Body	(PRINCIPAL ACTIONS are listed in CAPITAL LETTERS)
Blood and Circulatory System	BLOOD CLEANSER • BLOOD PURIFIER • DEPURATIVE (cleanses blood by promoting eliminative functions) • ANEMIA • lowers cholesterol • HIGH BLOOD PRESSURE • LOW BLOOD PRESSURE • dropsy (edema due to heart insufficiency) • hemorrhage • scurvy • spleen
Blood Sugar	pancreas • diabetes • HYPOGLYCEMIA
Body System	tonic (increases energy and strengthens the muscular and nervous system while improving digestion and assimilation, resulting in a general sense of well-being) • stimulates metabolism • ENDURANCE • stamina • energy • fatigue • lethargy • aging
Bones and Teeth	Fractures
Cancer	cancer • breast cancer • breast tumors
Digestive Tract	nutritive (supplies substantial amount of nutrients and aids in building and toning the body) • APPETITE STIMULANT • bitter (stimulates digestive juices and improves appetite) • heartburn • stomach • digestive disorders • dyspepsia (indigestion) • indigestion • bowel inflammation • ulcers • gas • flatulence (gas) • intestines • constipation • laxative (without purging)
Infections and Immune System	bacterial infections • flu • fevers • yeast infections • abscesses

Inflammation	ARTHRITIS • rheumatism • gout
Liver	LIVER CLEANSER • congestion in the liver portal system • LIVER DISORDERS • HEPATITIS • LIVER TOXICITY • JAUNDICE • CIRRHOSIS • GALLBLADDER • CHOLAGOGUE (promotes the flow of bile) • gallstones
Lungs and Respiratory System	ASTHMA • bronchitis
Muscle	leg cramps
Nervous System	mental fatigue • insomnia • senility
Reproductive System	*Female:* female organs • PMS • galactagogue (enhances lactation of nursing mothers)
Skin, Tissues and Hair	SKIN PROBLEMS • skin eruptions • dermatitis • ACNE • ECZEMA • psoriasis • EXTERNAL BLISTERS • boils • corns • warts • sores • AGE SPOTS
Urinary Tract	diuretic • water retention • URINARY TRACT INFECTIONS • KIDNEY INFECTIONS • kidney stones • bladder stones • lithotriptic (dissolves urinary stones) • deobstruent (removes obstructions) • bladder
Weight	WEIGHT LOSS

Key Properties:

HEPATIC	supports and stimulates the liver, gallbladder, and spleen, and increases the flow of bile
DIURETIC	increases the flow of urine without depleting potassium in the body
STOMACHIC	improves appetite and digestion
CHOLAGOGUE	increases bile flow
alterative	purifies the blood, cleanses and induces efficient removal of waste products, gradually detoxifying the spleen, liver, kidneys, and bowels
nutritive	supplies substantial amount of nutrients and aids in building and toning the body
tonic	increases energy and strength throughout the body
Primarily affecting	LIVER • gallbladder • BLOOD • KIDNEYS • STOMACH • pancreas

History	The Latin genus name Taraxacum is from the Greek 'taraxos', meaning disorder, and 'ako', meaning remedy. Dandelions have been purposely cultivated and widely used throughout history. The Celts introduced the herb to the Roman legions when Caesar invaded the north. The Anglo-Saxons and the Normans used it to prevent scurvy (a Vitamin C deficiency). In ancient Russia, dandelion was used for yellow spots (liver spots) of the skin and freckles. Arabic physicians introduced its use as a medicine to Europe in the 10th or 11th century, and it soon became valued as a medicinal herb. Monastery gardens used dandelion for both food and medicine in the Middle Ages. Herbalists used it for fever, boils, eye problems, diabetes, and diarrhea, and it has been largely cultivated in India as a remedy for liver complaints. The French called dandelion 'dents de lion', or 'lion's tooth,' in reference to the deeply jagged shape of the plant's leaves. In France, the roots are cooked as a vegetable and added to broth, and in Germany, they are sliced and used in salads. Germany has approved dandelion for digestive health, and the root is used in cases of bile flow disruption and when a diuretic is indicated. Native Americans used dandelion decoctions to treat kidney disease, swellings, skin problems, heartburn, and indigestion. Dandelion is still respected today as an expectorant, sedative, and one of the best tonic herbs for blood purifying, liver treatment, jaundice, gallbladder, skin conditions, and digestive disturbances.
Attributes *Nutrition*	**Key Components: (including, but not limited to)** Vitamins A (containing 7,000 units per ounce of herb) • B1 (thiamine) • B2 (riboflavin) • B3 (niacin) • B5 (pantothenic acid) • B6 (pyridoxine) • B9 (folic acid) • B12 (cobalamin) • Biotin • Choline • Inositol • PABA (Para-Amino Benzoic Acid) • C • Bioflavonoids • D • E • Boron • Calcium (a good source) • Cobalt • Copper • Iron (a good source) • Magnesium (a good source) • Manganese • Phosphorus • Potassium (a rich source) • Silicon • Sodium • Sulfur • Zinc • other Trace Minerals Sugars • Inulin • Mucilage • Bitter

General

Dandelion is a high-nutrient food and has been used as a valuable survival food. It is high in organic salts and minerals which build the blood, help correct anemia deficiencies, and restore the blood's electrolyte balance. It has also been noted dandelions can improve enamel health of teeth.

Dandelion acts as a tonic to the system. It cleanses acids and toxins from the blood and effectively builds and strengthens the liver and kidneys. The herb is also a mild stimulant for bowel elimination and is especially indicated in helping treat persistent constipation of the elderly.

By cleansing the blood and liver, dandelion is useful in the treatment of various oily and eruptive conditions of the skin such as acne, eczema, and sebaceous cysts. Dandelion is used for liver disease, jaundice, gallstones, diabetes, allergies and sensitivities, skin problems, water retention, urinary problems, swollen ankles, dropsy, gout, arthritis, and rheumatism.

Liver and Bile Flow

In Europe, many scientific experiments with the plant have confirmed its traditional use for liver health, and studies confirm that dandelion root stimulates the flow of bile.

The dandelion properties that open-and-cleanse help rid obstructions of the liver, gallbladder, and spleen. The first stages of cirrhosis of the liver have been known to be alleviated by consistent use of the herb, and dandelion also helps in cases of liver enlargement, hepatitis, and jaundice.

Inulin

Inulin (found in the dandelion root) is currently being studied extensively for its action on the pancreas and blood sugar balance and for its immune system stimulation properties.

Diuretic

Dandelion leaves have been found to increase the flow of urine and are useful in kidney formulas. Whereas most conventional diuretics deplete the body of its potassium, it does not generally decrease with dandelion use. Dandelion ideally pairs diuretic properties with an abundance of available potassium.

Dandelion has been used for water retention due to heart problems. It is a specific diuretic in cases of congestive jaundice, and it reduces uric acid in the system.

	When overweight individuals are losing weight, they can become over acidic. These acids in the blood are neutralized by dandelion.
Blood	Dandelion root and cedar berries have an excellent reputation for regulating blood sugar levels. Dandelion has been known to reduce serum cholesterol, equalize blood pressure, and build up the blood with nutrients and minerals that help with anemia, energy, and endurance. A cup of dandelion tea 30 minutes before meals acts as a tonic to the liver, stomach, blood, pancreas, and spleen.
	The continued use of dandelion helps detoxify the system, eventually cleansing out toxins and waste products, reducing stiffness in the joints and increasing mobility. The roots have been shown to be moderately anti-inflammatory, supporting their traditional use for arthritis, rheumatism, and gout.
Digestion	The 'bitter' component of dandelion helps stimulate digestive juices and improve appetite. In situations of severe vomiting, dandelion restores the gastric balance in patients. It acts as a gentle laxative and is invigorating and strengthening to the body in general.
Skin	Due to dandelion's blood and liver cleansing properties, the herb has been used effectively to treat skin diseases and eruptions, helping rid the body of accumulated toxins.
	Burdock and dandelion work especially well together to help cleanse and heal the skin.
Warts	The juice of a broken dandelion stem can be used to treat warts. When used on a daily basis (for about a week), it can dry them up. Dandelion juice from the broken stem is also useful to topically treat acne, blisters, corns, and calluses.
Cancer and the Immune System	In testing dandelion against cancer, it has been shown to be active against tumors and in stimulating macrophage (immune system) action. This further validates the historical Chinese use of dandelion for breast cancer and as a strong antibiotic in cases of lung infections for thousands of years.
Women	Dandelion has properties that improve lactation in nursing mothers and strengthen the female organs.

Herb Parts Used	The whole plant is used medicinally, especially the leaves and roots
Preparations and Remedies	The roots are pressed for juice and dried for use in various preparations. Fresh or dried leaves and roots are prepared in capsules, liquid extracts, tablets, and tinctures.
Fresh	The fresh buds and flowers are a cleansing and fortifying trail-side snack. Dandelion greens can be eaten fresh in green drinks and salads. The bitter taste is reduced by soaking the greens in salt water for 30 minutes before using as a spicy addition to a salad.
	Wart Juice: Rub the fresh juice from a broken dandelion stem on a callus or wart. It might take a while but, with persistence, the juice will work. Use an emery board or pumice stone every day to file off the dried, dead skin.
Powdered Formula	*Kidney Formula:* (see JUNIPER preparations)
Infusions	*Dandelion Tea:* Steep 1-2 teaspoons of the cut-and-sifted dried root or leaves in a cup of hot water for 10-15 minutes. Take twice a day (in morning and evening).
	Alkaline Formula: This formula can be made into a tea or a tincture as needed. It helps the body regulate stomach acidity and tone the digestive organs. 3 parts Dandelion leaves 3 parts Nettle 1 part Sassafras 1 part Peppermint 1/4 part Ginger Add a teaspoon of this mixture to 1 cup boiling water. Cover and steep for 20 minutes. Strain and drink. Take up to 3 cups daily to aid the liver and kidneys in ridding the body of excess acid. Also eat plenty of vegetables that contain chlorophyll.
	Liver/Jaundice Tonic: *1 part Yellow Dock Root* 1 part Barberry root 1 part Wild Yam 2 parts Dandelion Root

DANDELION — 127

	2 parts Dandelion Leaves 1/2 part Licorice root Mix together and simmer one ounce of the herb mix in a quart of water for twenty minutes. Strain and drink four ounces three times daily. *Kidney/Lower Back Tea:* (see UVA URSI preparations) *System Cleanse Tea:* (see CHAPARRAL preparations)
Safety	Dandelion root and leaves are believed to be quite safe, with no side effects or risks known other than rare allergic reactions. Dandelion is on the FDA's GRAS (generally recognized as safe) list. While handling the plant, the milky latex in cut stems and leaves of dandelions may cause contact irritation of sensitive individuals.
Plant Profile Description	*Natural Habitat:* Native to Greece, dandelions are now found growing abundantly in Europe, the United States, and in most temperate regions of the world. *Natural Habitat:* Native to Greece, dandelions are now found growing abundantly in Europe, the United States, and in most temperate regions of the world. The common dandelion, Taraxacum *officinale*, is considered by many to be a nuisance weed to lawns and landscapes, but it has redeeming features as a nutritious green for healthy eating and is a wonderful medicinal herb. The dandelion is easy to confuse with other plants such as sow thistle or false dandelion (also found commonly in lawns and gardens). Dandelion is the only one of the three that has single flowering heads on hollow, unbranched stalks, and long, hairless, jagged-toothed leaves. All three plants exude a milky fluid when they are cut. The long, jagged leaves radiate from the base to form a rosette lying close upon the ground. Each grooved leaf is constructed so all the rain falling on it is conducted straight to the center of the rosette and, thus, to the root.

The small (five to six inches in height) perennial (lives for more than two years) has a stout taproot with bright yellow flowers, followed by a spherical multiple-seed plant head. Seeds are light, gray-brown, and pinhead sized, with propeller-like tufts which easily disperse in the wind and weather.

Dandelions flower March through September and sporadically throughout the year. The flower opens in the morning, closes in the evening, and remains closed all night and in cloudy weather. All parts of the plant contain a milky, bitter juice which exudes when broken or wounded, but the more powerful juice of the root is the part of the plant most used for medicinal purposes. The juice of the root is thin and watery in the spring; milky, bitter, and tends to coagulate in the latter part of summer and autumn; and sweet and less bitter in the winter when affected by the frost.

Growing Dandelion

If newly harvested seeds are planted in the spring, they will come right up. When planting in the fall, or if using last year's seed in the spring greenhouse, dormancy is a real problem, and the seeds do not readily come up. It may take multiple cycles to germinate. All this has survival advantage for the plant but is frustrating for growers. The growing cycle for cultivating dandelion is to seed in the spring and harvest the plants the following spring after a full year's growth.

Harvesting

Leaves are harvested before the flowering season, and the root is collected when it is mature from July through September. When harvesting the greens and flowers for use throughout the year, leave the roots for new plant growth in the spring.

Echinacea

Latin Name: *Echinacea angustifolia, E. purpurea, E. pallida*

Also known as: Purple Coneflower, Coneflower, Black Sampson, Rudbeckie, Sampson Root, Snake Root

Scientific Classification
Three of the nine echinacea species are used medicinally:
E. angustifolia, *E. purpurea*, and *E. pallida*

Family:	Asteraceae – aster, daisy and sunflower family Compositae – in earlier classifications
Genus	Echinacea – purple coneflower
Species	*E. angustifolia* – narrow-leaf coneflower, Black Sampson Echinacea *E. purpurea* – eastern purple coneflower *E. pallida* – pale purple coneflower

Influence on the Body	(PRINCIPAL ACTIONS are listed in CAPITAL LETTERS)
Blood and Circulatory System	BLOOD PURIFIER • BLOOD BUILDER • BLOOD CLEANSER • DEPURATIVE (cleanses blood by promoting eliminative functions) • BLOOD DISEASES • BLOOD POISONING • circulation • hemorrhage
Body System	stimulant (strengthens metabolism and circulation)
Cancer	cancer • tumors
Digestive Tract	sialagogue (promotes an increase flow of saliva) • digestion • carminative (brings warmth and circulation, relieves intestinal gas discomfort, promotes peristalsis) • peritonitis (inflammation of abdominal cavity) • parasiticide (kills parasites and worms)
First Aid	WOUNDS • BITES • STINGS • POISONOUS BITES • ANTISEPTIC
Infections and Immune System	INFECTIONS • IMMUNE DEFICIENCY • IMMUNE REGULATOR • ANTIBIOTIC • INFECTION prevention • EAR INFECTION • FEVERS • COLDS • flu • GLANDS • LYMPHATIC SYSTEM • LYMPHATIC CONGESTION • CONTAGIOUS DISEASES • DIPHTHERIA • typhoid fever • GANGRENOUS CONDITIONS • peritonitis (inflammation of abdominal cavity)

Lungs and Respiratory System	MUCUS • catarrhal conditions (mucous drainage and discharge) • bronchitis • EMPHYSEMA
Mouth, Nose and Throat	SORE GUMS • pyorrhea (gum disease) • gingivitis • MOUTH SORES • bad breath • sore throat • GARGLE • TONSILLITIS • laryngitis
Reproductive System	syphilis • gonorrhea *Male:* PROSTATE GLAND
Skin, Tissues and Hair	SKIN ERUPTIONS • ACNE • abscesses • septic sores • BOILS • carbuncles • ECZEMA • diaphoretic (promotes perspiration, increasing elimination through the skin)
Urinary Tract	bladder infection • edema

Key Properties:

IMMUNE REGULATOR	*increases resistance to infection*
ANTI-MICROBIAL	*specifically bacterial, viral and fungal; it is also considered to be a prebiotic (helps good bacteria grow and flourish in the intestines, keeping pathogenic bacteria from proliferating)*
ALTERATIVE	*cleanses toxins from blood, lymph, and eliminative organs*
ANTI-INFLAMMATORY	*protects mucous membranes and relieves inflammation*
Primarily affecting	IMMUNE SYSTEM • BLOOD • LYMPH • mucous membranes

History	Relatively new to most of the world, echinacea was first used by Native Americans. The Sioux used the fresh, scraped root for snake bites and septicemia (a serious bacterial infection of the blood). Before antibiotics were discovered, American physicians widely used echinacea for difficult infectious conditions such as gangrene, tuberculosis, and diphtheria. Its use dwindled for a time (when sulfa drugs appeared in the 1920's, and penicillin became popular in the early 1940's), but it has experienced a dramatic resurgence of interest in recent years. Germany began reporting their scientific-based 'phytomedicine' (plant based) studies regarding echinacea in the 1930's and the plant has become widely used by German physicians from that time. It has been reported German physicians prescribed echinacea over 2.5 million times in the year 1994 alone.

Today, Echinacea *angustifolia* is traded at a higher price than the other two plant species, as it is mostly wildcrafted (harvested from the wild), and populations are declining. Because Echinacea angustifolia brings a higher price on the market, many growers are jumping on board, and it is becoming much more readily available at a better price. The challenge to medicinal herb growers is finding a reliable source of seed true to the particular species, since echinacea easily cross-pollinates. I recommend 'Horizon Herbs' out of Oregon as a reliable source of quality-certified, organic plants and seeds.

E. *angustifolia* tolerates hot and dry conditions and can adapt to desert conditions like Nevada's Las Vegas Valley when artificial stratification methods (pre-chilling for seed germination) are used. See *Growing Echinacea* section.

Echinacea is the first real herb I was exposed to after I left home and started raising a family of my own. A 'crazy herb lady' I met gave me a tincture of Echinacea she made from plants growing in her backyard. I started to use it, and I felt better. I was suffering from immune symptoms associated with lupus. I had sun sensitivity, butterfly rashes on my face, pain, and low energy. I was only twenty-five years old, and I felt horrible. Within days of taking this Echinacea tincture, I felt much better.

Subsequently, all of my symptoms disappeared. This makes me wonder why the medical establishment in the United States tells people with Lupus not to take Echinacea. I, for one, have found out for myself the majesty of this life-saving herb.

Regarding Media Reports

Most of the supportive scientific studies on echinacea were done several years ago in Germany with E. *purpurea*. Recently, there have been conflicting accounts in the media about studies regarding echinacea having good, little, or no effect on healing colds or flus.

Given the vast, positive, out-of-the-country information on echinacea, along with personal experiences with the herb, I'm left to wonder, 'What is wrong with the study? Which species of the plant did they use? What part of the plant was used? Was it dried or fresh? Was it properly prepared? Were active components extracted, or was the herb left in its whole state? Did they use enough of the herb to be effective? What chemical fillers were added?'

What we do know is many of these studies used only 120 mg of Echinacea purpurea (the weakest of the Echinaceas) per day. An average capsule holds 500 mg. These studies were set up to fail. The recommended dose of Echinacea is at least 5000 mg per day. We must also ask, "Who is doing the study and what are their motives?"

Without fully understanding the nature of herbs, 'studies' may come up with misleading conclusions. I encourage the research of herbs. There is much that still can be learned. It would be the ideal circumstance to combine the disciplines of science and herbalism in this endeavor. Until that occurs, I recommend further investigation when contrary information about healing herbs is reported in the media.

Attributes	**Key Components:** (including, but not limited to)
Nutrition	Vitamins A • C • E • Copper • Iron • Potassium • Sulfur • Mucilage
	While echinacea is popularly known for its ability to limit and prevent infectious diseases, it has other healing qualities which include cleansing the blood and lymph system, protecting mucous membranes, and soothing inflammations in the body.
Immune System	Echinacea has been approved by the German Federal Health Agency as supportive therapy for upper respiratory tract infections, urogenital infections, and wounds.
	The immune system comprises multiple processes that recognize and neutralize pathogens in the body. Extensive research on echinacea has revealed it supports and enhances the actions of the immune system in several ways:

- It increases killer T-cell production. T-cell lymphocytes are types of white blood cells that recognize foreign substances and initiate the immune response. Without recognition, pathogens are free to invade and destroy tissues unhindered.
- It enhances production of alpha-1 and alpha-2 gamma globulins which contain the antibodies used by the body to identify and neutralize foreign matter (such as bacteria and viruses).
- It is a natural antibiotic. Echinacea is said to work like penicillin without adverse side effects. It is one of the best

- remedies for septicemia (blood poisoning). It has been shown to inhibit staphylococcus bacteria and is helpful in typhoid and other fevers.
- It is a natural prebiotic, keeping beneficial bacteria healthy and crowding out pathogenic bacteria. Echinacea does not kill the good bacteria.
- It is an antiseptic, combating and neutralizing pathogenic bacteria and preventing infection. Echinacea assists in healing wounds by fighting infection and stimulating cell growth. It helps with skin infections like impetigo, boils, and carbuncles. Studies show that echinacea has been used successfully to treat psoriasis and eczema. It has also been used as a mouthwash for gum problems.
- It has antifungal properties and has been used successfully to treat candida (a persistent yeast-like fungal infection). In one study, patients treated with an antifungal cream and echinacea extract were less likely to suffer a recurrence than those treated with the anti-fungal cream alone.
- It enhances the properdin/complement system, a system of proenzymes that participate in phagocytosis (engulfing and destroying bacterial and viral invaders) and helps to neutralize some viruses. Echinacea speeds resolution of colds, flu, bronchitis, and all kinds of upper respiratory infections.
- It inhibits hyaluronidase enzyme activity. Microbes (especially viruses) produce hyaluronidase to penetrate tissues and spread infection.
- It increases interferon levels. Interferons are proteins that prevent the reproduction of viruses. In 1978, a study in *Planta Medica* showed a root extract of echinacea destroyed both herpes and influenza viruses.
- It inhibits tumor growth. In vitro, echinacea stimulates the production of cytokines (immune proteins). Based on these findings, echinacea is currently being investigated as a possible antineoplastic (anti-tumor) agent.

Echinacea is one of the most potent herbs that support and strengthen immune system function. Because of this, it has been theorized that echinacea should be avoided in cases of autoimmune disorders (illnesses that occur when tissues of the body are attacked by elements of its own out-of-control immune system). There has not been any scientific evidence to support this supposition. It has been our experience that echinacea modulates and regulates activities of the immune system in cases of autoimmunity.

Cleansing

Echinacea is useful in all diseases which involve impurities in the blood such as boils, carbuncles, gangrene, persistent sores, cellular abscesses, snake bites, spider bites, and more. It is called the 'King of Blood Purifiers' for its ability to stimulate the efficient removal of waste and toxins from the body.

Echinacea improves lymphatic filtration and drainage, and it accelerates healing of lymph gland infections like strep throat and other lymph gland ailments. It has benefited headaches accompanied by vertigo (dizziness characterized by a spinning sensation) and a confused mental state when caused by toxemia (an accumulation of toxins throughout the system).

Once the blood is cleansed, the body proceeds to purge toxins from its cells, tissues, and organs, gradually detoxifying the lymphatic system, spleen, liver, kidneys, bowels, and skin. Echinacea promotes peristalsis (intestinal contractions), cleanses morbid matter from the stomach, and expels poisons and toxins. Echinacea can increase elimination through the skin by inducing perspiration. Over time, digestion and nutrient assimilation are improved, energy increases, and organ systems (including the skin) can become cleansed and healthy.

Anti-inflammatory

Echinacea assists in the healing of synovial membranes (connective tissues that line joint cavities) by enhancing the production of hyaluronic acid (a viscous slippery substance that lubricates the joints, maintains the shape of the eyeballs, and is a key component of connective tissue).

As a mucilage (complex sugar molecules that are soft and slippery), it soothes and protects mucous membranes and inflamed tissues. Science confirms its cortisone-like activity eases the pain of inflammation. It is invaluable as an external lotion for swellings.

Reproductive Health

Some have found it to be helpful for an enlarged and weakened prostate gland and, historically, it has been used for syphilis and gonorrhea.

Herb Parts Used	The medicinal parts of echinacea are typically the roots and leaves. The whole plant may also be used in various stages of development (usually fresh). Echinacea *angustifolia* root has the highest potency (fresh or dried) of the echinaceas.
Preparations and Remedies	
Fresh	A small piece of the fresh or recently-dried root may be held in the mouth and slowly chewed. This is very effective. Fresh leaves and flowers are as potent as the root but lose some of their vitality in the drying process.
Powdered	Leaves may be dried and powdered, but they are not as potent in this state as the dried root. Leaves are used as a general tonic to the system, rather than for a specific action. Once the root has been thoroughly dried, it may be powdered and added to herbal preparations or put into capsules. *Infection Formula:* (see GOLDENSEAL preparations)
Tinctures / Extracts	Tincturing is the process of extracting, concentrating, and infusing the active constituents of an herb into a liquid. The basic recipe calls for four parts liquid to one part powdered herb or four parts liquid to two parts cut or whole herb. (To use fresh herbs, fill the jar with the newly harvested herb and then cover with liquid). *Echinacea Tincture:* 1 part powdered Echinacea *angustifolia* root (or 2 parts cut or whole herb) 2 parts Vegetable Glycerin 2 parts Distilled Water *Optional:* Replace half the herb with goldenseal root. Echinacea and goldenseal work synergistically together, multiplying (not just adding) the quality of the end product. First, sterilize containers and utensils that will be used by rinsing them with hydrogen peroxide. Mix the measured ingredients together in a clean glass bottle. With the lid on, shake well. Label the bottle and then store it on the counter. Shake two times a day for ten to fourteen days.

After two weeks, finish the tincture by separating the infused liquid from the herb-powder residue. Sterilize all of the containers and utensils that will be used by rinsing them with hydrogen peroxide. Strain the extract mixture through a clean, unbleached, muslin cloth. Return the used herb powder to the earth or throw it away, as the medicinal qualities have been infused into the liquid. Keep the infused tincture in a closed, light-proof (preferably amber) bottle. It is important to label the tincture bottle with both the name of the tincture and the date. Tinctures will store with good potency for about three years if kept from light and heat. Keeping the tincture in the refrigerator will increase its longevity.

General use: Three squirts (about a half teaspoon) two to three times a day (or more as needed).

Poultices	*Poultice for boils and abscesses:* 4 parts Comfrey 1 part Lobelia 1 part Slippery Elm powder 1/8 part Cayenne Echinacea tea (as needed) Make a tea of echinacea leaves and add to the herb mixture until a peanut butter consistency is achieved. Apply the poultice fresh two times daily for four days. *Alternative 1:* Use ground flaxseed, lobelia, slippery elm powder, and a small amount of cayenne with echinacea tea. *Alternative 2:* Add comfrey and plantain to these for additional benefit and healing. *Slippery Elm Poultice:* (see SLIPPERY ELM preparations)
Enema / Douche	*Red Raspberry Enema / Douche:* (see RED RASPBERRY preparations)
Safety	No health hazards or side effects are known. No serious side effects have been reported in the prescribed use by millions of individuals in Germany and more than a century of use in the United States. If needed, echinacea is beneficial during pregnancy. German guidelines discourage use of echinacea for more than eight weeks, as it is thought prolonged, habitual use may suppress immunity. Although reasonable as a precaution, there

has been no convincing empirical evidence to support or refute this contraindication.

Plant Profile

Natural Habitat:
Echinacea is native to North America. It was introduced to European countries in the early 1900s. E. *angustifolia* grows naturally in the western United States; E. *purpurea* and E. *pallida* originated in the middle and eastern United States. All three species are now cultivated in Europe as well.

Description

E. *angustifolia* root (fresh or dried) has the most potent medicinal qualities of all the echinacea species. Fresh leaves and flowers are as powerful as the dried roots but more difficult to come by year-round. E. *purpurea's* effects have been most widely studied, and the plant is a viable choice for health care. E. *pallida* has not been as well studied and seems to be the least potent of the three.

Echinacea *angustifolia* (or narrow-leaved, purple coneflower) is a North American perennial (after tops die down in the winter, the plant grows back from a persistent rootstock in the spring) that is indigenous to the central plains. It grows on road banks, prairies, fields, and in dry, open woods. It is also called snake root, because it grows from a thick black root that Native Americans traditionally used to treat snake bites.

The plant grows two to three feet high, with single, stout, bristly stems and leaves that are rough, hairy, and three to eight inches long with narrowing tips.

The single, large, flower head appears from July through October and has a prominent, cone-shaped center surrounded by pale to deep purple ray petals. The genus name is taken from the Greek 'echino', meaning spiny or hedgehog, due to the flower's prickly center. The taste of the flower and leaves is slightly sweet, then bitter, leaving a tingling sensation on the tongue. The plant is faintly aromatic.

Growing Echinacea

Echinacea prefers well drained, limey soil in a sunny location.

Planting

Raised beds are highly recommended. The plant may be grown from seeds or transplants. Echinacea requires light and cold stratification (pre-chilling for seed germination). In climates that do not have cold enough winters to accomplish this, stratification may be done artificially with refrigeration in the following manner.

Stratification

Using containers deep enough to allow for good root development, fill with prepared soil mix and plant seeds by barely covering them with soil. Space seeds 2 inches apart. Moisten, cover, and put in the refrigerator at 40-50° F for 30 days. After stratifying, expose the plants (still in their containers) to warmer temperatures to allow for the emergence of seedlings. Germination generally occurs 10-20 days after the stratification process. When plants are several inches tall (usually 2-3 months after germination), transplant them into well-prepared, permanent, planting beds in the spring. Space plants 8-15 inches apart, making rows 18-30 inches apart. Weed control is very important, as echinacea does not compete well with weeds. The plants benefit from the use of mulch.

Harvesting

Echinacea Root:
The root is harvested in the fall after the plant has gone dormant, usually the second to fourth growing season. After the plant has died back, the energy of the plant will be in the root. A spading fork or other digging tool may be used. Be careful not to damage or break the taproot as roots are pulled out of the planting beds.

Harvesting is best done in the early morning just after the dew has evaporated or in the late evening (after the heat of the day has passed, but before the night air has a chance to deposit moisture on the plants). Picking in the heat of the afternoon sun results in a wilted plant that is depleted of its natural oils, making it a less effective product. Shake the roots free of dirt and put in the shade until the harvesting is complete. The root takes seven years to completely mature, but it may be taken earlier with good effect.

Leaves and Flowers:
The leaves and flowers are best harvested at the time of peak flowering with leaves in good condition. Once picked, wash plants and gently shake out excess moisture. The fresh flower and leaves are highly valued as they have the rich oils that harbor the greatest strength.

Seeds:
Seeds may be harvested when the plant is dying. Cut the flowering tops off, tie the stems together and place upside-down in a brown paper bag. Tightly tie or tape the bag closed and allow it to dry in a warm place. Collect the seeds by shaking the bag or rubbing the flower heads between the palms of the hands to release the seeds.

Drying Herbs

Screen Drying:
You may dry whole leaves, chopped roots, or sectioned flower heads. Carefully wash and brush the roots. Process soon after washing to minimize oxidation and deterioration. Place onto non-aluminum screens over a shallow collecting pan to catch scattered pieces and leaves of the herb as it dries.

Whole Plant Drying:
Before drying, first wash and air dry the plant. Gather five to eight stems of the plant together and tie them into a bundle. Place them in a brown paper bag with the stems extending out of the open end. Hang the bag with the plant upside-down in a dark, warm place (70-80° F). It will take two to four weeks for the herbs to become completely dry, depending on plant size, temperature, and moisture.

Drying Time:
The length of time for herbs to dry varies, depending on the plant part being dried. Flowers should be light and dry but not so dry they crumble into powder with handling. Leaves should be brittle enough to break between the fingers but not crumble. Stems and stalks should be breakable but not bendable. Bark and roots should be dry enough to snap if they are thin or chip easily with the blow of a hammer if they are thick.

Storage

Heat, light, air, and infestation will dissipate the healing properties of herbs, as will exposure to some types of plastics and metals. It is recommended that herbs are stored in light-proof containers (preferably amber bottles) or, otherwise, out of the light. Stored correctly, dried herbs will last for 10 years, retaining up to 90 percent potency.

Eyebright

Latin Name: *Euphrasia officinalis*

Also known as: Red Eyebright, Eyewort, Clear Eye, See Bright

Scientific Classification

The genus Euphrasia is a complex plant group with up to 170 named species, many separated by minute technical details. E. officinalis is represented most often in literature. Other species seem to be similar in their chemical makeup and are generally considered by herbalists collectively as Euphrasia officinalis

Family: Scrophulariaceae – figwort family

Genus Euphrasia – eyebright

Species E. officinalis – common eyebright

Influence on the Body	(PRINCIPAL ACTIONS are listed in CAPITAL LETTERS)
Blood and Circulatory System	BLOOD CLEANSER
Blood Sugar	DIABETES
Body System	tonic (increases energy and strength throughout the body) • astringent (increases the tone and firmness of tissues, lessens mucous discharge from the nose, intestines, vagina, and draining sores)
Digestive Tract	bitter (stimulates digestive juices and improves appetite) • digestive disorders • ulcers
Ears	EARACHE • middle ear problems
Eyes	EYE strengthening • EYE STRAIN • VISION AID • EYE INFECTIONS • PINK EYE • dissolves styes • EYE DISORDERS • CONJUNCTIVITIS • CATARACTS • GLAUCOMA
Infections and Immune System	ALLERGIES • COLDS • hay fever
Inflammation	anti-inflammatory
Liver	LIVER STIMULANT • jaundice
Mouth, Nose and Throat	anti-catarrh (helps heal inflamed mucous membranes with discharge, especially affecting the nose and throat) • congestion

	• coughs • RUNNY NOSE • sinus congestion • SNEEZING • sore throat
Nervous System	memory • headache

	Key Properties:
ALTERATIVE	*cleanses the blood and induces efficient removal of waste products*
astringent	*tightens and constricts tissues, reduces swelling*
antiseptic	*prevents the growth of disease-causing microorganisms*
bitter	*stimulates digestive juices and improves appetite*
tonic	*increases energy and strength throughout the body*
Primarily affecting	EYES • MUCOUS MEMBRANES • liver • blood

History	The word 'Euphrasia' is of Greek origin, derived from 'euphrosyne', meaning gladness. It is believed the plant acquired this name because of its reputation for curing eye ailments. It brought much gladness by preserving the eyesight of the sufferer. Though known and named by the Greeks, there is little history of its medicinal use until the 1300's, when it was ascribed to cure 'all evils of the eye.'
	Euphrasia was regarded as a treatment in diseases of the eyes by the great herbalists of the 1500's (Tragus, Fuschsius, Dodoens, etc).
	The 'Doctrine of Signatures' was a popular theory during the 1500's and 1600's. It was believed the way a plant looked indicated the ailments for which it should be used in herbal medicine. With the flower's spots and stripes, eyebright became known, under this discipline, for resembling bloodshot eyes, initiating or adding to its traditional use as an herbal aid for the eyes.
	In Queen Elizabeth's time (1533-1603), there was a type of ale called 'Eyebright Ale.' In *'Paradise Lost'* (published in 1667), the poet Milton relates the Archangel Michael used eyebright to cure Adam of the eye infliction caused by his eating the forbidden fruit.
	'Eyebright,' says Salmon (1671), 'clears the sight and strengthens

the head, eyes, and memory.' Nicholas Culpeper (English botanist, herbalist, physician, and astrologer, 1616-1654) extolled the herb's virtues as being neglected. If people had been using it more, there would be much less need for spectacles.

For centuries, eyebright has been depended upon as an herb of choice for various eye disorders.

In Iceland, the expressed juice is used for most ailments of the eye. In Scotland, the Highlanders make an infusion of the herb in milk for weak or inflamed eyes.

Herbalists continue to use eyebright as an herb of choice for a wide variety of eye disorders, sinus, and cold infections.

Attributes	**Key Components: (including, but not limited to)**
Nutrition	Vitamins A • B1 (thiamine) • B2 (riboflavin) • B3 (niacin) • B5 (pantothenic acid) • B6 (pyridoxine) • B9 (folic acid) • B12 (cobalamin) • Biotin • Choline • Inositol • PABA (Para-Amino Benzoic Acid) • C• D • E • Copper • Iron • Zinc • other Trace Minerals
	Bitter • *Tannic Acid* • *Flavonoids* • *Iridoid Glucosides (*including *Aucubin)* • *Volatile Oils*
	Some of these compounds have antibacterial and anti-inflammatory effects.
Eyes	Eyebright is used for relieving red, itchy, or inflamed eyes and for healing styes. When it is used as an eyewash, it tends to prevent excessive secretion of fluids, relieves discomfort from eye strain and minor irritation, and rejuvenates tired eyes.
	It is excellent for weak eyesight. Eyebright strengthens and soothes the eyes, often improving eyesight (even in advanced years), and retards or reverses cataracts.
	Eyebright is excellent for acute or chronic inflammations of the eyes, including over-sensitivity to light. It helps with eyes that are cloudy and irritated with mucous lacrimation (excessive tearing), and has antiseptic properties that fight eye infections.
	Poultices and eyewashes of eyebright are used for eye complaints associated with conjunctivitis (inflammation and the

	mucous membranes covering the eyeball and inside the eyelids) surrounding blood vessels and as a preventive measure against mucus build up. Taken internally, eyebright supports and strengthens eye health and healing.
Mucous Membranes	Eyebright is used with excellent results for problems relating to mucous membranes of the nose and sinuses. It works as a vaso-constrictor and astringent to nasal and conjunctiva (around eyes) mucus. It brings relief in frequent sneezing bouts. A concentrated tincture every two hours is specific for acute nasal and sinus congestions, attacks of hay fever, and colds. Eyebright is used in all mucous diseases accompanied by increased discharge and for coughs, hoarseness, ear-aches, and headaches associated with head colds. It has been used to clear a foggy head and improve memory.
Liver	Eyebright is known to stimulate and detoxify the liver and clean the blood. It is used in Europe as an astringent tonic in the treatment of jaundice. Eyebright is high in iridoid glycosides such as aucubin. In several laboratory studies, aucubin has been found to be hepatoprotective (liver protective) and possess antimicrobial activity. (1)(2)(3)
Anti-inflammation	Several iridoid glycosides have been isolated from eyebright (particularly aucubin), which possess anti-inflammatory properties comparable to those of Indomethacin (a nonsteroidal anti-inflammatory drug). (4)
Herb Parts Used	The entire above-ground plant
Preparations and Remedies	The dried herb is used whole, cut, and sifted, for infusions, in tinctures, and powdered to put into capsules, tablets, and other preparations.
Infusions	The tea may be used as an eyewash or taken internally. It is particularly effective in combination with other herbs and often used with goldenseal. *Eyebright Tea:*

Steep a heaping teaspoonful of the leaves into a cup of boiling water for half an hour. When cold, drink one or two cups a day. Four fluid ounces of the infusion taken every morning on an empty stomach and every night at bedtime has been found successful in relieving epilepsy.

Eyewash

For all preparations that go directly into or on the eyes, it is essential to keep utensils, containers, and preparations clean and sterile.

Simple Eyewash:
This eyewash is for tired, strained eyes. It cleanses the tear ducts and stimulates circulation.

1 tablespoon Eyebright herb
1 cup distilled water

Boil water and remove from heat. Add eyebright and let steep (covered) for ten minutes. Strain through a muslin cloth or unbleached coffee filter. Cool until lukewarm. Fill sterile eyecup with cooled solution. Tip your head back, letting the solution wash the eye as you blink several times.

Always discard used solution and refill eyecup with fresh solution. Apply to the same eye three separate times, re-sterilize eyecup (to avoid cross-contamination infections from eye to eye), and repeat procedure on the other eye. The eyewash should be made fresh each application, as it does not store well in the refrigerator.

Eyebright – Goldenseal Eye Wash:
 (see GOLDENSEAL preparations)

Fomentations

Eye Wash or Fomentations:
Use eye herbs in a tea. Strain and then use as an eyewash or fomentation (towel soaked in infusion and placed on affected area). Use alternating hot and cold fomentations over the eyes several times daily. This eyewash has been used for babies who have clogged tear ducts and by people with cataract problems.

When there is great discomfort, it is considered desirable to use a warm infusion rather more frequently for inflamed eyes until resolved. In most cases, the cool application is sufficient.

Eye Compress

Soothing Eye Compress:

1 tablespoon Eyebright herb
1/2 tablespoon powdered Comfrey root

1/2 tablespoon Goldenseal root powder
1 pint distilled water

Make a tea by stirring comfrey and goldenseal into the water and bringing to a boil. Turn down heat to simmer (keeping covered) for ten minutes, remove from heat, and add eyebright. Leave lid on and steep for ten more minutes.

In cases of tired or inflamed eyes, a compress can relieve symptoms, relax the eye muscles, and improve vision. Prepare the compress by putting cotton into a bowl with a wooden spoon and wrapping it with gauze. Strain the tea, dip the spoon into it, and apply it to the eye. In the case of styes, the mixture may be applied while still fairly warm (to tolerance) and alternated with cold applications to encourage drainage of the infection. For this procedure, separate the tea into two vessels; leave one covered to stay hot and put ice cubes in the other.

Safety	No health hazards or adverse side effects are known
Plant Profile	*Natural Habitat:* Native to Europe and some parts of western Asia, eyebright grows wild in grasslands, meadows, and pastures. It is now cultivated in North America as well
Description	Eyebright is a low creeping annual (must grow from new seed each year) with a rising black-green stem that is one to nine inches in height (depending on growing conditions and species), fanlike, bristle-toothed leaves, and several flowers. The leaves are downy and appear opposite each other in two's, alternating below and above. The small, whitish flowers are two-lipped (with the top lip/petal being slightly hooded). The petals have a yellow throat with marked purple stripes. Flowers appear June through September and are followed by an oblong pod filled with numerous seeds. The plant essentially lacks odor but has a bitter, salty, astringent taste. The root is long, small, and thready at the end, with suckers that spread out and attach to surrounding grass plant roots to share in their nutrients as a semi-parasitic symbiote. The grass thus preyed upon does not suffer very much. Penetration is slight, and there is no permanent drain of strength, as eyebright dies out each year.

Earlier herbal literature sometimes describes a red-flowered eyebright, which is now considered to be a different, though related, plant.

Growing Eyebright

The plant prefers full sun to part shade and rich, moist soils. It draws on the strength of other plants (particularly grasses), but some species are less dependent than others. To plant, press seeds firmly into the surface of soil in fall or very early spring. A period of cold, moist conditioning improves germination. The seed produces a low germination rate the first year, achieving a better rate the second year. There is a survival advantage to splaying germination out over a couple of years, and extended dormancy of this sort is fairly common with wild (undomesticated) seeds.

Harvesting

Eyebright is best gathered when it is in flower and cut just above the root.

Flaxseed

Latin Name: *Linum usitatissimum*

Also known as: Flax, Common Flax, Linseed, Lint Bells

Scientific Classification

Flax seeds come in two basic varieties, brown and yellow (or golden), with several species having similar nutritional values and equal amounts of short-chain, omega-3 fatty acids. The exception is a type of yellow flax called Linola or solin, which has a completely different oil profile and is very low in omega-3's

Family: Linaceae – flax family

Genus Linum – flax

Species L. usitatissimum – common flax

Not to be confused with Linum catharticum – Mountain Flax, which has much stronger purgative qualities.

Influence on the Body	(PRINCIPAL ACTIONS are listed in CAPITAL LETTERS)
Blood, Heart, and Circulation	CHOLESTEROL • HIGH BLOOD PRESSURE • atherosclerosis
Blood Sugar	Diabetes
Cancer	breast cancer • endometrial cancer (inner layer of the uterus) • colon cancer prevention • mouth cancer • skin cancer
Digestive Tract	inflamed digestive MUCOUS MEMBRANES • antacid • CONSTIPATION • GASTRITIS • DIVERTICULITIS (inflammation of out-pouches of the bowel wall) • DYSENTERY (colon inflammation with pain, cramping, and diarrhea) • MILD LAXATIVE (softens stool without purging) • LAXATIVE CORRECTIVE • enemas • hemorrhoids
Infections and Immune System	Fevers
Inflammation	INFLAMMATION • rheumatism • gout
Lungs and Respiratory System	inflamed respiratory MUCOUS MEMBRANES • coughs • bronchitis • asthma • pleurisy (inflammation of the chest cavity)
Nervous System	Memory
Reproductive System	*Female:* menstrual problems • menopausal symptoms

FLAXSEED — 148

Skin, Tissues and Hair	SKIN IRRITATIONS • EMOLLIENT (softens and soothes) • BOILS • SORES • SCALDS • BURNS
Urinary Tract	inflamed urinary tract MUCOUS MEMBRANES • renal irritation • bladder irritation • bladder infection • KIDNEY STONES
Industrial Uses	animal feed • linen thread and cloth (from stem) • linseed oil (in paints, varnishes, stains, furniture polish, linoleum flooring product, and concrete preservatives)

Key Properties:

MILD LAXATIVE	softens stools without purging
NUTRITIVE	supplies substantial amount of nutrients and aids in building and toning the body
MUCILAGE	soothes inflammation
DEMULCENT	soothes inflammation of mucous membranes
EMOLLIENT	softens and soothes skin externally and mucous membranes internally
Primarily affecting	DIGESTIVE TRACT • BLOOD VESSELS • MUCOUS MEMBRANES • lungs

History	Brown flax can be consumed as readily as yellow and has been for thousands of years. Flax seeds produce a vegetable oil known as flaxseed or linseed oil, which is one of the oldest commercial oils. Flaxseed has been cultivated first by the ancient Mesopotamians (about 3,000 BC) and then by the Egyptians. Burial chambers depict flax cultivation and clothing from flax fibers, and the Egyptians wrapped their mummies in linen. Greeks ate roasted flax seeds and baked them in bread. Hippocrates (ancient Greek physician, ca. 460-370 BC) wrote about using flax for the relief of abdominal pains. In the same era, Theophrastus recommended the use of flax mucilage as a cough remedy. Tacitus (Roman senator and historian, ca. 56-117 AD) praised the virtues of flax. Mucilaginous properties of the oil are mentioned by early Roman authors, who reported flaxseed's use for colds, urinary tract inflammations, and

lung conditions. They were probably responsible for spreading the use of flax as a crop plant throughout Europe. Its slender stalks are a source of strong, supple fibers used for countless centuries to make rope, nets, sacks, bowstrings, sails and, of course, linen fabrics.

Emperor Charlemagne (ca. 742-814 AD) was so convinced of the therapeutic properties of flax, he demanded his subjects eat flaxseed regularly to maintain good health. After Charlemagne, flaxseeds became widely appreciated throughout Europe.

Hildegard von Bingen, German abbess, naturalist, herbalist, and poet (ca. 1098-1179 AD), used flax meal in hot compresses for the treatment of both external and internal ailments.

Flax was widely used as poultices (made from the boiled, crushed seeds) applied to swellings, burns, boils, and other skin eruptions and to ease aches and pains in muscles and joints. A thick, mucilaginous liquid extracted from the seeds was also applied as a poultice to burns and other types of inflammation.

Native Americans used flax for skin and eye problems, stomach disorders, kidney disease, urinary infections, coughs, and diseases of the lungs.

In the American colonies, flax was a main source of fabric in the form of homemade 'linsey-woolsey' made from linen and wool.

Later, the coming of two world wars increased the demand for flax as a source of oil for many products in the home and factory, and commercial production in North America expanded substantially.

During the 1950's-60's, flax products were widely used throughout the world. Oil-based coatings enhanced and protected wood and concrete surfaces, and durable linoleum became a popular flooring material. Flax breads and other baked goods were commonplace. Farmers and animal breeders fed flax to their livestock for maintenance of a healthy coat and to improve animal digestion.

Today, the seeds are commonly used as a mild, lubricating laxative to relieve Irritable Bowel Syndrome (IBS) diverticulitis, gastritis, enteritis, and joint discomfort, and is a great source of nutrients such as omega 3.

Attributes

Nutrition

Key Components: (including, but not limited to)
Vitamins B1 (thiamine) • B2 (riboflavin) • B3 (niacin) • B5 (pantothenic acid) • B6 (pyridoxine) • B9 (folic acid) • C • E • Calcium • Copper • Iron • Manganese • Magnesium • Phosphorus • Potassium • Selenium • Sodium • Zinc Sugars • Mucilage • Dietary Fiber • Fat • high in Omega-3 Fatty Acids (an alpha-linolenic acid, ALA) • Lignans (phytoestrogens) • Protein

Flaxseed is 30-40 percent linseed oil (55 percent of the linseed oil is ALA and about 6 percent is mucilage).

Flaxseed is a superfood, high in fiber, proteins, omega-3 fatty acids, and good fats (which can help lower cholesterol, reduce swellings, and soothe inflammation). Flax is excellent for helping to build muscle and bone tissues and for losing excess weight.

Digestion

Germany's Commission E authorizes the use of flaxseed for various digestive problems including chronic constipation, irritable bowel syndrome, diverticulitis, and general stomach discomfort.

The mucilaginous fiber in the seeds is not digested in the stomach. It absorbs water in the colon and swells to form a soothing gel that softens the stool. Flaxseed stimulates peristalsis (intestinal contractions that propel contents onward) and relieves intestinal irritation and inflamed conditions. The laxative effect produces a bowel movement (may take a few days).

This mild laxative is non-habit forming and is used in cases when purgative laxatives have been overused and bowels are sluggish. Its mucilaginous qualities make it effective for all types of intestinal inflammation, chronic constipation, irritable colon, diverticulitis, gastritis, and enteritis (inflammatory disease of the digestive tract).

Flaxseed tea enemas may be used to help loosen a heavy mucous coat of the inner intestinal walls. People with painful, bleeding hemorrhoids experience easy bowel movements without irritation when the enema tea is used every day.

In a double-blind study, those taking flaxseed had significantly fewer problems with constipation, abdominal pain, and bloating than those taking psyllium.

Ground flaxseed is excellent for diets which are low in fiber. A teaspoon of flaxseed in a warm cup of water or juice before meals will stop excessive food cravings and assist the dieter in losing weight.

Blood Sugar

As a high-fiber food, flaxseed slows down glucose absorption, leading to better control of blood-sugar levels.

In a study conducted by the University of Toronto, participants who ate flaxseed bread had blood-sugar levels 28 percent lower an hour after eating than their counterparts who ate bread made with wheat flour.

Omega-3 Health Benefits

The body cannot make the essential fatty acids Linoleic (omega-6) or Linolenic (omega-3). They must be consumed as part of the daily diet. In proper balance, omega-3 and omega-6 fatty acids work to form the walls of every cell in the body, play a vital role in the active tissues of the brain, and control the way cholesterol works in the body.

The American diet has high levels of omega-6 (found in most of the oils used in food processing, the fat of meat, butter, cheese, egg yolks, etc.) and not enough omega-3's. This has caused health problems resulting in increased incidence of blood clotting (leading to heart attack and stroke), elevated blood pressure, suppressed immune system, and accelerated cancer cell growth.

The richest sources of omega-3 fatty acids are flaxseed oil and fish oil. Flaxseed contains ALA (alpha-linolenic acid), one of the three types of omega-3's which can be converted in the body into the other two longer-chain omega-3 fatty acids DHA (Docosahexaenoic acid), and EPA (Eicosatetraenoic acid).

Fish oil contains DHA and EPA omega-3's, but it does not contain sufficient quantities of vitamin E for the diet if taken alone. Flaxseed is an excellent plant source of omega-3's, as well as a source of vitamin E with its abundant antioxidant properties.

Research shows that omega-3 oils can reduce blood pressure, decrease the risk of heart attack and disease, lower cholesterol, stimulate the immune system, and protect against inflammation, kidney diseases, and some types of cancer.

At the conclusion of a 12-week study, both systolic and diastolic blood pressures were significantly lower in participants using omega-3-rich flaxseed oil.

Research has shown that flaxseed reduces cholesterol, platelet aggregation (which may lead to blood clots, heart attack and stroke), and inflammation. It also protects against degenerative diseases.

In a study comparing daily consumption of ground flaxseed with the use of statin medications (cholesterol lowering drugs), participants receiving flaxseed did just as well as those given statin drugs. Significant reductions were seen in total cholesterol, LDL (Low Density Lipoprotein, the 'bad' cholesterol), triglycerides, and the ratio of total cholesterol to HDL (High Density Lipoprotein, the 'good' cholesterol) in both groups.

Brain Function

Research notes that a diet rich in omega-3 fatty acids is important for brain development. DHA also acts as a mood boosting agent that is essential for the proper function of brain cells. Participants in one study saw a decreased risk of Alzheimer's from eating a diet high in omega-3 fatty acids. Flax is the richest source of omega-3's in the plant kingdom.

Urinary Tract

Preliminary research indicates potential benefits in treating kidney and bladder congestion, inflammation, and diseases with a flaxseed decoction (strong infusion).

Respiratory System

An old poultice recipe uses a thick flaxseed paste to relieve pain and congestion in peritonitis (inflammation of the tissues lining the inner wall of the abdomen and pelvis), pneumonia, pleurisy, and so forth. The tea taken internally is also good for coughs, asthma, and pleurisy.

Skin

Mixed in poultices, ground flaxseed is one of the best remedies for sores, boils, carbuncles, inflammations, and tumors of the skin. Adding slippery elm bark and comfrey to the poultice adds to the benefits and is particularly effective for boils, pimples, and oozing sores and burns.

Eyes

An old folk remedy for removing foreign bodies from the eye is to take a single, moistened flaxseed and place it under the eyelid. The foreign body will stick to the mucous secretion of the seed.

Women	Lignans, found abundantly in flaxseed, act as phytoestrogens (compounds from plants that mimic estrogen in the body) and help balance a woman's hormone levels. Flaxseed can promote normal ovulation (improving fertility) and extend the second, progesterone-dominant half of the cycle (restoring hormone balance). This lowers the risk of suffering from estrogen-dominant imbalances, including irregular menstrual cycles, breast cysts, headaches, sleep difficulties, fluid retention, anxiety, irritability, mood swings, weight gain, lowered sex drive, brain fog, fibroid tumors, heavy bleeding, peri-menopausal / menopausal symptoms, and estrogen-dominant cancers. One study showed a 50 percent decrease in frequency of hot flashes after subjects took 1.4 ounces of crushed flaxseed every day for 6 weeks. Flax is one of the most concentrated known sources of plant lignans. The seeds contain 100-800 times the amount found in other plants.
Cancer	Observational studies suggest that people who eat more lignan-containing foods have a lower incidence of breast, and perhaps, colon cancer. Preliminary research indicates flaxseed lignans may also fight cancer by acting as an antioxidant. Flaxseed can offer protection against breast cancer without interfering with estrogen's role in normal bone maintenance. The lignans in flaxseed can hook onto the same receptor sites as estrogen. When estrogen is abundant, lignans may reduce the hormone's effects by displacing it from cells. In this manner, they may help prevent estrogen-dependent cancers from starting and developing. This is how soy is believed to work in breast cancer prevention (although soy uses isoflavones as phytoestrogens instead of lignans).
Industrial Uses	Linen cloth is made from fibers found in the sturdy flax stalk. Linseed oil (from flax seeds) rapidly absorbs oxygen from the air and forms (when laid in thin layers) a hard, transparent varnish. This has been used in the manufacture of paints, varnishes, stains, furniture polish, linoleum flooring products, and concrete preservatives.
Herb Parts Used	Seed and its oil *Oil Extraction:*

The oil is obtained by expressing the seeds which contain about 30-40 percent oil. On a large scale, seeds are usually roasted before being pressed to destroy the gummy matter contained in their coating. This frees the oil from the mucilage but results in a darker colored, acrid oil. Flaxseed oil to be used for health food purposes should be processed by cold expression without heat. It is a yellowish, oily liquid having a peculiar odor and a bland, slightly nutty taste. When exposed to air, it gradually thickens, darkens in color, and acquires a strong odor and taste. It becomes rancid quickly and should be used as soon after expression as possible and always refrigerated.

Do not use boiled flaxseed oil for medicinal or nutritional purposes. Heat produces undesirable by-products in the oil. When flaxseed oil is heated and processed, it is used as a paint binder and wood finishing product and is then called linseed oil.

Preparations and Remedies

Quality Testing:
When ground flaxseed is carelessly preserved, it is subject to insect infestation and rancidity. Flaxseed should be free of parasites and unpleasant odor.

Storage

Flax seeds are stable while whole. Milled or ground flaxseed can be stored for four months at room temperature with minimal to no change of taste, smell, or rancidity. Storing sealed containers of flaxseed in the refrigerator or freezer will keep ground flax from becoming rancid for even longer.

Flaxseed oil is especially perishable and should be purchased in opaque bottles that have been kept refrigerated. Flaxseed oil should have a sweet, nutty flavor. Never use flaxseed oil in cooking. Add it to foods only after taking from heat.

Nutritional Food

Drink a cup of water when taking flaxseed. The fiber needs the water to swell and form the mucilage which soothes the intestinal tract and stimulates peristalsis.

Grind flaxseeds in a coffee or seed grinder to enhance their digestibility and nutritional value. If adding ground flaxseeds to a cooked cereal or grain dish, do so at the end of cooking, since the soluble fiber in the flaxseeds will thicken liquids if left too long.

Sprinkle flaxseed meal on cereals or mix it with oatmeal, yogurt, water (similar to Metamucil), or any other food item where a nutty flavor is appropriate. Flaxseed sprouts are edible and have a slightly spicy flavor.

Egg Substitute

Use one tablespoon ground flaxseeds and three tablespoons water to serve as a replacement for one egg in baking. However, it may somewhat alter the texture of the finished product.

Flax Paste

Seeds can be soaked overnight and then blended into a thick paste for eating. Add garlic, cayenne, olive oil, apple cider vinegar, or any herbs or spices to taste. Flax paste can heal a severe case of diarrhea or intestinal upset just by going on a bland diet of it for a day until the problem resolves.

Flaxseed Oil

Laxative Oil:
Taken internally, flaxseed oil is sometimes given as a laxative. It is excellent for kidney stones and has been used for pleurisy with great success.

Infusions

Flaxseed Tea:
A teaspoon of the ground seed mixed in a cup of hot water or juice, taken three times a day, can help ease ulcers and inflammations. The tea is also good for coughs, asthma, and pleurisy.

Syrup

Cough Syrup: (see LICORICE preparations)

External Applications

Flax is an excellent pulling herb to draw out pain, swelling, splinters, infection, and poisons. To retain freshness, grind seeds only as needed.

Poultices

Ground Flaxseed Poultice:
Grind one or two tablespoons of flaxseeds to a powder in a seed grinder or blender and stir into two to four ounces of hot water. Let soak until it forms a slimy gel. At this point, you may add other herbs to enhance healing such as goldenseal root or comfrey. Spread the gel onto a small piece of cloth and apply to boils and sores. You can also spread the paste directly on the injured area, cover with a piece of clean cloth, then a layer of plastic, and finally, with a towel.

An old poultice recipe uses a thick flaxseed paste, spread at least half an inch in thickness upon muslin or flannel, and applied as hot as possible (without burning) every two or three hours, in order to relieve pain and congestion in peritonitis (inflammation of the tissues lining the inner wall of the abdomen and pelvis), pneumonia, and pleurisy.

Inflammation Wrap:
To help ease the pain of inflammation, simmer flaxseeds (one teaspoon to a cup of water) for five minutes. Spread the seed and some of the tea on a cloth. Wrap it around swollen joints, cover with a towel, and keep it on all night.

Skin Irritations:
1 oz. Goldenseal
9 oz. Flaxseed oil

Mix thoroughly. Apply freely to the skin as needed for itching, burning, or rashes of the skin (also used topically for the rash that accompanies smallpox, measles, and scarlet fever).

Burns:
Pulverize a raw potato and mix with powdered flaxseed or slippery elm and aloe vera gel. Spread mixture on unbleached muslin cloth and apply to burns.

Boils and Abscess Poultice: (see ECHINACEA preparations)

Safety

Like other sources of fiber, flaxseed should be taken with plenty of fluids. No health hazards or adverse side effects are known.

Plant Profile

Natural Habitat:
Thought to be a native of Europe and Asia, flax is cultivated worldwide in temperate and tropical regions, including North America.

Description

Flax is pretty in the garden, with the added advantage of yielding a valuable seed crop. Homegrown organic flaxseed is very tasty as an addition to breads and cereals. Since rancidity can be a problem after it is ground, it is nice to grow and have a fresh supply close at hand.

Flax is a slender annual (plant that must be grown from new seed each year) that grows quickly up to one to two feet. The plant has an erect stalk with narrow, gray-green leaves and branches at the top, terminating with five petaled, sky-blue-to-white flowers (June and July). Seed capsules follow (in August) that contain small, glossy, flattened, brown (or golden) seeds. Inside the seed is olive-green, with a mildly odorous oil which has a nutty flavor and is very mucilaginous (sticky and viscous).

Growing Flax

In addition to referring to the plant itself, the word 'flax' can refer to the unspun fibers used to make linen thread and cloth. For extracting the flax fibers contained in the durable stalk, the plant is cut when it is mature. Seeds are collected when they are ripe and sold whole or pressed to extract their oil. Crude flaxseed oil is called linseed oil. It has a wide variety of industrial uses (a component of paints and the original linoleum tiles) and can be prepared for sale in health food stores.

Flax is easy to grow. To plant an area of good soil in the spring, strew seeds on the surface, work them into the soil with the fingers, pat down soil surface, and water. The plant grows best in a self-supporting patch and not in carefully defined rows. The distinctive sprouts appear quickly and tend to out-distance weeds. Within 6 weeks of sowing, the plant will reach 4-6 inches in height. It continues growing an inch or more a day (under optimal growth conditions), reaching its full height within another 15 days.

Garlic

Latin Name: *Allium sativum*

Also known as: Clove Garlic, Stinking Rose, Poor-Man's-Treacle (treacle is a middle English term for a medicinal syrup used for poisons, snakebite, and various ailments)

Scientific Classification

There are many varieties of garlic, each differing in size, pungency, and color, but the most known are the white-skinned American, Creole (pink or purple Mexican, Italian garlic), and the larger, Tahitian garlic. Elephant garlic is a variety of garlic with a large bulb which has a relatively mild flavor and lacks many of the healing qualities.

Family: Liliaceae – lily family
Genus: Allium – onion
Species: A. sativum – cultivated garlic
Sister plants: onion, leek, chives

Influence on the Body	(PRINCIPAL ACTIONS are listed in CAPITAL LETTERS)
Blood and Circulatory System	HEART • heart palpitation • ALTERATIVE (cleanses and stimulates efficient removal of waste products) • BLOOD CLEANSER • BLOOD PURIFIER • POOR CIRCULATION • HIGH BLOOD PRESSURE • ARTERIOSCLEROSIS • BLOOD POISONING • dropsy • anemia
Blood Sugar	diabetes • hypoglycemia
Body System	TONIC (increases energy and strength throughout the body) • stimulant (increases internal heat and strengthens metabolism and circulation) • physical endurance • anti catarrhal (eliminates mucous conditions) • insomnia • restlessness • antispasmodic • ANTIOXIDANT • aging • diaphoretic (promotes perspiration)
Cancer	CANCER (prevention) • CANCERS (particularly gastro-intestinal) • TUMORS
Digestive Tract	aromatic (contains volatile essential oils which aid digestion and relieve gas) • improves appetite • heartburn • DIGESTIVE DISORDERS • cramps • stomach ulcers • ulcers • diverticulitis • FLATULENCE (gas) • CARMINATIVE (relieves intestinal gas discomfort, promotes peristalsis) • colic • diarrhea • INTESTINAL INFECTIONS • COLITIS • parasiticide (kills and expels parasites and worms)

Ears	EAR INFECTIONS
Endocrine System	helps regulate glands
Eyes	inflamed eyes • eye catarrh (mucous membrane inflammation with discharge)
First Aid	WOUNDS • VULNERARY (promotes healing of wounds by protecting against infection and stimulating cellular growth) • leg ulcers • insect bites • bee stings • poisonous bites and stings • lead poisoning • metal poisoning • nicotine poisoning
Infections and Immune System	INFECTIONS • abscesses • COLDS • COUGHS • FEVER • chills • swollen glands • FLU • allergies • ANTIBIOTIC • ANTI-STAPH • ANTI-STREP • ANTI-VIRAL • YEAST INFECTIONS • CANDIDA ALBICANS • ANTI-FUNGUS • athlete's foot • ringworm • ANTISEPTIC (fights pathogenic bacteria and helps prevent infection) • IMMUNO-STIMULANT • childhood diseases • INFECTIOUS DISEASES • CONTAGIOUS DISEASES • smallpox • CHOLERA • SPINAL MENINGITIS • rabies • typhoid fever • WHOOPING COUGH • PLAGUE • leprosy
Inflammation	ARTHRITIS • osteoarthritis • rheumatism
Liver	gallbladder • cholagogue (promotes the flow of bile) • detoxifies LIVER
Lungs and Respiratory System	EXPECTORANT (loosens and removes phlegm in the respiratory tract) • ANTI-CATARRHAL (eliminates mucous conditions) • mucus • RESPIRATORY CONGESTION • CHRONIC BRONCHITIS • LUNGS • ASTHMA • pneumonia • emphysema • TUBERCULOSIS
Mouth, Nose and Throat	TOOTHACHE • rhinitis (clogged and running nose) • sinus problems • sinus congestion • sore throat • pharyngitis
Muscles	lumbago • muscle cramps
Nervous System	nervine (improves nerve function) • neuralgia pains • migraine headaches • dizziness • epilepsy • paralysis
Reproductive System	*Male:* PROSTATE GLAND problems *Female:* emmenagogue (promotes menstrual flow)
Skin, Tissues and Hair	acne • chapped and chafed hands • necrosis (death of cells or tissues) • eczema • psoriasis • WARTS • carbuncles • diaphoretic (promotes perspiration, increasing elimination through the skin)

GARLIC — 160

Urinary Tract	promotes kidney function • diuretic (increases urine flow) • bladder weakness
Other Uses	NATURAL INSECTICIDE

Key Properties:

ANTI-MICROBIAL	kills or limits the growth of bacteria, virus, fungus, and counteracts poisons
IMMUNO-STIMULANT	stimulates the body's defense system
EXPECTORANT	loosens and removes phlegm from the respiratory tract
ANTI-CATARRHAL	diminishes excessive mucous conditions
CLEANSING and ELIMINATION	cleanses blood, lymph, skin (through perspiration), digestion, increases urine output
HEART and CIRCULATION	reduces blood platelet adhesion, thins blood, lowers elevated blood pressure, improves circulation, protects blood vessels, lowers cholesterol, removes plaque
DIGESTIVE AID	improves appetite, relieves gas, promotes intestinal elimination, and expels parasites and worms
ANTIOXIDANT	protects blood vessels and other tissues from degradation and aging
TONIC	reduces muscular spasms, convulsions and cramps, and stimulates and nourishes nerves
Primarily affecting	IMMUNE SYSTEM • LUNGS • MUCOUS MEMBRANES • HEART • BLOOD • BLOOD VESSELS • NERVES

History	According to a 3,500-year-old Egyptian scroll, healers believed garlic could help a person fight cancer. Garlic was thought to be bestowed with sacred qualities and was placed in the tombs of pharaohs. It was given to slaves that built the pyramids to enhance their endurance and strength. This strength-enhancing quality was also honored by the ancient Greek and Roman civilizations, whose athletes and soldiers, respectively, ate garlic before sporting events and going off to war.
	The Roman naturalist Pliny the Elder (ca. 23-79 AD) declared, "Garlic has powerful properties and is of great benefit against changes of water and residence." He recommended it to treat asthma, suppress coughs, expel intestinal parasites, and as an antidote for snake bites and certain poisons.

Dioscorides (ca. 40-90 AD) was a surgeon and physician for the Roman army. He described garlic with regard to the Doctrine of Signatures (the belief that medicinal properties are revealed symbolically by the plant's outward appearance). Thus, a plant such as garlic, with a long hollow stalk, would be good for diseases of the windpipe. He also wrote of garlic's ability to "clear the arteries."

Garlic was first noted in Chinese literature in the *Collection of Commentaries on the Classic of the Materia Medica* (500 AD). It was traditionally used in China for fevers, colds, tuberculosis, dysentery, intestinal parasites, and had beneficial effects on circulation and the heart.

When the plagues ravaged Europe, it was discovered garlic was an effective preventive and treatment. The Black Death is estimated to have killed 30-60 percent of all Europeans in the 1400's, reducing the world's population from an estimated 450 million to between 350-375 million.

Garlic formed the principal ingredient in the 'Four Thieves' Vinegar', used successfully at Marseilles for protection against the plague when it prevailed there in 1722. It is said this formula originated with four thieves, who confessed that while taking the aromatic vinegar liberally, they were protected as they plundered the dead bodies of victims of the plague.

During an outbreak of infectious fever in certain poor quarters of London, the French priests (who constantly used garlic in their meals) visited the worst cases without harm, while the English clergy caught the infection and, in many instances, fell victim to the disease.

In an 1858 study, Louis Pasteur, the French microbiologist, demonstrated garlic's antiseptic activity. Albert Schweitzer (ca. 1875-1965) used the herb to treat amoebic dysentery in Africa. Garlic oil was so popular in Russian medicine, it was referred to as 'Russian penicillin.' Their hospitals and clinics have used volatile garlic extract treatments in the form of vapors and inhalants.

During World War I, garlic was used as an antiseptic for wound care. In 1916, the British government issued a general plea for the public to supply it with garlic in order to meet wartime needs.

Throughout the millennia, garlic has been a beloved plant in many cultures for both its culinary and medicinal properties. Over the last few years, it has gained popularity, as researchers have scientifically validated many of its numerous health benefits.

When I first discovered the virtues of garlic, I used it for everything. In the beginning, I didn't understand the importance of using fresh garlic. Needless to say, I fed my family the cheapest garlic oil capsules I could find. When my husband would come home from work, he would open the door to the stale smell of rancid garlic. He was not a fan! My five-year-old son would chew up the capsules straight. He called them 'footballs.' I am sure it did him some good but, fortunately, a short time later, I realized fresh garlic was infinitely more potent and effective.

The problem was how to get my family to eat it raw? Over time, I found some simple ways to get raw garlic into my family. One way was to give them a garlic shooter (see GARLIC preparations). You see, garlic is best when used fresh. Garlic shooters help get the garlic down without it being so hot or pungent to the taste.

I remember one time when I had a bunch of scouts and their leaders over for a cooking class. I introduced them to garlic shooters. They loved them! However, one of the leaders ate so many, his wife made him sleep on the couch that night. You can get away with one garlic shooter and still be okay in public, but more than that, you definitely smell of the stinking rose. The solution to this problem is simple: we all eat it together!

I can't talk with you about the virtues of garlic without mentioning garlic enemas (see GARLIC preparations). We have used this method when nothing else seemed to work. We used it for severe allergic reactions, appendicitis, severe strep infections, high fevers, and, yes we even saved a dog dying of parvo. I always tell my kids they need to take their herbs by mouth, or they will have to take them another way.

I for one am grateful for this incredible herb that has surely saved many lives. I highly recommend the book '*Garlic: Nature's Super Healer*' by Joan and Lydia Wilen. Every home library should have this great book on hand.

Attributes

Key Components: (including, but not limited to)

Nutrition

Vitamins A • Lutein (yellow carotenoid pigment) • B1 (thiamine) • B2 (riboflavin) • B3 (niacin) • B5 (pantothenic acid) • B6 (pyridoxine) • Folate • Choline • C • E • K • Organic Aluminum (needed by the brain and protects the body from inorganic aluminum) • Calcium • Chlorine • Copper • Germanium • Iron • Magnesium • Manganese • Phosphorus • Potassium • Selenium • Sodium • Sulfur • Zinc • Protein • Enzymes • Allicin • Allicetoin I and II • S Allylcysteine

Garlic has measurable amounts (more than any other herb) of germanium, a mineral which strengthens the immune system.

Allicin is a sulfur-containing amino acid formed when alliin comes into contact with the enzyme alliinase. This happens when a garlic clove is crushed, bruised, chopped, or heated.

Allicin is responsible for the strong, characteristic aroma of garlic. The odor lingers because the aromatic compounds are exhaled from the lungs (and sometimes excreted through the skin) throughout digestion. Chewing parsley, basil, mint, or thyme helps counteract the intense odor.

Garlic preparations in which allicin has been removed (as in the 'odorless' garlic preparations) lose most of the antimicrobial effects.

General

Garlic is warming to the digestive and respiratory tracts, has stimulating and rejuvenating effects on the body, helps to regulate menstrual flow, and is an important antibiotic, anti-viral, and antiseptic remedy for colds, flu, bronchitis, pneumonia, and other infections. Garlic is famous for killing and clearing intestinal parasites. Garlic's ability to protect the blood and cardiovascular system and its anti-cancer activity have been researched extensively. With regular use, the herb can help lower high blood pressure, reduce high cholesterol, and help prevent and reverse atherosclerosis.

Anti-Microbial

Raw garlic kills a wide variety of microorganisms by direct contact, including fungi, bacteria, viruses, and protozoa. It is excellent for wound healing and infectious diseases. The juice, oil, or powder may be used on open wounds for this purpose. It protects wounds from infection and stimulates cell growth. In India, garlic is used to wash wounds and ulcers.

In research studies, allicin has been shown to be effective against common infections like staphylococcus and E. coli bacteria colds, flu, stomach viruses, and Candida yeast. It also impedes powerful pathogenic microbes such as tuberculosis and botulism. Studies have found garlic to be a potent antibiotic, even against drug-resistant bacteria.

It stimulates the immune system, rejuvenates the spleen, and strengthens the body's defenses against allergens and infections.

One source reports a garlic necklace or small bag containing garlic may be worn around a child's neck to make body parasites disappear. Garlic is that powerful.

Respiratory Tract

Garlic nourishes and disinfects the lungs, loosens mucus, and is a superior expectorant. It is effective in treating asthma, bronchitis, and other respiratory conditions, and it has been used in cough remedies for centuries. The odor is so readily diffusible, when a fresh garlic preparation is applied to the soles of the feet, in seconds, it is exhaled by the lungs and detected on the breath.

Successful treatments of tubercular consumption by garlic have been recorded. The sufferer inhales the freshly expressed juice, diluted with an equal amount of water. Bruised and mixed with oil (like extra virgin olive oil), then rubbed on the chest and between the shoulder blades, it has relieved whooping cough.

Cleansing and Detoxification

Garlic has a powerful detoxifying effect on all the body systems and provides protection against pollutants and heavy metals. Garlic purifies the blood by promoting eliminative functions, thus cleansing, and efficiently removing waste products. It stimulates the lymphatic system to move waste materials and promotes perspiration, allowing for toxin elimination through the skin. Garlic increases the secretion and flow of urine, protects the liver, and promotes digestive evacuation.

Anti-inflammation

Garlic, like onion, contains compounds that inhibit enzymes that activate the inflammatory response, thus markedly reducing inflammation. These anti-inflammatory compounds protect against severe asthma attacks and help reduce the pain and inflammation of osteoarthritis and rheumatoid arthritis.

Digestion

Garlic improves the appetite, stimulates gastric secretions and bile flow (helping digest fats), increases the mobility of stomach walls, promotes peristalsis (contractions that propel contents onward) of the intestines, and relieves gas and painful distension. It destroys infectious bacteria without destroying the natural flora (beneficial bacteria) and rids the bowels of harmful parasites and worms.

Inserting one clove of garlic in the rectum can relieve the discomfort of hemorrhoids by helping to shrink hemorrhoid tissue.

Heart and Blood Vessels

Garlic helps to control disorders of the blood and strengthen the heart, blood vessels, and circulation in several interrelated ways. Extensive research with garlic in this area of health has shown allicin, Vitamin C, Vitamin B6, Vitamin E, selenium, and manganese all play an integral part in cardiovascular health.

Blood Thinner - Stickiness
Garlic contains an anticoagulant which normalizes blood platelet adhesion by reducing the 'stickiness' of the blood and its tendency to clot. This increases fluidity and thins the blood. Eating one garlic clove a day for several months will significantly thin the blood.

Relaxes and Enlarges Blood Vessels
Allicin activates sensory nerve endings which induce the relaxation and enlargement of blood vessels, lowering blood pressure, improving blood circulation, and reducing the formation of atherosclerotic plaque. Garlic is excellent for both high and low blood pressure, though it is especially useful in lowering hypertension.

Protects Blood Vessel Walls
Allicin inhibits coronary artery calcification laid down by the body in areas that have been damaged. In a year-long study, patients given daily, aged, garlic extract showed an average calcium level score of 7.5 percent compared to 22.2 percent in the placebo group.

Reduces Plaque Formation – by Lowering Cholesterol
Atherosclerotic plaque develops when blood cholesterol is damaged by oxidation. Garlic's antioxidant properties (with Vitamin C, Vitamin E, selenium, and allicin) limit the amount of free radicals in the bloodstream, protect blood vessels from the deleterious effects of free radical damage, and reduce the oxidative damage of serum low-density lipo-proteins (LDLs – 'bad

cholesterol'). Vitamin E defends the fat-soluble areas, and Vitamin C protects the water-soluble areas, from oxidation.

Clinical studies have shown garlic lowers total serum cholesterol by about 9-12 percent, principally by inhibiting cholesterol absorption from food. It lowers levels of LDL's in the blood and triglycerides, in comparison to high-density lipoproteins (HDL's – so called 'good cholesterol'). This shift helps the liver metabolize fat substances in the blood, rather than allow them to be deposited in tissues.

A German study indicates the allicin in garlic greatly reduces plaque deposition and size by up to 40 percent by preventing the formation of the initial complex that develops into an atherosclerotic plaque. It hinders the docking of LDL cholesterol to its receptor sites in blood vessels and existing plaques. Researchers suggest garlic can help prevent and potentially reverse atherosclerotic plaque formation.

Breaks Down Existing Plaque
Garlic has soft oils that help emulsify plaque, loosen it from arterial walls, and help dissolve calcifications such as uric acid crystals found in arteriosclerosis. In a double-blind, placebo-controlled study that followed 152 individuals for 4 years, standardized garlic powder at a dosage of 900 mg daily significantly slowed the development of atherosclerosis, as measured by ultrasound. They also showed less evidence of damaged arteries.

Purifies the Blood
Garlic purifies the blood and enhances a physiological process called fibrinolysis, which works to remove plaque and clots from blood vessels.

Heart Attack Reduction
Garlic oil given over a period of three years to 432 individuals who had suffered an initial heart attack resulted in a significant reduction of second heart attacks and an average 50 percent reduction in death rate among those taking garlic regularly.

Blood Sugar

Garlic lowers high blood-sugar levels and assists the body to normalize glucose tolerance in cases of both hypoglycemia and hyperglycemia (diabetes).

Studies have shown allicin in garlic combines with Vitamin B1 (thiamine) and, in the process, stimulates the pancreas to begin releasing insulin.

Rejuvenating Effects

Garlic is a stimulating tonic. It builds endurance, enhances energy, and strengthens all systems. As an antioxidant, the herb protects blood cell walls, nerves, and tissues of the body from degradation and aging.

Brain and Nervous System

Research in China has shown that S allylcysteine (a sulfur compound present in garlic), prevents degeneration of the frontal lobes of the brain.

Garlic nourishes the nerves and is a valuable nervine tonic and anti-spasmodic. An infusion of bruised cloves, given before and after every meal, has been effective in epilepsy. Garlic acts as an anti-stress agent. When sniffed into the nostrils, it will revive sensibility to someone suffering with hysteria. It is excellent for relieving nervous headaches.

Cancer

Substances found in garlic, such as allicin, germanium (an anti-cancer agent), selenium, and Vitamin C have been shown to protect colon cells from the toxic effects of cancer-causing chemicals and to stop the growth of cancer cells once they develop. Studies show garlic helps white blood cells in the body to protect and fight against cancer cells.

Researchers at Loma Linda University have found substances in garlic that activate enzymes in the liver which destroy alpha-toxins, a potent carcinogen. Alpha-toxins are claimed to be a leading cause of liver cancer.

In Russia, garlic was found to retard tumor growth. Several large studies strongly suggest a diet high in garlic can prevent cancer. 41,837 women were followed for four years. Results of the study showed women whose diets included significant quantities of garlic were approximately 30 percent less likely to develop colon cancer.

A large data set of case-control studies of Southern European populations were reported by Galeone C, Pelucchi C, et al, in the *American Journal of Clinical Nutrition*. When compared to those eating the least amount of garlic, study participants consuming the most garlic had a reduced risk for cancer of the oral cavity and pharynx of 39 percent; esophageal cancer, 57 percent;

	colorectal cancer, 26 percent; laryngeal cancer, 44 percent; breast cancer, 10 percent; ovarian cancer, 22 percent; prostate cancer, 19 percent; and renal cell cancer, 31 percent.
Insect Repellant	Garlic is an effective insect repellant, primarily due to its thiamine (Vitamin B1) content. It helps repel mosquitoes and relieves the discomfort of insect bites. Take garlic internally with liquid capsules of Vitamins B1 and B12 one hour before going outside and/or apply garlic oil to the skin. In the garden, garlic discourages insects that might prey on plants.
Herb Parts Used	The whole plant
Preparations and Remedies	Garlic is highly digestible and elements enter the bloodstream rapidly. Grated garlic placed near the most virulent bacteria will kill them in five minutes
Selection and Storage	Garlic is freshest in summer when the bulbs are firm and the cloves harder to peel. Soft, shriveled, moldy or sprouting garlic are all indications of decay that will cause a rancid flavor and inferior quality. Buy garlic that is plump, firm, compact, solid, and heavy for its size. The papery, outer skin should be taut and unbroken.
	Store fresh garlic in either an uncovered or a loosely covered container in a cool, dark place away from exposure to heat and sunlight. This will help maintain its maximum freshness and help prevent sprouting (which reduces its flavor and causes excess waste). It is not necessary to refrigerate garlic. Some people freeze peeled garlic, but it reduces its flavor and changes its texture.
	Depending upon its age and variety, whole garlic bulbs will keep fresh for two weeks to two months. Inspect the bulb frequently and remove any cloves that appear to be dried out or moldy.
	To store peeled cloves, place them in a jar and cover with olive oil. Close the jar and refrigerate for up to two weeks. The garlic flavored oil may be used for cooking.
Types of Preparations	*Raw Garlic and Fresh Juice:*
	Fresh garlic is thought to be the most effective form of garlic for antibiotic and antifungal activity. Garlic is nature's antibiotic. It can

heal almost any infection including the plague. Those who eat fresh garlic regularly rarely get sick.

Garlic Oil – There are two types of garlic oil:

- *Garlic Infused Oil:* Extra virgin olive oil infused with the healing properties of garlic cloves.

- *Garlic Essential Oil:* Isolated by distilling raw garlic. Essential oils are highly concentrated and may irritate unprotected skin. Garlic essential oil can be particularly harsh on unprotected skin. First, apply a carrier oil (like extra-virgin olive oil) on the skin or dilute the essential oil within a carrier oil.

Cooked Garlic:
When garlic is heated, enzymes are denatured and activity significantly reduced. Cooked garlic adds flavor to food but reduces its antibiotic properties.

Dehydrated Garlic Powders:
Prepared by dehydrating garlic cloves then grinding them into powder. A large portion of the allicin content is lost, losing some of the antibiotic and antifungal action of garlic (though not all of it). Dried garlic can still have therapeutic properties and benefits.

Aged Garlic Extract:
A cold-aging process where garlic is sliced, placed in an alcohol based extracting solution, and naturally cold-aged for up to twenty months without heat. Allicin decomposes, producing an odorless garlic that does not agitate the stomach of sensitive individuals and is readily digested. Many health benefits are retained, but it loses its antibiotic and antiviral activity.

Fresh Clove

When a sliced clove of garlic is rubbed over a cut, it will clean and sterilize the wound.

For rheumatism, take a clove or two of crushed garlic with honey two or three nights in a row.

Garlic may also be used as an arthritic rub with one part chopped garlic mixed with two parts camphor oil.

For hemorrhoids, insert a clove of garlic into the rectum before bed (be sure to first protect the skin with a layer of extra virgin olive oil).

Hold a piece of garlic on each side of the mouth (between the teeth and cheek) at the onset of a cold. Colds will disappear within a few hours or a day. This is also good for coughs and sore throats.

Take up to twelve or more raw cloves per day for acute cases such as pneumonia, strep throat, or other serious diseases. When taken internally, garlic effectiveness for lowering blood pressure is increased by adding cayenne.

Garlic Shooter:
from the Gilroy Garlic Festival Cookbook

Freshly squeezed juice of ½ Lemon (1-2 tablespoons)
1-2 tablespoons Water (optional)
1 clove Garlic, crushed

Put lemon juice and water into a cup. Add freshly crushed garlic clove. Immediately swirl cup to achieve a circling motion and drink in one gulp. The 'shooter' experience may be followed by an immediate feeling of rejuvenation called the 'shooter rush'.

Note:
Once the garlic is crushed, it should be used within ten minutes for best potency. Upon contact with the liquid, the garlic begins to 'heat'. If swallowed fast enough, the shooter can be taken without tasting garlic (it will still produce lung-healthy 'garlic breath' and great healing benefits).

Pickled Garlic:
There are lots of wonderful pickled garlic recipes out there, but most of them use heat in the cooking process. Heated garlic still has some of its medicinal properties, but they are greatly diminished.

One recipe my mom came up with was to take the leftover brine or juice from her favorite pickles and pour it over whole cloves and let it sit for two to four weeks. This gave it enough time for the brine to get into the clove, sweeten it up, and lessen the amount of heat of the straight, raw garlic. The best thing about it is that all the benefits of raw garlic are retained, plus it tastes great! When my mom opens a jar around my kids, it's gone in no time. They love it!

Decoction	*Mullein Decoction:* (see MULLEIN preparations)
Syrup	*Sore Throat and Coughs:* Take the freshly expressed garlic juice, mixed with honey, (optional: add a small amount of cayenne, to tolerance) for coughs and sore throats.
Tea	*Garlic Water (Tea):* Crush one to four cloves of garlic and put in a cup of hot water. Leave to steep (covered) overnight. In the morning, filter and discard the pulp and drink the garlic-infused water for colds, fevers, tuberculosis, and blood diseases. Use the tea as an enema for worms and bowel infections.
Infused Oil	*Garlic Oil:* Crush approximately 20 cloves of fresh garlic and put in a glass jar. Cover with 4 ounces extra-virgin olive oil and stir. Top with a lid. The oil may be used within 3 hours, however, for best potency, solar macerate (soak in liquid to soften and release constituents in the sun) for 2 weeks by shaking daily and putting the jar in the sun for a few hours each day over the first 3 days. Water and garlic juice will sink to the bottom of the jar. Separate carefully by pouring the oil off without retaining any of the watery pulp. The finished oil must not contain water droplets. Filter the infused oil through several layers of clean, dry cheesecloth. (Left-over pulp is great for garlic bread, soups, etc.) Properly label and store oil in tightly closed amber bottles in a cool, dark place. Store in the refrigerator for six months to a year in this manner. Throw away if mold begins to form. *On Food:* Use the oil on fresh salads. It may also be used for cooking, but it will lose most of its medicinal properties when heated. *Earaches:* Put two to three warmed drops (to body temperature) in the ear, one to three times daily. Keep the ear up for a few minutes to let the oil absorb. Use a clean cotton ball in the ear if needed. *Infections:* The oil may also be taken internally to kill infection. Take one teaspoon every hour in a little lemon juice or water for fevers, intestinal infections, mucus of the stomach, colds, and flu.

Take two teaspoons three to four times daily for chronic colitis or ulcerated stomach conditions.

Rashes, Aches, Sore Muscles:
For skin problems, rub the oil directly onto the skin. It is also good for aches, sprains, rheumatic pains, sore muscles, and chapped or chafed hands.

Acne:
Rub pimples several times daily with garlic oil. Eruptions will disappear without leaving a scar, but this does not remove the cause. Purify the skin by cleansing the blood and colon internally.

Athlete's Foot:
Wash infected areas in hot, soapy water. Rinse and dry well. Massage in the garlic oil two or three times daily. Continue to apply once a week to prevent recurrence.

Raw garlic may irritate or even burn skin if left on it for a length of time. To prevent this, rub extra-virgin olive oil on the skin prior to applying garlic preparations.

Poultices

Garlic Poultice:
Crush fresh garlic and add warm water and flour. Good for aches, pus, and infections. After covering the area with olive oil, use on the chest for chronic bronchitis. Apply a poultice of freshly grated garlic to ringworm.

Yeast Infection:
Blend one clove of garlic in one pint of water. Strain, and add one or more pints of water, and use as a douche.

Garlic Enema:
Blend 10 cloves garlic with one cup of hot water. Cool, strain, and use as an enema. Hold in as long as possible (usually a very short amount of time). Garlic kills germs and parasites, improves peristaltic action (intestinal contractions that propel bowel contents onward), and pulls mucus.

Optional:
Add catnip tea, chamomile, or organic coffee. These herbs help pull mucus, soothe colon cramping, and alleviate a lot of the burning sensation.

My family lovingly calls garlic enemas "the ring of fire." It is not comfortable but it is extremely effective. When nothing else works at our house, we use garlic enemas. This technique has never failed us.

Catnip and Garlic Enema: (see CATNIP preparations).

Insecticide

Garlic Spray for the Garden:
12-15 chopped Garlic cloves
2 tablespoons Mineral Oil
1/4 ounce Soap
9 cups Water
Soak chopped garlic in mineral oil for 24 hours. Dissolve soap in water and slowly add it to the garlic mixture. Strain mixture through fine gauze before storing in a glass container. When using, dilute 1 part garlic mixture to 50 parts water. Use garlic spray for aphids, mites and small caterpillars. It provides plants some fungicide protection.

Safety

Direct topical application of garlic may cause skin irritation and even blistering. It is recommended to put on a layer of extra virgin olive oil before applying garlic preparations directly to skin.

Garlic thins the blood. This should be taken into account prior to surgery and when taking blood thinning medications.
Garlic is on the Federal Drug Administration's (FDA's) generally regarded as safe (GRAS) list, including during pregnancy, lactation and childhood.

Common side effects include garlic breath and possible body odor. Initial stomach discomfort has also been reported. When garlic is not well-tolerated by the stomach, it is often due to having inflamed or ulcerated mucous membranes of the digestive tract. It is possible to ease discomfort by thoroughly chewing garlic or use garlic water as a substitute until the stomach is healed.

Plant Profile

Natural Habitat:
A native of central Asia, garlic is cultivated worldwide (although it does not flourish in cold climates).

Description

Garlic is a perennial herb (the plant grows back from a persistent rootstock in the spring) with a tall central stalk (2-3 feet) and long, narrow, flat, grass-like leaves that extend from the ground to the middle of the stem. The most utilized part of the plant is the segmented bulb, which breaks apart into 10-16 cloves. Mature bulbs are 2-3 inches in diameter. Garlic tastes somewhat like an onion but stronger, with its own distinctive flavor. Once the cloves are crushed or cut, the odor is intensely pungent.

In early summer, white to light purple flowers bloom in a cluster at the end of the plant's stalk, contained within a sheath. The sheath also contains the bulb. Small black seeds are later produced in wild garlic. Seeds do not mature in cultivated varieties (cloves are used to replant).

Growing Garlic

Planting:
Garlic grows well in sunny locations where the soil is rich, sandy, and kept relatively moist. Separate individual cloves from the bulb just prior to planting in October or early spring for harvesting the following summer. Space cloves (base side down, pointy side up) six to eight inches apart and one to two inches deep. For largest bulbs at harvest time, prune away flowering stems that shoot up in early summer and add compost in early spring to fertilize (avoid planting after heavy applications of fresh manure).

To minimize bulb diseases, do not over-water. Newly planted garlic needs moisture for its developing roots but does not do well in sodden conditions. If rain does not fall, water deeply once a week. Gradually reduce watering as the weather warms up in the spring. Garlic needs a hot, dry summer to mature the bulbs.

Harvesting and Storage

Dig bulbs after the tops have died down. Place in a single layer in a shaded spot to dry, then either cut away the tops (leaving about a two-inch stem) or plait the tops of the plants together. Hang plaits or loose bulbs in nets from the ceiling in a cool, dark place.

Ginger

Latin Name: *Zingiber officinale*

Also known as: African Ginger, Jamaica Ginger, Black Ginger

Scientific Classification

The ginger family is a tropical group, especially abundant in Indo-Malaysia, consisting of more than 1200 plant species in 53 genera. The genus zingiber includes about 85 species of aromatic herbs from East Asia and tropical Australia.

Family: Zingiberaceae – ginger family

Genus Zingiber – ginger

Species Z. officinale – garden ginger

Ginger is cultivated in great quantities in Jamaica. Though it is the least pungent and most delicate of the gingers, it is still very useful in medicinal applications. The root from the West Indies is considered to be the best. Ginger is also imported from Africa.

There are several varieties known in commerce. Jamaican and the White African have short rhizomes (underground roots) with a light-brown color and a very pungent taste. Cochin have short rhizomes that are a red-gray color. Green ginger is just the immature, undried rhizomes.

Influence on the Body	(PRINCIPAL ACTIONS are listed in CAPITAL LETTERS)
Blood and Circulation	POOR CIRCULATION • hemorrhage
Body System	TONIC (increases energy and strength throughout the body) • ENERGY • FATIGUE • endurance
Digestive Tract	APERITIVE (improves the appetite) • AROMATIC (has a spicy taste and volatile elements which aid digestion and relieve gas) • sialagogue (promotes an increase flow of saliva) • HEARTBURN • DIGESTIVE DISORDERS • DYSPEPSIA (discomfort after eating) • STOMACHIC (strengthens stomach function) • INDIGESTION • helps prevent MOTION SICKNESS • NAUSEA • settles the STOMACH • antacid • VOMITING • COLIC • GAS • CRAMPS • cholagogue (promotes the flow of bile) • colon spasms • antispasmodic • bowels • COLITIS • constipation • DIARRHEA

Infections and Immune System	COLDS • COUGHS • FEVERS • FLU • influenza • CHILDHOOD DISEASES • chicken pox • mumps • WHOOPING COUGH • cholera
Inflammation	osteoarthritis • gout
Lungs and Respiratory System	CHRONIC BRONCHITIS • pneumonia • lung hemorrhage
Mouth, Nose and Throat	sinus congestion • sinusitis • TOOTHACHE • SORE THROAT • tongue paralysis
Muscles	positively inotropic (increases the strength of muscular contractions)
Nervous System	nervine (improves nerve function) • neuralgia (nerve pain) • HEADACHE • DIZZINESS • shock • LEARNING PROBLEMS • analgesic (relieves pain) • anodyne (relieves pain and reduces nerve excitability)
Reproductive System	pelvic circulation *Female:* MORNING SICKNESS • menstrual cramps • emmenagogue (promotes menstrual flow) • vagina
Skin, Tissues and Hair	boils • RUBEFACIENT (increases blood flow to the skin causing local reddening) • DIAPHORETIC (promotes perspiration when taken hot, increasing elimination through the skin)
Urinary Tract	kidneys • diuretic (increases urine flow)

Key Properties:

ANTIEMETIC	*settles stomach, helps prevent vomiting*
DIGESTIVE AID	*spicy elements stimulate digestive juices and bile flow, settle stomach, relieve griping*
CARMINATIVE	*brings warmth and circulation, relieves intestinal gas discomfort, and promotes peristalsis*
ENHANCES ELIMINATION	*promotes PERSPIRATION (when taken hot), advances digestion, increases urine output*
STIMULANT	*increases internal heat, dispels internal chill, and strengthens metabolism and circulation*
Nervine **anti-inflammatory** **anti-catarrhal**	*eliminates mucous conditions*

GINGER — 177

CATALYST HERB — *enhances effectiveness and improves circulation of other herb combinations*

Primarily affecting STOMACH • INTESTINES • CIRCULATION • NERVES • JOINTS • MUSCLES

History	The English botanist William Roscoe (1753-1831) gave ginger the binomial Latin name 'Zingiber officinale' in an 1807 publication. In Latin, zingiber means 'horn-shaped', referring to the shape of the herb's rhizomes.
	Ginger has been cultivated for so long, its exact origin is unclear. China and India have raised it for millennia, and it reached the West at least two thousand years ago. Chinese medical texts from the 4th century BC mention ginger as being used in treating nausea, vomiting, diarrhea, stomachache, cholera, toothache, bleeding, and rheumatism.
	Chinese herbalists later used ginger to treat a variety of respiratory conditions, including coughs and the early stages of colds. Most of the thousands of prescriptions in Traditional Chinese Medicine are combinations of many herbs, and ginger is used in nearly half of them to mediate the effects of other ingredients, stimulate the appetite, and calm the stomach.
	In traditional Chinese and Indian medicines, fresh and dried ginger are considered to be two different medicines.
	In general, fresh ginger is used for its warming qualities to promote sweating and stimulate circulation in the spleen, stomach (alleviating vomiting), and lungs (to stop coughs).
	Dried ginger is used for 'cold' pains of the pelvic region, rheumatism, poor appetite, vomiting, diarrhea, listlessness, chills, and a weak pulse.
	Arabic and Indian Ayurvedic (traditional) medicines also used ginger to treat inflammatory joint diseases like rheumatism and arthritis. Arabian traders carried ginger root from China and India to be used as a food spice in ancient Greece and Rome.
	More than 4,000 years ago, the Greeks wrapped ginger in bread and ate it after meals as a digestive aid. Ginger was quite common in ancient Rome, where it was used medicinally to alleviate eye problems (including cataracts) and as a way to prevent or eliminate parasites.

In fact, ginger was so popular, the government started to tax it, which made it much more expensive. Records show ginger as a subject of Roman tax in the 2nd century, after being imported via the Red Sea from Alexandria, Egypt.

Ginger was known in England before the Norman Conquest (begun in 1066), and it is commonly found in the 11th century Anglo-Saxon leech books. Tariff duties appear in the records of Marseilles in 1228 and Paris by 1296.

Ginger was expensive in many parts of the world. In England, one pound of ginger cost nearly the price of a sheep. During that time, ginger was prescribed to promote perspiration, warm the stomach, improve circulation to the extremities (hands and feet), and treat colds, flu, and bronchitis.

Spaniards introduced the Americas to ginger in the early 1600's. The herb impacted Europe and the Americas, where it established itself as a helpful medicinal herb and became popular as a soothing drink for stomach ailments (ginger ale, ginger beer, and ginger tea).

Originally, ginger was widely used in its powdered, dried, crystallized, or preserved forms, which could be purchased from other countries, but as Asian, Indian, and Middle Eastern cuisine spread throughout the world, fresh and cultivated ginger became increasingly available. It can now be purchased year-round.

In the early 1980's, Scientist D. Mowrey noticed ginger-filled capsules reduced his nausea during an episode of the flu. He then performed the first double-blind study on ginger. Germany's Commission E subsequently approved ginger as a treatment for indigestion and motion sickness. Ginger has continued to be studied for its varied medicinal uses.

Attributes	
Nutrition	**Key Components: (including, but not limited to)** Vitamins A • B1 (thiamine) • B2 (riboflavin) • B3 (niacin) • B5 (pantothenic acid) • B6 (pyridoxine) • B9 (folic acid) • B12 (cobalamin) • Biotin • Choline • Inositol • PABA (Para-Amino Benzoic Acid) • C • Calcium • Iron • Magnesium • Phosphorus • Potassium • Sodium • Zinc • Sugars • Dietary Fiber • Fat

• Protein • Gingerols • Shogaols • Zingerones • Zingibain (counteracts inflammation)

Gingerols are responsible for the pungent spiciness of ginger. When ginger is dried and stored, gingerol rapidly converts to zingerones and shogaols. Shogaols are twice as pungent as its parent compounds, making properly dried ginger much 'hotter' than fresh ginger. Chemically, gingerol is similar to capsaicin (found in cayenne peppers).

Digestion and Nausea

Gingerol and its derivatives stimulate the flow of saliva, bile, and gastric secretions, settle stomach upsets, and encourage gentle muscle contractions that move food through digestion. They are also responsible for ginger's anti-nausea effects. They have abilities to curb diarrhea and inhibit violent muscle spasms in the digestive tract.

Ginger has been found in multiple studies to be effective in the treatment of morning sickness during pregnancy, motion sickness, seasickness, and nausea from anesthesia and chemotherapy (studies suggest ginger reduces the severity and duration of nausea during chemotherapy, but not the vomiting).

A Denmark study concluded ginger can significantly reduce the nausea and vomiting often associated with pregnancy. In another study of 80 novice sailors (prone to motion sickness), when compared to subjects taking a placebo, those who took powdered ginger experienced less vomiting and cold sweating.

Ginger has the ability to mildly stimulate and strengthen the stomach and intestines, and it has been used as a natural treatment for colds, stomach flu, and food poisoning.

Ginger is spicy, yet it is kind to the digestive system. The volatile oils that are so pungent stimulate digestive juices and bile secretions. Ginger is able to absorb and neutralize toxins and stomach acid. It tones the bowels, helps prevent griping and cramping, and soothes the stomach and spleen.

Ginger has long been used for treating dyspepsia, including relief from heartburn, bloating, flatulence (gas), and nausea.

Blood Vessels

Ginger is a blood-vascular stimulant that improves blood circulation and warms the body, starting with capillaries in the extremities (hands and feet).

Gingerol (an active ingredient in ginger) has proven to be effective in preventing recurrences of 'mini strokes.' It is believed gingerol inhibits an enzyme that causes blood cells to clot. Danish researchers at Odense University found ginger's blood thinning effects to be more effective than those found in garlic or onion.

Studies indicate ginger reduces cholesterol absorption in the blood and liver. Research conducted at Cornell University Medical College concluded ginger may help prevent strokes and hardening of the arteries.

Cleansing

When fresh ginger is taken in a warm infusion, it acts as a diaphoretic. Sweating provides an outlet for toxins, cools the body, and reduces fevers. Ginger is a kidney stimulant that increases kidney filtration and urine output (especially when taken as a hot infusion), cleansing the kidneys and bowels.

Lungs

Ginger is an excellent herb to use for strengthening and healing the respiratory system, helping remove phlegm and fight off colds and flu. It lowers congestion in the sinus cavities (especially when combined with cayenne), relieves headaches and body aches, and soothes sore throats and coughs. It is often used in gargle preparations and cough syrups. In China, ginger is often used in the first stages of the common cold.

Body System

Ginger is a warming stimulant to the body. It can raise body temperature when taken frequently.

Ginger is also an alkalizer, which is very healthy for the body. Pollution, the common American diet, and lifestyle often raise the acidic level in the body. This makes the body more susceptible to illness and disease. Ginger helps neutralize acidic buildup in the body.

Nervous System

Research shows ginger may provide migraine relief by its ability to stop prostaglandins (which are known to cause pain and inflammation in blood vessels) without the side effects found in most headache medications.

One study suggests ginger may protect nerve cells in the brain against Alzheimer's disease.

Ginger works well as a catalyst in nervine and sedative herbal formulas. Ginger is helpful in cases of learning disabilities and problems.

Anti-inflammation	The active compound zingibain (an enzyme found in ginger) counteracts inflammation. Ginger extract has long been used for osteoarthritic pain and inflammation. Ginger heats the joints and exhibits pain relieving and anti-inflammatory properties. In a study of 261 people with osteoarthritis of the knee, those who received a ginger extract twice daily reported less pain and required fewer pain-killing medications than those who received a placebo.
Women	When taken hot, ginger helps arrest excessive menstrual flow and eases menstrual cramping. A hot ginger tea is also good in conditions of suppressed menstruation and scanty urine. The most effective and concentrated way to take ginger for morning sickness is in capsules. Ginger is packed with minerals and is very healthy for both mother and baby.
Antiseptic	Ginger exhibits antiseptic action that may be used to reduce fevers and recovery time of those suffering with a cold or flu.
Catalyst Herb	Ginger is often used in herb formulas that affect the lower abdominal and colon areas. Because of its abilities to stimulate and improve circulation, ginger enhances the effectiveness of other herb combinations and is considered to be a catalyst herb (an herb that helps other herbs work better in the body).
Herb Parts Used	Fresh or dried root
Preparations and Remedies	Ginger root is used fresh, pickled, candied, dried, or powdered, and is included in many herbal preparations. Fresh, dried, and preserved gingers all taste different. They have hints of each other but are unique in taste and in qualities.
Types of Preparations	*Fresh Ginger and Juice*: Unless it is very fresh, ginger is usually peeled before being grated or sliced. Ginger is at its best when it is young, juicy, has a tender skin, and a sweet, peppery flavor. As the root matures and becomes larger, the flavor strengthens and the flesh becomes more fibrous, grainy, pithy, and woody, but it is still very effective in healing at this stage. As a food, ginger helps digest proteins in meat dishes, and is a common ingredient in Asian cuisine. When using dried ginger in

cooking, bruise it well before grinding or grating to release the full flavor. Ginger becomes hotter as it is cooked. Ground ginger loses its aromatic principles quickly, so it is always best to use freshly ground ginger whenever possible.

Preserved and Crystallized:
Pieces of ginger are boiled in sugar syrup to preserve them. Crystallized ginger results when it is finally removed from the syrup. Use this ginger in baking and drizzle the syrup on ice cream or fruit.

Pickled:
Thin slices of young ginger may be pickled and was, at one time, dyed pink and eaten as a palate cleanser between pieces of sushi. The color of ginger in sushi changed back to natural when that particular dye became illegal in the United States just a short time ago.

Essential Oil:
Ginger's essential oil is isolated by a distillation process. Essential oils are highly concentrated and may irritate unprotected skin. First apply a carrier oil (like extra virgin olive oil) to the skin or dilute the essential oil within a carrier oil before applying.

Ground (powdered):
As a food, powdered ginger is mainly used in baked goods such as gingerbread, ginger cake and ginger snap cookies. As an herb, powdered ginger is used in many preparations and herb formulas.

Fresh or dried ginger has been chewed for paralysis of the throat and tongue, and for lung hemorrhage.

Herbal Preparations

Powdered

Slippery Elm Gruel: (see SLIPPERY ELM preparations)

For morning sickness take ginger capsules first thing in the morning when getting out of bed, then every couple of hours for severe nausea. The idea is to take the capsules before even feeling the nausea. Ginger is more effective when taken with this in mind. Take as many as needed. The nutrients in ginger are healthy for mother and baby.

Infusions

Ginger Tea:

Put 5 or 6 thin slices of fresh ginger root for every cup of hot water, or put a teaspoonful of the dried and powdered root in a pint of hot water. Cover and let steep for 30 minutes.

Tea stimulates elimination and can be used for internal warmth. It is excellent for digestion, chills, nausea and menstrual cramps. Dilute for babies and young children.

Strong Ginger Tea:
Simmer several slices of the fresh root or one teaspoon of the cut and sifted dried herb for every cup of water.

Tea for Difficult Menstrual Period:
Make a warm infusion of equal parts squaw vine, red raspberry leaves, blessed thistle and ginger. Use one teaspoonful of the combined herbs for each cup of water. Take one cup three times a day for difficult menstrual periods.

Alkaline Formula Tea: (see DANDELION preparations)
Urinary Tract Infections Tea: (see UVA URSI preparations)
Kidney/Lower Back Tea: (see UVA URSI preparations)
Pregnancy Decoction: (see WILD YAM preparations)

Syrup

Ginger Cough Syrup:
1/4 teaspoon Cayenne
1/4 teaspoon Ginger
2 tablespoon Honey
2 tablespoon Raw Apple Cider Vinegar or fresh squeezed Lemon juice
Use as needed. It is great for coughs and relieving congestion. Add a tablespoon or two of hot water for a soothing effect.

Slippery Elm Cough Syrup:
    (see SLIPPERY ELM preparations)

Foot Bath

Simmer a half pound or more of freshly grated ginger in one quart of hot water; then dilute as needed, to fill the foot bath container. Soak feet in water and keep water hot. Use for colds, flus, fevers, chills, poor circulation, and headaches.

Bath

Ginger Bath:
Simmer a piece of fresh ginger root in a pan of water. Heat until water turns yellow. Strain and add to bath water.

Alternative method:

Add a half cup of ground ginger powder with a half cup of Himalayan Salt or Real Salt to a very warm bath.

A ginger bath is very soothing. It helps relax and relieve tired, achy muscles after over-exercising. By opening pores and promoting perspiration, ginger relieves congestion and fevers, and rids the body of wastes and toxins. It can also be used for the

burn and itch of rashes and dermatitis. If using the ginger bath for cleansing, rinse in a tepid-water shower afterwards. Cleansing baths may be used two or three times a week while on a cleansing diet.

Fomentations

Ginger Fomentation:
Grate 5 ounces of fresh ginger root and simmer in 2 quarts distilled water for 10 minutes. Use as a fomentation (towel soaked in infusion or decoction and placed on affected area) and cover with a heavy towel to keep in the heat. Repeat procedure when fomentation cools. Fomentations may be left on for 1 or 2 hours if necessary.

Use for painful joints, arthritis, gout, menstrual cramps, strains, sprains and sore backs.

A cool ginger tea fomentation is effective for easing the pain of minor burns and rashes.

A ginger fomentation of alternating hot and cold packs can relieve the pain of excess gas and stimulate the kidneys. Alternate back and forth as needed, for 30-60 minutes.

Soothing Fomentation: (see LOBELIA preparations)

Oil

Ginger Oil:
Mix ginger juice with extra virgin olive oil or sesame oil and massage it into the skin. This oil may also be applied to the scalp as a remedy for dandruff or put on a cotton ball and inserted into the external ear canal to help an earache.

Essential Oil

The essential oil of ginger is useful against colds, coughs, sore throats, arthritis, and has even been used as an aphrodisiac. Use a few drops to inhale or put in a carrier oil and apply where needed. Combine ginger essential oil within a carrier oil to the bottoms of the feet for distribution throughout the body.

Safety	Ginger is beneficial during pregnancy. It is an excellent remedy for morning sickness and has lots of minerals for mother and baby.
	Ginger is on the Federal Drug Administration's GRAS (generally recognized as safe) list as a food.
	Ginger has anti-coagulation and blood thinning qualities that should be considered when taking blood thinning medications. British research indicates that ginger is unlikely to cause adverse effects when taken before or after surgery.
Plant Profile	*Natural Habitat:* Ginger is indigenous to Southeast Asia, and is cultivated in the United States, India, China, West Indies and tropical regions. It is a native of tropical lowland rain forests.
Description	Ginger is a creeping perennial (after dying back in the winter, plant grows back in the spring from a persistent rootstock) with a thick tuberous rhizome (underground root). The odor and taste of ginger are characteristic, aromatic and pungent. In the spring, the root sends up a green reed, like a stalk (2-5 feet high), with narrow grass-like leaves (8-12 inches long and almost an inch wide).
	Ginger rarely flowers under cultivation. In the wild, it produces dense cone-like spikes on a stalk, from which a white, yellow-green or purple flower grows in the summer. The rhizome is a knobby, beige-colored root.
Growing Ginger	*Planting:* Plants may be started from a section of fresh root ginger purchased from a fruit market. Cut the rhizome in sections about three inches long, ensuring that each has a pointed growth bud. Allow the cut ends to dry for a few days before planting horizontally three to four inches below the surface. Water thoroughly. In tropical areas, ginger is best planted in the fall. In other areas, mid spring is better. Fertilize. Don't plant too closely together (especially in the tropics), as ginger is a spreading plant that needs space.
	For cooler climates, grow ginger in pots placed outdoors during the warm season. Plant rhizomes in a mix containing peat, sand, and compost. Keep the plant indoors or in a greenhouse during the winter, moving the pots outdoors in warm summers. For

healthy growth, keep the soil moist during the hot summer months.

Harvesting

Dig the plant up after a year's growth (in January or February), when the stems have withered. Remove the leaf stems, cutting away as much root as you need and replant the remaining root.

Storage

Clean carefully to avoid bruising. Refrigerate the harvested roots in tightly wrapped paper towels inside a plastic bag, for up to one month. Dry, shaved bits of the root may be stored in airtight containers in the refrigerator. Ginger is not suitable for freezing.

Goldenseal

Latin Name: *Hydrastis canadensis*

Also known as: Yellow Root, Yellow Puccoon, Orange Root, Ground Raspberry, Wild Curcuma, Turmeric Root, Indian Dye, Eye Root, Eye Balm, Indian Paint, Jaundice Root, Warnera, Indian Plant, Golden Thread, Seal-all, Brown Raspberry, Hydrastis

Note: Herbalists use the spelling Goldenseal and Golden Seal interchangeably

Scientific Classification

Family: Ranunculaceae – buttercup family
Genus Hydrastis – hydrastis
Species H. canadensis – goldenseal

Influence on the Body	(PRINCIPAL ACTIONS are listed in CAPITAL LETTERS)
Addictions	chronic alcoholism
Blood and Circulatory System	CIRCULATION • heart trouble • BLEEDING • INTERNAL HEMORRHAGE
Blood Sugar	INSULIN • DIABETES
Body System	MUCOUS MEMBRANES • ANTI-CATARRHAL (eliminates mucous conditions) • general cleanser • depurative (cleanses body by promoting eliminative functions) • astringent (increases tone and firmness of the tissues and diminishes mucous discharge from the nose, intestines, vagina, and draining sores) • swelling
Digestive Tract	bitter (stimulates digestive juices and improves appetite) • aperitive (improves the appetite) • dyspepsia (indigestion) • digestive disorders • antacid • nausea • stomach problems • gastritis (inflammation of the lining of the stomach) • enteritis (inflammation of the intestinal tract) • bowel problems • INTESTINES • constipation • COLITIS • COLON INFLAMMATION • DIARRHEA • laxative • vermifuge (expels or repels intestinal worms) • HEMORRHOIDS
Ears	Earaches
Endocrine System	swollen glands • PANCREAS • low thyroid
Eyes	EYE INFECTIONS • EYE WASH • conjunctivitis

GOLDENSEAL — 188

Infections and Immune System	allergies • hay fever • ANTIBIOTIC • ANTISEPTIC • FUNGAL INFECTIONS • ringworm (fungal disease) • INFECTIONS • COLDS • COUGHS • fever • stomach flu • CONTAGIOUS DISEASES • MEASLES • CHOLERA • TYPHOID FEVER • chicken pox • diphtheria • scarlet fever • smallpox • malaria • anti-periodic (prevents regular recurrence of symptoms or disease) • immuno-stimulant • lymph glands • spleen
Inflammation	INFLAMMATION
Liver	LIVER PROBLEMS • liver • hepatitis • gallbladder • cholagogue (promotes the flow of bile)
Lungs and Respiratory System	respiratory • asthma • BRONCHITIS
Mouth, Nose, and Throat	GUM DISEASES • PYORRHEA (gum disease) • MOUTH SORES • CANKERS • TOOTH EXTRACTION infection • breath freshener • hoarseness • NASAL PASSAGES • NOSEBLEEDS • SINUS CONGESTION • SINUSITIS • SORE THROAT • tonsillitis
Muscles	antispasmodic (relaxes muscle spasms and cramps)
Nervous System	nervous disorders • nerves • spinal nerves • spinal meningitis
Reproductive System	genital herpes • venereal disease • GONORRHEA • syphilis *Male:* PROSTATE GLAND *Female:* regulates excessive MENSTRUATION • EMMENAGOGUE (promotes menstrual flow) • VAGINITIS • DOUCHE • uterus • morning sickness
Skin, Tissues, and Hair	acne • boils • carbuncle • SKIN DISORDERS • skin ulceration • erysipelas (streptococcal infection of the skin) • seborrhea (skin disease) • eczema • psoriasis • rash • lupus erythematosus (skin disease typically having facial 'butterfly' rash) • itching • SKIN CANCER • poison ivy • poison oak • WOUNDS • burns
Urinary Tract	KIDNEYS • kidney disease • KIDNEY INFECTION • water retention • diuretic (increases urine flow) • urethritis • BLADDER INFECTIONS • BLADDER PROBLEMS
Weight	obesity • weight loss

Key Properties:

MUCOUS MEMBRANE ALTERATIVE
cleanses mucous membranes and stimulates efficient removal of wastes

ANTIBIOTIC, ANTISEPTIC, AND ANTIFUNGAL DIGESTIVE AID
improves appetite, induces the flow of digestive juices and bile, reduces nausea and the urge to vomit, cleanses and eliminates the congestion of mucous waste, intestinal parasites and worms

TONIC
increases energy, strengthens the muscular and nervous system, and improves digestion and assimilation, resulting in a general sense of well-being

Primarily affecting
MUCOUS MEMBRANES • LIVER • EYES • IMMUNE SYSTEM • STOMACH • INTESTINES

History

The American Thomsonian herbalists gave goldenseal its present common name, referring to the color of the root and its seal-like scars. Its Latin name 'Hydrastis' comes from two Greek words, one signifying 'water' and the other 'to accomplish', possibly given for goldenseal's effect on the mucous membranes.

Goldenseal grows primarily in the eastern parts of North America. It is found most plentifully in the woods of Ohio, where the Native American Cherokee introduced goldenseal as a cure for cancer and as a treatment for ulcers and arrow wounds. The Iroquois used goldenseal for liver disorders, fever, sour stomach, and diarrhea.

Native Americans also used goldenseal as a yellow dye. The juice was used to stain skin and clothing. It was also mixed with indigo to produce green-colored dyes.

Pioneers followed the Native American's example in using goldenseal to treat watering eyes, wounds, and rashes. They also chewed it to relieve mouth sores.

Goldenseal was on the endangered species list in the year 2000, largely due to over-harvesting practices, insufficient cultivation, and the commercial farming of other food crops encroaching on natural habitats. Wild-harvest collection became increasingly difficult and high priced. Start-up goldenseal cultivation projects were initiated in the 1990's to increase availability. This was a very successful project. Now, cultivated goldenseal is readily available, and the price has started to come down a little.

My Mom used to mix goldenseal root in a little water and make us drink it. If we complained about it, she would mix in a spoonful of honey to make it taste better. It didn't! To this day, the smell of goldenseal root makes my cheeks tighten up and my saliva glands run.

I have found very few herbs that match the infection-fighting power of goldenseal root. When it was put on the endangered list, many people, including myself, looked for alternatives (without much success, I might add). I feel we should continue to use this amazing herb in cultivated form from farmers. We are not only supporting family farms: but we also will not further deplete goldenseal from the wild. If we don't support the goldenseal farmers, they will grow something else, people will go back to wildcrafting, and we might lose this great herb.

My favorite way to take goldenseal root is in a tincture made with echinacea angustifolia root, yarrow, and a little stevia or licorice (for blood sugar balance). See formula below. The tincture assimilates quickly into the bloodstream and is tolerated by most, including children. It also can be used topically with great success. This is a formula everyone should have in their cupboards. It lasts a long time without refrigeration.

Attributes	
Nutrition	**Key Components: (including, but not limited to)** Vitamins A • B1 (thiamine) • B2 (riboflavin) • B3 (niacin) • B5 (pantothenic acid) • B6 (pyridoxine) • B9 (folic acid) • B12 (cobalamin) • Biotin • Choline • Inositol • PABA (Para-Amino Benzoic Acid) • C • E • Calcium • Copper • Iron • Manganese • Phosphorus • Potassium • Zinc Starches • Alkaloids including: Berberine (yellow) • Hydrastine (white) • Canadine • Bitter Berberine is antibacterial, antifungal, antiprotozoa, antimalarial, and antipyretic (reduces fever); it also has antispasmodic qualities. Hydrastine acts as a uterine hemostatic (stops bleeding) and antiseptic. Canadine acts as a sedative and muscle relaxant.
Catarrh	Mucous membranes are naturally moist internal surfaces that ease movement and absorption and are a protection for the body against pathogens and toxins. Mucus is a thick, sticky fluid secreted by mucous membranes and glands. It can trap intruding toxins and eliminate them from the body. Inflamed mucous

membranes and thickened, discolored, or excessive mucous congestion (beyond what the body can efficiently expel) are conditions known as 'catarrh.'

Catarrh can be problematic throughout the body. It is typically seen in the eyes, nose, sinuses, throat, bronchi, lungs, digestive tract, and urogenital organs. Catarrh can cause sore throats, colds, flu, pneumonia, fevers, swollen glands, and congestion in all the eliminative systems of the body. The problem contributes to such diseases as arthritis, asthma, hay fever, bronchitis, sinusitis, cystitis, vaginal infections, kidney stones, jaundice, etc. If catarrh collects in the bloodstream and obstructs circulation, it can cause high blood pressure and stroke.

Along with pathogenic parasites, catarrh may be caused by eating processed foods, eating starches in excess, poor circulation, poor elimination, and lack of sunshine, fresh air, or exercise. Along with proper diet, exercise, fresh air, and herbs can help rid the body of congestive catarrhal conditions.

Anti-catarrhal Mucous Membranes

Goldenseal is an anti-catarrhal herb that affects the mucous membranes throughout the body. Mucous membranes line internal structures of the body, including the respiratory system, digestive system, reproductive organs, urethra, etc.

Goldenseal is referred to as the 'King of the Mucous Membranes', because of its remarkable ability to heal, cleanse, and tone the mucous membranes of the body.

It can be used at the onset of upper respiratory infections. Some believe it is better employed once redness, swelling of the membranes, or excessive discharge of thick yellow or green mucus begins to occur. We have seen amazing success with both methods. Goldenseal helps both in cases of dry, parched mucous membranes and those with profuse thickened discharge.

Take as needed internally *and* topically as a fomentation (towel soaked in infusion or decoction and placed on affected area), gargle, ear drops, and nasal or eye wash.

Goldenseal is excellent as an antiseptic mouthwash for pyorrhea or as a drink and gargle for tonsillitis and other throat problems. For nasal catarrh, goldenseal root may be snuffed up the nose, or drops of goldenseal extract may be put in the nose for sinus infections. It is especially indicated when mucous discharge is abundant or during an asthma attack.

Goldenseal is useful in superficial disorders of the eyes, and conjunctival inflammations, particularly when a catarrhal discharge is present. Used as an eyewash, goldenseal is mildly antibiotic and astringent. It is used to strengthen the eyes and reduce eye inflammation and infection.

Goldenseal may be used for all types of congestion and chronic inflammation of the respiratory and urogenital tracts. It is used for catarrh of the bladder and induces the flow of urine to speed pathogenic elimination. Ulceration of the internal coat of the bladder and other indolent (non-healing) ulcers may be repaired with the use of goldenseal. A full-strength infusion makes a healing vaginal douche for infections.

The liver may become congested, as the body eliminates overabundant mucus and irritants. Goldenseal can help to soothe, support, and heal hepatic (liver) congestion.

Use goldenseal in cases of catarrh of the intestines. When it is used with the herb cascara sagrada, goldenseal is an effective bowel tonic. Myrrh and goldenseal together are used to help treat ulcers of the stomach. Goldenseal will help reduce swollen hemorrhoids when used as a retention enema.

Goldenseal promotes respiratory function by increasing lung capacity, cleansing mucous membranes, and fighting infection. It stimulates the respiratory and circulatory systems, increasing their tone and power.

Goldenseal is helpful for general debility and convalescence from diseases with excessive mucous discharges, protracted fevers, inflammation, nervous prostration, or where hemorrhaging has occurred.

Heart and Circulation

Goldenseal taken with cayenne helps strengthen the heart. The tone imparted to the heart muscle is permanent (rather than intermittent), and muscular nutrition is increased. Goldenseal is one of the few herbs that tones and sustains venous circulation.

Muscles

Goldenseal reduces muscular tenderness and soreness. It relaxes muscles, is antispasmodic, and relieves tension headaches.

Blood Sugar	Goldenseal is a source of natural insulin and lowers blood sugar. It is useful in treating stress and anxiety due to high blood sugar. It also reduces swelling caused by high sugar levels.
	Note: Individuals with low blood-sugar disorders could either take goldenseal with real licorice (counteracts goldenseal's low blood sugar effect), or substitute myrrh for goldenseal.
Women	Goldenseal can be used for female problems related to inflammation of the vagina, uterus, and the urethra. It normalizes profuse menstruation. Goldenseal may cause uterine contractions; therefore, ***it should not be used until the last few weeks of pregnancy.***
	Goldenseal was listed in the 1934 British Pharmaceutical Codex as being useful in controlling uterine hemorrhage. Midwives use goldenseal to stop hemorrhaging after birth and to induce uterine contractions to return the uterus to its normal size.
Skin Breaks and Wounds	Goldenseal heals fissures and cracks in the skin, including those occurring on the breasts when nursing. Sprinkle goldenseal powder directly on any break in the skin, or make a paste by mixing with water or extra-virgin olive oil to apply to the affected area.
	Goldenseal is an antiseptic used to cleanse boils, wounds, and ulcers. When the powder is applied topically, it helps prevent pitting of the skin from smallpox and heals ringworm without leaving a scar.
	Goldenseal helps stop internal and external bleeding, reduces swelling, and speeds wound healing. Skin diseases, rashes, and eruptions all benefit from goldenseal.
	Acne, seborrhea, lupus erythematosus, boils, carbuncles, and ulcers can be helped by the internal use alone, but topical use, at the same time, hastens healing.
Immune System	Berberine (an active ingredient in goldenseal) strengthens the immune system and has antimicrobial activity. Goldenseal activates macrophages (white blood cells that ingest pathogens and foreign material in the blood) and increases the blood supply to the spleen (produces white blood cells). Goldenseal shows tumor-inhibitory action and has also been used for skin cancers.

Digestion	Goldenseal is bitter to the taste and induces secretions of the salivary glands. It sharpens the appetite and aids digestion. It is indicated in gastric disorders and ulcerations, especially those with mucus or pus. It relieves irritation and, afterward, restores the tone of the tissues.

Goldenseal is used for chronic gastritis and enteritis. It is a remedy for obstinate constipation. The intestines are gently stimulated to normal activity. |
| *Drugs* | Because of the popular, though false, perception that goldenseal can mask illicit drug use in urine tests, drug screening labs have begun checking for the presence of hydrastine (a component of goldenseal) in the urine as well. If found, hydrastine is considered possible proof the person being tested is a drug user. |
| **Herb Parts Used** | The medicinal parts are the air-dried rhizome (underground stem) and root fibers. The leaf is not as potent (it contains approximately one-tenth the amount of active alkaloids), and is used principally as a general tonic. |
| **Preparations and Remedies**

Powder and Tincture | Infusions, extracts, salves, and capsules are made from the dried and powdered root.

Wounds:
Powdered goldenseal root may be dusted directly onto wounds as an antibacterial dressing. Goldenseal tincture may be applied full strength for treating infected wounds, eczema, hemorrhoids, and skin ulcerations. Salves may be similarly employed.

Pyorrhea (gum disease):
Dip moistened toothbrush into goldenseal powder and brush teeth.

Ringworm:
Use one level teaspoonful of powder in a half cup of warm water. Sweeten to taste and drink (dilute for children). Also apply powder topically as a salve or paste (mixed with extra-virgin olive oil).

Infection Formula:
4 parts Goldenseal Root
3 parts Echinacea Angustifolia Root
2 parts Yarrow Flower
1 part Lobelia Herb |

Combine herbs and encapsulate or use to make a tincture. This formula is very powerful and gets results.

The herbs in this formula have been used for hundreds of years to help alleviate colds, flu, and other infections. They are highly regarded by many, due to their incredible healing properties. The combination of these herbs is extremely effective, more so than the herbs taken individually.

Drops of goldenseal extract may be put in the nose for sinus infections. For middle ear infections and earaches accompanied by inflammation, warm goldenseal extract (to body temperature for comfort) and drop into the ear. The ear may also be cleansed with a goldenseal tea wash.

Kidney Formula: (see JUNIPER preparations)

Infusions

Goldenseal Tea:
Place one teaspoonful of powdered root into a pint of boiling water. Let stand until cold. Drink one or two teaspoonfuls three to six times a day. For ulcers of the mouth and throat, use a goldenseal infusion as a gargle.

Urinary Tract Infection Tea: (see UVA URSI preparations)
Pregnancy Decoction: (see WILD YAM preparations)

Fomentations

As a fomentation (towel soaked in infusion or decoction and placed on affected area), use externally on open sores, inflammations, eczema, ringworm, erysipelas, and itchy skin afflictions.

Eye Wash

It is essential to keep utensils, containers, and ingredients clean and sterile for all preparations that go directly on or into the eyes.

Eye Wash Tea:
Great for tired and irritated eyes, infections, and sties.
1/2-1 teaspoon Goldenseal root, cut or powdered 1/4-1/2 cup distilled Water, hot *(not boiling)*
Recommended alternative:
Add 1/2-1 teaspoon each:
Eyebright herb, Goldenseal root, and Raspberry leaves
Pour hot water over the herb(s). Steep and cool for about ten minutes. Run infusion through a cloth to filter out any grit. Keep

unused liquid refrigerated and make a new batch every two to three days to avoid contamination.

Use a sterile eyedropper or glass eyewash cup to wash eyes with liquid two to three times a day. After using the eyecup on one side, clean thoroughly before using for the other eye to prevent spreading infection from eye to eye. A tea-saturated cotton ball may also be used to apply to closed eyes. Use tea both internally and externally.

Alternate Method:
Use (non-alcohol based) goldenseal root tincture diluted in distilled water.

Optional:
Add a pinch of cayenne. It will sting a lot, but it is remarkably effective for helping the body heal cataracts. Wash eyes with milk if burning sensation becomes intolerable. The fat in the milk will dilute the 'heat' of the cayenne.

Soothing Eye Compress: (see EYEBRIGHT preparations)

Nasal Douche

For treating sinusitis, use a goldenseal root cold infusion at full strength once daily. Put into a sinus wash syringe, or a neti pot, and rinse.

Vaginal Douche

Use a goldenseal tincture in two cups of warm water twice daily or goldenseal root warm infusion (full strength) twice daily.

Enema / Douche: (see RED RASPBERRY preparations)

Poultices

Flaxseed Poultice: (see FLAXSEED preparations)
Slippery Elm Poultice: (see SLIPPERY ELM preparations)

Oil

Goldenseal Oil:
1 ounce Goldenseal root
8 ounces Flaxseed oil or Extra-Virgin Olive Oil
Mix thoroughly and let stand for 24 hours. Strain through clean, unbleached muslin. Apply freely as needed for burns, itching, and skin-eruptive diseases (smallpox, measles, scarlet fever, etc.).

Salve

Goldenseal / Myrrh Antiseptic Salve:
This is a wonderful antiseptic salve for scrapes and closed wounds. It is best to let wounds drain and close on their own before sealing them off with the salves of any kind. Use the powder alone or as a poultice for open wounds.

GOLDENSEAL — 197

	1 oz. powdered Goldenseal 1 oz. powdered Myrrh gum 4 oz. Extra-Virgin Olive Oil 1/4 oz. Beeswax Essential oil(s) if desired *Note: It is possible to make more than one batch at a time* Measure oil into a crock pot and bring the temperature no higher than 80-100° F by heating on the 'warm' setting. Stir in herbs and maintain this temperature (with lid on) for 24 hours, stirring occasionally. When mixture is ready (partially determined by the loss of herb color and smell), line a colander with two layers of unbleached broadcloth or muslin. Place the colander inside a collector bowl and pour in the contents of the crock pot. Strain and squeeze out all possible oil into the collector bowl (use gloves while squeezing). The herbs (left inside the cloth) become dry and powdery. Return them to the soil or discard. Return the herb-infused oil to the wiped-down, clean crock pot. Cut in the beeswax and slowly heat until melted (beeswax liquefies at 148.4° F). Once melted, turn off the heat. To determine if enough beeswax has been added, spoon a small amount onto a plate to cool. The room temperature consistency should be gel-like without liquefying. In warmer climates, it is necessary to add additional beeswax to set up properly. When satisfied, mix in essential oils (if used) and pour mixture into clean ointment jars (one to two ounce jars are a convenient size for single or family use). This salve lasts up to three years in the refrigerator or for several months when stored at room temperature.
Ointment	*Skin Ointment:* (see LICORICE preparations)
Safety	Goldenseal is generally considered safe. For those who have low blood sugar, goldenseal should be taken with true licorice, or it can be replaced with myrrh. Goldenseal may cause uterine contractions. Its use is not recommended for pregnancy until the last few weeks.
Plant Profile	*Natural Habitat:*

Description

Goldenseal is native to the moist woods and damp meadows of eastern North America and cultivated elsewhere.

Goldenseal is a low, herbaceous perennial (after tops die down in the winter, the plant grows back from a persistent rootstock in the spring), characterized by an erect, purplish, hairy stem (6-12 inches tall) and small, greenish-white flowers that bloom in early spring and subsequently become clusters of red berries. The berries are inedible and contain 1 or 2 hard, glossy, black seeds.

The plant has several three-to-seven-lobed leaves and a thick, yellow, knotty, and twisted rhizome (underground stem) one or two inches long, out of which grow yellow root fibers (a foot or more in length).

Younger rhizomes are well marked on the upper surface with cup-like depressions (looking something like a seal, from which it gets its common name) showing where the stems of the previous years have grown, died, and broken off. These marks become less noticeable as the rhizome ages.

Harvesting

The fresh root is a vivid yellow color, both within and without, but the outside becomes dull brown upon drying. The best rhizomes have a large amount of yellow juice, which may leave the interior yellow or orange-yellow after drying. Upon fracture of the dried root, the interior is lemon-yellow. With age, the yellow pigment breaks down and the color turns greenish-yellow or even brown. These should be rejected as being of inferior quality.

Goldenseal is considered to be a 'bitter' herb. The taste is quite bitter, and the smell is strong, characteristic, and disagreeable. Once the herb is dried and powdered, it has a distinctive yellow color which stains when mixed with liquid.

Optimum plant development requires approximately five years from seed and three to four years from root bulbs. After the plant seeds ripen in the autumn, sufficiently aged roots are harvested, washed, and air dried in partial shade. Leaves and stems are collected in the late summer for drying and preserving.

Hawthorn

Latin Name: *Crataegus laevigata*

Also known as: Hawthorne, English Hawthorn, Mayflower, May Bush, Mayblossom, Quickset, Whitethorn

Scientific Classification

Species in the Crataegus genus readily hybridize (mutate, crossbreed). Species identification is difficult, even for experts. If the berry contains two or fewer seeds, it is probably a wild-form hawthorn. If it contains more than two seeds, it is more likely a cultivated strain.

Several wild-form species are considered to have medicinal qualities, notably the English Hawthorn (*C. laevigata*, also known as *C. oxyacantha* in earlier literature) and the One-Seed Hawthorn (*C. monogyna*), most widely used in the West. In China, *C. pinnatifida* (Shen-Za) is used

Family: Rosaceae – rose family

Genus Crataegus – hawthorn

Species C. laevigata – smooth hawthorn
C. oxycantha – in earlier classifications, was often confused with C. laevigata. They are currently used interchangeably

Influence on the Body	(PRINCIPAL ACTIONS are listed in CAPITAL LETTERS)
Blood and Circulatory System	HEART TONIC • HEART WEAKNESS • CARDIAC SYMPTOMS • ANGINA PECTORIS (chest pain) • ARRHYTHMIAS (irregular heartbeats) • IRREGULAR HEARTBEAT • heart fibrillation • HEART PALPITATIONS • ENLARGED HEART • hypertrophy (enlargement of the heart muscle due to increased workload) • weak or inflamed HEART MUSCLE • CONGESTIVE HEART FAILURE (CHF) • DROPSY (edema due to heart insufficiency) • EDEMA • astringent (increases the tone and firmness of tissues) • HEART DISEASE • HEART VALVES • CIRCULATION • blood clots • ARTERIOSCLEROSIS • HARDENING OF THE ARTERIES • HYPERTENSION • HIGH BLOOD PRESSURE • LOW BLOOD PRESSURE
Blood Sugar	Hypoglycemia
Body System	vibrancy • endurance • energy • stress • sleeplessness • restlessness • insomnia • sedative
Digestive Tract	Stomach

Endocrine System	adrenal weakness
Infections and Immune System	sore throat
Inflammation	arthritis • rheumatism
Liver	Liver
Nervous System	nerves • antispasmodic
Reproductive System	*Female:* menopause • emmenagogue (promotes menstrual flow)
Urinary Tract	nephritis (inflammation of the kidneys) • diuretic (increases urine flow)

Key Properties:

CARDIAC TONIC — *helps prevent hardening of the arteries, increases circulation in the extremities, relaxes and opens blood vessels, improves blood flow to the heart, rejuvenates the heart, strengthens and tones the heart muscle*

Primarily affecting   HEART • CIRCULATION • nerves

History	The Latin name, 'Crataegus' is derived from the Greek word 'kratus' for strength, probably referring to the hardness of the wood. The Greek physician Dioscorides (ca. 40-90) mentioned beneficial actions of hawthorn on the heart in his writings. Roman physicians used it as a heart drug in the 1st century AD, but most of the literature from that period focused on its symbolic use for religious rites and political ceremonies. A Chinese herbal dating 659 AD mentions hawthorn, which has been used in China for centuries to treat high blood pressure, arteriosclerosis, and heart pain. The hawthorn tree has been regarded as sacred by Christians. Tradition holds the crown of thorns placed on the head of Christ was from the hawthorn tree. A grove of hawthorn trees still stands outside of Jerusalem on the Mount of Olives. The spiny tree was used as a living, thorny, hedge fence in much of Europe. Besides protecting estates from trespassers, hawthorn

was used medicinally as a cure for scurvy (a Vitamin C deficiency disease) and for various stomach ailments.

During the Middle Ages, hawthorn was used for the treatment of dropsy (now considered to be congestive heart failure) and other heart ailments. It was also used to treat a sore throat. Branches were hung over doorways to keep away evil spirits.

Native Americans used hawthorn to treat stomachache, diarrhea, dysentery (bowel inflammation), female diseases, and cramps; as a diuretic for kidney and bladder ailments; and a cardiac strengthener to improve circulation. The Kwakiutl chewed hawthorn leaves and used them as a poultice for wounds and sores.

Native American groups ate the fruit as food and used the thorns to pierce and drain boils and to probe ulcers and wounds. Thorns were also inserted like acupuncture needles into joints with arthritic pain and sometimes burned as a form of moxibustion. Inserted thorns were ignited and allowed to burn down near the skin.

By the early 1800's, American doctors recognized the herb's medicinal properties and began using it to treat circulatory disorders and respiratory illnesses. Hawthorn soon became a common therapy to strengthen the heart. Hawthorn was considered a cardiotonic and used to treat irregular heartbeat, high blood pressure, chest pain, hardening of the arteries, and heart failure.

Attributes	**Key Components: (including, but not limited to)**
Nutrition	Vitamins B1 (thiamine) • B2 (riboflavin) • B3 (niacin) • B5 (pantothenic acid) • B6 (pyridoxine) • B9 (folic acid) • B12 (cobalamin) • Biotin • Choline • Inositol • PABA (Para-Amino Benzoic Acid) • C • Iron • Phosphorus • Sodium • Zinc • other Trace Minerals
	Flavonoids • Oligomeric Procyanidins (OPC's) • Pectin
	Flavonoids help dilate blood vessels, improve blood flow, and protect the blood vessels from damage. Both flavonoids and OPC's have potent antioxidant effects.

Heart

The berries, flowers, bark, and leaves are all restorative to the heart. Hawthorn preparations lower blood pressure, clear blood vessels, and are antispasmodic. Hawthorn works best when used on a regular basis. It may take four to eight weeks to reach a therapeutic effect. This regimen is used to prevent and treat coronary heart disease. Hawthorn is also used for long-term recovery from heart attacks and coronary surgeries.

Hawthorn is used effectively as a cardiac tonic and is valuable for the improvement of cardiac weakness, sighing respiration, nerve depression, or unexplained chronic fatigue. There is evidence it improves heart action in cases of mitral regurgitation (a heart valve defect).

Hawthorn helps prevent hardening of the arteries, inflammation of the heart muscle, arteriosclerosis, and is useful in cholesterol reduction.

Hawthorn flower and leaf extracts improve circulation to the extremities by reducing resistance in the arteries (in general, the less elastic the arteries, the greater the arterial resistance).

Hawthorn preparations relax blood vessels, dilate coronary arteries, and permit a freer flow of blood and oxygen to the heart muscle. Active ingredients in the herb inhibit the release of angiotensin (a substance which activates an enzyme known to cause high blood pressure). The herb regulates both high and low blood pressure and promotes a general sense of well-being.

Hawthorn extract was recently used effectively in a study for hypertension in patients with Type 2 diabetes. Patients took 1,200 mg of hawthorn extract, or a placebo daily for 16 weeks. Those taking hawthorn had lower blood pressure than those taking the placebo.

Hawthorn is excellent for feeble heart action, valvular insufficiency, and irregular pulse. It is a cardiac tonic with antispasmodic properties that ease angina pectoris. Hawthorn has several antioxidant constituents and is especially good for weakened heart muscle caused by age degeneration.

Individuals who received a hawthorn preparation in one study experienced improved blood flow to the heart. They were able to exercise for longer periods of time without suffering chest pain. Hawthorn increases myocardial (heart muscle) enzyme metabolism and improves oxygen utilization by the heart. It is used to reduce a sensation of pressure or anxiety in the heart area and difficulty in breathing due to ineffective heart action. Hawthorn alleviates hypertrophy and fibrillation of the heart.

Numerous studies have shown that hawthorn berry extract improves blood flow to and from the heart by strengthening its muscle contractions. The heartbeat becomes more regular, and each contraction is more efficient, pumping more blood throughout the body with less effort.

Hawthorn is safer to use than the well-known heart herb 'foxglove' from which the drugs Digoxin, Digitoxin, and Digitalis are derived. In addition to improving the heart's pumping ability, foxglove and its derivatives make the heart more irritable and liable to dangerous irregularities of rhythm.

In contrast, hawthorn both strengthens the heart and stabilizes it against arrhythmias by lengthening what is called the refractory period (the short period following a heartbeat during which the heart rests). Many irregular heart rhythms begin with an early beat. Hawthorn protects against such potentially dangerous breaks in the heart's even rhythm.

Hawthorn is widely regarded in modern Europe as a safe and effective treatment for the early stages of congestive heart failure (CHF), a long-term heart condition with persistent symptoms including rapid or irregular heartbeat, shortness of breath with exertion, reduced ability to exercise, and edema in legs, ankles, and feet. The cumulative results of several studies on hawthorn performed between 1981-1994 suggest hawthorn is an effective treatment for congestive heart failure.

One study found hawthorn extract (900 mg/day) taken for 2 months was as effective as low doses of Captropril (a leading heart medication) in alleviating symptoms of heart failure.

A large study of 952 patients with heart failure (a condition in which the heart is unable to pump adequate amounts of blood to other organs in the body) observed differences in the use of conventional medications alone, patients using only hawthorn, and those using hawthorn in addition to conventional heart drugs.

Other Uses	After two years, the clinical symptoms of heart failure (palpitations, breathing problems, and fatigue) decreased significantly in the groups taking hawthorn. It was also noted patients taking both hawthorn and traditional medications were able to take fewer conventional drugs for their condition. Hawthorn tea helps relieve nervous conditions, restlessness, and insomnia. A decoction of the berries is used for sore throats and acid conditions of the blood. Hawthorn also produces a natural adrenalin-like effect that gives an extra boost during stressful situations.
Herb Parts Used	In the spring, leaves and flowers harvested in the early flowering stage are used fresh or dried. Berries harvested when mature, after the first frost, are used fresh or dried.
Preparations and Remedies *Dried Berries*	Fresh berries are delicious and may be used in season to fortify the heart (probably the mildest way to take the herb). Reconstitute whole dried berries in large quantities with pure water, blend, and strain. In all cases of heart disease, consume two or three bowls of the thick sweet mucilage daily as a heart and circulatory tonic. Dried berries may be powdered (including the seed) and used in heart preparations and formulas.
Tinctures	It is difficult to maintain a liquid tincture of fresh hawthorn berries because of its high pectin content. The smashed berries clump together, and the finished tincture is prone to crystallization.
Infusions	Infusions are made with dried leaf and flower, or dried berries. *Tea:* Steep one teaspoon herb in a cup of hot water for ten to fifteen minutes. *Yarrow and Calendula Tea (alternative Hawthorn):* (see YARROW preparations)
Decoction	*Decoction:* Simmer dried berries in water on low heat for 5-15 minutes.
Syrup	Hawthorn Syrup:

Combine one part (by volume) strong decoction of dried berries and two parts (by volume) raw honey. Combine and heat gently (stirring constantly) until ingredients mix thoroughly. Remove from heat, and pour into sterilized canning jars. Cap tightly with sterilized lids. Label and store in a cool, dry place out of the light. Keep opened containers refrigerated. Syrup made in this manner has an expected shelf life of one year. Discard syrup if mold appears on the surface.

This syrup carries the active constituents of the herb. It is fully preserved but is subject to crystallization. If this occurs, re-liquify the syrup by setting the jar in a pan of hot (not boiling) water.

Safety	No health hazards or adverse side effects are known with the proper use of hawthorn. Eye scratches from its thorns can seriously impair eyesight.
Plant Profile	*Natural Habitat:* The plant is indigenous to northern temperate zones of Europe, Asia, and North America. It grows in open woodlands and pastures in sun to partial shade.
Description	Hawthorn is a thorny shrub or small tree that grows up to five feet tall on hillsides and in sunny wooded areas throughout the world. It has small, beautiful, white, red, or pink rose-like flowers (usually with five petals) that grow in clusters in the spring, followed by berries (also called haws) in the fall. The fruit is usually red (sometimes black) when ripe, containing one to five hard seeds. The flowers have an unpleasant smell (likened to the odor of decaying fish) and a slightly bitter taste. The fruit is dry and mealy with a sour taste. Hawthorn leaves are shiny and grow in a variety of lobed edges, wedge shapes, and sizes, depending on the species. Branches and trunk are studded with sharp-tipped thorns, typically a half to an inch long (although up to four and a half inches in one species), giving haw (fruit) + thorn its common name. The name may also be a corruption of the Anglo-Saxon or German names for 'hedge thorn'.

Juniper

Latin Name: *Juniperus communis*

Also known as: Dwarf Juniper, Ground Juniper, Juniper Berry

Scientific Classification

There are between 50-67 classified species of juniper.

Family: Cupressaceae – cypress family

Genus Juniperus – juniper

Species J. communis – common juniper
Note: other species also exhibit medicinal qualities

Influence on the Body	(PRINCIPAL ACTIONS are listed in CAPITAL LETTERS)
Blood and Circulatory System	heart • shortness of breath • blood • blood purifier • DROPSY (edema due to heart insufficiency) • arteriosclerosis • BLEEDING • scurvy
Blood Sugar	DIABETES • HYPOGLYCEMIA
Body System	catarrhal conditions (inflamed mucous membranes with discharge, especially affecting the nose and throat) • mucus • lymph cleansing
Digestion	aromatic (has a spicy taste, contains volatile oils which aid digestion and relieve gas) • improves appetite • digestive tonic (increases energy and improves digestion and assimilation) • digestion • dyspepsia (indigestion) • stomach • gas • colic • carminative (brings warmth, circulation, relieves intestinal gas discomfort, and promotes peristaltic movement) • bowel • dysentery (bowel inflammation) • expels worms • parasiticide (kills parasites and worms)
Endocrine System	PANCREAS • ADRENAL GLANDS • adrenal weakness
Eyes	OPTIC NERVE weakness
First Aid	abrasions • bee stings • poisonous insect bites • poisonous snake bites
Infections and Immune System	allergies • hay fever • coughs • COLDS • INFECTIONS • FUNGAL INFECTIONS • destroys FUNGI • disease

	preventative • contagious diseases • cystic fibrosis (childhood disease characterized by glandular secretion failure) • plague • leprosy
Inflammation	arthritis • rheumatism • swollen joints • bursitis • gout
Lungs	Tuberculosis
Mouth, Nose and Throat	bleeding gums • mouth sores • sore throat • gargle
Nervous System	strengthens nerves • anodyne (relieves pain and lessens the excitability of nerves) • pain • sciatica • brain • memory • convulsions • epilepsy • ANTISPASMODIC • palsy
Reproductive System	gonorrhea (a venereal infection affecting the urethra) *Male:* prostate gland *Female:* cramps • emmenagogue (promotes menstrual flow) • vaginal discharge • leukorrhea (vaginal discharge due to infection) • douche
Skin, Tissues and Hair	boils • pimples • acne • itching • eczema • chapped skin • hair loss
Urinary Tract	KIDNEYS • kidney stimulant (increases internal heat, dispels internal chill, and strengthens metabolism and circulation) • astringent (increases the tone and firmness of tissues, lessens mucus) • urinary antiseptic (fights pathogenic bacteria and prevents infection in the urinary tract) • cystitis (bladder inflammation) • kidney inflammation • NEPHRITIS (kidney inflammation) • KIDNEY INFECTIONS • KIDNEY STONES • URIC ACID buildup • RENAL DROPSY (edema) • DIURETIC (increases urine flow) • WATER RETENTION • lithotriptic (dissolves urinary stones) • URINARY PROBLEMS • burning urination • BLADDER PROBLEMS • incontinence • BEDWETTING

Key Properties:

KIDNEY SUPPORTIVE HERB	*Stimulates, tones, and cleanses kidney and bladder, increases circulation, urine flow, and pathogenic elimination, dissolves stones, fights infection, relieves pain and inflammation*
DIGESTIVE AID	*improves digestion and assimilation, relieves indigestion and gas, kills and expels parasites and worms*

Primarily affecting   KIDNEYS • BLADDER • stomach

History

In biblical times, junipers were valued for their protection from evil spirits and bad luck. There are many references in the Bible to people using juniper trees for shelter. Branches were also burned in temples as a purifying herb.

Juniper berries were used by the ancient physicians of Greece, Arabia, and Rome. Roman naturalist and philosopher Pliny the Elder (23-79 AD) wrote of its ability to relieve the aches and pains of rheumatism. Roman physicians prescribed preparations of the berries for stomach and chest pains, flatulence, coughs, colds, tumors, and uterine disorders.

In England, branches of juniper were often strewn on floors to sweeten the smell of a room and to cleanse the air of infection and disease. The scent of juniper was believed to ward off the plague in Europe.

The 15th and 16th century herbalists highly praised the use of junipers. Juice from the berries was recommended against the bitings of vipers, the plague, and pestilence. Nicholas Culpeper (herbalist and physician, ca. 1616–1654) suggested the use of ripened berries for asthma and sciatica and to speed childbirth.

Native Americans believed in juniper's cleansing and healing powers. Boughs were often used as a fumigant in sweat lodges, and berries were used to keep away infection, relieve arthritis, and cure various wounds and illnesses. Leaf tea was taken before women went into labor to relax muscles and ease delivery. Convulsions were treated by rubbing scorched twigs on the body. Chewed berries or berry teas were used as a laxative, diuretic, douche, and female contraceptive. It was used to help treat fevers from the flu. Western tribes combined the berries of juniperus communis with berberis root bark in an herbal tea to treat diabetes.

Juniper berries have a long history of use as a diuretic. In the early 1900's, juniper was often prescribed as a diuretic for treating edema, cystitis, kidney problems, gonorrhea, ringing in the ears, and hay fever. In external ointments, it was a remedy for eczema and chapped skin.

Attributes	Key Components: (including, but not limited to)
Nutrition	Vitamin C • Cobalt • Copper • Sulfur • other Trace Minerals Flavonoids • Tannins • Juniperin (a bitter which stimulates digestive juices and improves appetite) • Volatile Oil (having more than a hundred constituents)
	All parts of the plant contain a volatile oil, which imparts a distinctive scent and flavor. The active diuretic principles of juniper berries are in the volatile oil. It increases urine flow, helps remove excess fluid in edema or congestive heart failure cases, and washes out pathogenic bacteria in urinary tract infections.
Urinary Tract	In cases where acid has been retained in the body, juniper helps prevent uric acid crystallization in the kidneys, keeping it dissolved to pass easily in the urine. Juniper also helps to dissolve and wash out kidney stones and prostate sediment.
	The kidneys and adrenals are stimulated by the action of juniper berries, increasing filtration and urine flow. Earlier literature suggests diseased and inflamed kidneys may be overstimulated and irritated in this way, but there is no real evidence to back up these claims.
	Juniper relieves pain and heals the kidneys, urinary passages, and bladder. Science confirms its antiseptic, anti-inflammatory and spasm-reducing activity.
	Juniper berries are effective as a tea for helping to alleviate water retention, bladder problems, and catarrhal congestion of the bladder and kidneys. Juniper is one of the best diuretics known. It is especially beneficial in eliminating congestion of the kidneys resulting from water retention (renal dropsy). It assists the body in removing waste products and cleansing the bloodstream through the urinary tract.
Circulation	Juniper is an excellent blood and lymph cleanser. It has the ability to tone the pancreas and helps to reduce the body's susceptibility to diseases. It works well in rheumatic disorders that are caused by diminished circulation and general toxicity.
	Being a moderate circulatory stimulant, juniper relieves congestions throughout the body that result from heart problems. Medieval physicians wrote, 'If juniper boughs are burnt to ashes, and the ashes put into water, a medicine will be obtained that has cured the dropsy in an advanced stage.' Dropsy is known today as congestive heart failure (CHF).

Infections

Sebastian Kneipp, in *My Water Cure* (1897), says this of juniper berries:

> 'Those who are nursing patients with serious illness as scarlet fever, smallpox, typhus, cholera, etc. and are exposed to contagion by raising, carrying, or serving the patient, or by speaking with him, should always chew a few juniper berries (six to ten a day). They give a pleasant taste in the mouth and are of good service to the digestion, they burn up as it were, the harmful miasmas, exhalations, when these seek to enter through the mouth or nostrils.'

The berries, boiled and used as a spray, will disinfect rooms used by patients with infectious diseases. The spray kills fungi and is excellent for disease prevention.

As a poultice, juniper bark or fruit may be applied directly onto wounds to prevent infection. A berry tea can be used on insect bites and bee stings, it is an antidote for poisonous snake bites.

Because of its blood-cleansing properties, juniper taken internally helps wash out infections from the body. It is often included in other herb combinations for its ability to flush out infections and remove acid and toxic wastes.

Digestion

The berries can improve impaired digestion and strengthen weak stomachs. It is an excellent digestive tonic. Juniper decoction or oil taken internally is used when there is putrefaction and gas in the stomach and intestines. Obstinate stomach troubles have been relieved by releasing pressures that cause stomach tissue weakness, indigestion, and poor assimilation.

Juniper increases appetite, aids digestion, expels wind, and kills worms and parasites. Juniper teas are approved in Germany for stomach complaints and to stimulate appetite.

Nervous System

Juniper can strengthen brain, memory, and optic nerves. It helps heal epilepsy.

Lungs

Juniper helps dilate the bronchial tubes and has been used effectively for coughs, shortness of breath, and tuberculosis.

Blood Sugar

Juniper naturally helps produce usable insulin, aids in the healing of the adrenal glands, and aids in the prevention or alleviation of diabetes and hypoglycemia.

Women	Clinical studies have verified the effectiveness of juniper as a treatment for insulin-dependent diabetes. It triggers insulin production in the body's fat cells & stabilizes blood sugar levels. Juniper tea is effective for leukorrhea and gonorrhea. It makes an excellent douche for vaginal infections and can be used for suppressed menstrual flow.
Herb Parts Used	Usually, the berries are used medicinally, as well as the leaves and bark. Juniper essential oil is distilled from berries and wood.
Preparations and Remedies	Juniper berries are used as a spice in a wide variety of culinary dishes. Juniper berry sauce is a popular flavoring choice for quail, pheasant, veal, rabbit, venison, and other meat dishes.
Chew Berries	Juniper is a good disease preventative. When exposed to contagious diseases, chew the berries or use as a gargle in a strong infusion form. *For a weak stomach:* Chew 5 softened berries a few days in succession, increasing the amount 1 a day until 15 berries are taken a day. Then decrease the amount by 1 berry a day for 5 more days.
Powdered Formula	*Kidney Formula:* The herbs in this formula have been used to nutritionally support the body in strengthening the bladder, kidneys, and lower back. They have also historically been used to alleviate water retention. 2 parts Juniper Blue berries 2 parts Parsley root 2 parts Dandelion root 2 parts Uva Ursi leaves 1 part Buchu 1 part Ginger root 1 part Althea root (Marshmallow) ½ part Goldenseal root ½ part Astragalus Use encapsulated powdered herbs or make a glycerin extract.
Infusions	*Juniper Tea:* 1 ounce Juniper berries (or leaves), cut or crushed 1 pint distilled water

To make an infusion, soften several tablespoonfuls of the berries by soaking. Drain and add 1 pint of boiling water and steep for 15-30 minutes. Cool and take the infusion in 2 fluid-ounce doses every 3-4 hours (or 1 tablespoon doses for children).

Urinary Tract Infection Tea: (see UVA URSI preparations)

Essential Oil:

Essential Oil	Juniper berries are steam distilled to produce an essential oil that may vary from colorless to yellow or pale green. It works as a detoxifier and cleanser, is beneficial for the skin, and assists with nerve regeneration. Use as a spray for fumigation. Apply topically for skin irritations, depression, fatigue, sore muscles, rheumatism, urinary infections, fluid retention, and wounds.
Safety	No adverse side effects are known with proper dosages. Avoid during pregnancy, as juniper has strong vasodilating and diuretic effects.
Plant Profile *Description*	This common shrub grows in dry woods, on hills and mountain slopes in North America, Europe, Asia, and North Africa. *Natural Habitat:* Junipers are evergreen shrubs or small trees that vary in shape and size (2 to 20 feet tall) with needle-like leaves and numerous seed cones. The female seed cones are very distinctive with thin, waxy-coated scales which fuse together to form a fleshy, berry-like structure. These contain 1 to 12 hard-shelled seeds. Berries do not ripen until the second year, changing from green to the mature-blue-to-dark-purple color (red-brown or orange in some species). The berries are usually aromatic, sticky when crushed, and initially taste sweet and pleasant then bitter. The male cones are similar to other cypress, with 6 to 20 scales. Most shed their pollen in early spring (in autumn for some species).
Harvesting *Storage*	Do not use first-year berries, which are green and acidic. Only use second-year berries, which are dark blue to deep purple. Juniper berries may be preserved for longer periods of time by drying them or by preparing a tincture.

Kelp

Latin Name: *Laminaria digitata (kelp)*
Fucus vesiculosus (bladderwrack)

Also known as: Kelpware, Bladderwrack, Bladder Fucus, Seawrack, Seaweed, Tangleweed, Black-tang, Kombu

Scientific Classification

Kelp is not a true plant but a type of brown algae seaweed. Worldwide, there are about 1500-2000 species of brown algae. The designation 'seaweed' loosely describes any type of vegetation growing in the ocean, including many types of algae and plants.

Brown algae that are of particular use herbally are kelp and bladderwrack. They are placed in different order classifications but have similar physical and nutritional makeup. In herb texts, the names are often used interchangeably, as their herbal use is similar. They also work synergistically with each other.

Two distinctions are:

1) Physically, kelp plants (Laminaria genus) do not have air sacs called bladders. Plants of the bladderwrack genus (Fucus) usually have bladders, but not always.
2) Nutritionally, laminaria plants contain ten times the amount of iodine and are preferred when commercially harvesting for iodine.

Class	Phaeophyceae – brown algae
Order	Laminariales
Family:	Laminariaceae
Genus	Laminaria
Species	*L. digitata* – true kelp
Class	Phaeophyceae – brown algae
Order	Fucales
Family:	Fucaceae
Genus	Fucus
Species	*F. vesiculosus* – bladderwrack, also called kelp by some

Influence on the Body	(PRINCIPAL ACTIONS are listed in CAPITAL LETTERS)
Blood and Circulatory System	anemia • CLEANS ARTERIES • alterative (cleanses and purifies the blood and facilitates efficient removal of waste products) • arteriosclerosis • high blood pressure • heart disease
Blood Sugar	Diabetes

Body System	ENERGY • stimulant (increases internal heat, dispels chill, and strengthens metabolism and circulation) • tonic (increases energy and strength throughout the body) • low vitality • debility • muculent (a soft and slippery sugar molecule that protects mucous membranes and inflamed tissues) • DEMULCENT (softens and soothes inflammation of mucous membranes) • BIRTH DEFECT PREVENTION
Bones and Teeth	Fractures
Cancer	TUMORS • cancer
Digestive Tract	NUTRITIVE (supplies substantial amount of nutrients) • poor digestion • nausea • COLITIS • gas • expels worms and parasites
Endocrine System	GLANDULAR BALANCE • THYROID IMBALANCE • LOW THYROID • HYPOTHYROIDISM • GOITER (swelling of the thyroid gland related to iodine deficiency) • enlarged glands • low thyroid fatigue • ADRENAL GLAND WEAKNESS • ENDOCRINE GLANDS • PITUITARY GLAND • pancreas
Infections and Immune System	INFECTION • antibiotic • antiseptic
Inflammation	arthritis • bursitis
Liver	Gallbladder
Lungs and Respiratory System	expectorant (loosens & removes phlegm in the respiratory tract)
Muscles	leg cramps
Nervous System	headaches • neuritis (inflamed and weakened nerves)
Poisoning	RADIATION POISONING • lead poisoning
Reproductive System	*Male:* tones prostate gland
	Female: MENOPAUSE • hot flashes • MORNING SICKNESS • PREGNANCY • hypermenorrhea (excessive menstruation) • dysmenorrhea (painful or difficult menstruation) • endometriosis
Skin, Tissues and Hair	emollient (softens and soothes skin when applied externally and mucous membranes when taken internally) • COMPLEXION • ACNE caused by thyroid imbalance • ECZEMA • psoriasis • FINGERNAILS • NAIL PROBLEMS • HAIR LOSS
Urinary Tract	kidneys • water retention • diuretic (increases urine flow)
Weight	OBESITY • weight distribution
Other Uses	fertilizer • cattle feed

	Key Properties:
SUPPORTS GLANDULAR BALANCE	*strengthens, tones, and provides nutrients for endocrine system balance and health (particularly thyroid, adrenal, pituitary, and reproductive glands)*
alterative	*cleanses, purifies, and detoxifies the spleen, liver, kidneys, and bowels, improves digestion, assimilation, and skin health*
NUTRITIVE	*Tonic*
Primarily affecting	*THYROID • ENDOCRINE GLANDS • BRAIN • KIDNEYS*

History	People of Japan, China, and Korea have eaten kelp as a 'vegetable from the sea' for thousands of years. The Chinese have recommended it for treating thyroid disease and lowering blood pressure. The Japanese bathe with strips of kelp to help ease nervous disorders.
	Kelp was discovered in 1811 as an original source of iodine and then used extensively to treat goiter. In the 1860's, kelp and bladderwrack were marketed for their ability to increase the metabolic rate for the obese. They have since been featured in numerous weight-loss products.
Attributes	**Key Components:** (including, but not limited to)
Nutrition	Vitamins A • B1 (thiamine) • B2 (riboflavin) • B3 (niacin) • B5 (pantothenic acid) • B6 (pyridoxine) • B9 (folic acid) • B12 (cobalamin) • Biotin • Choline • Inositol • PABA (Para-Amino Benzoic Acid) • C • E • Calcium • Chlorine • Chromium • Cobalt • Copper • Fluorine • Iodine • Iron • Magnesium • Manganese • Phosphorus • Potassium • Selenium • Sodium • Sulfur • Vanadium • Zinc • other Trace Minerals
	All eight Essential Amino Acids • Algin (a carbohydrate commercially used as a thickening agent) • Mannitol (a very sweet type of sugar) • Mucilage
	Mannitol is sometimes used as a sweetener in diabetic foods.
	Kelp abounds in calcium, chlorine, magnesium, potassium, and especially iodine. It is also a good source of folic acid.
General	Kelp promotes glandular balance and health, which, in turn, affects many systems of the body. It offsets the effects of stress, aids digestion and respiration, guards against sickness, and generally promotes healthy function and balance in the body.

Nutritive

Kelp is well known for its healthful qualities, and many use it alone. I have found when bladderwrack is taken along with kelp, the combination is even more powerful.

As a product of the ocean, kelp has numerous elements the ocean contains. The brown algae seaweed has minerals and vitamins that stimulate the body's metabolism and strengthen and tone organs such as the thyroid gland.

Kelp helps build cell membranes and contributes to the healthy growth of hair, skin, and nails. Kelp is especially useful during pregnancy and for ailing and convalescent patients who need concentrated nutrients that are easy to assimilate.

Thyroid and All Endocrine Glands

Kelp has a high content of natural plant iodine, which is absorbed much more slowly (and, therefore, more safely) than chemical iodine. Iodine is necessary for the proper function of the thyroid gland and production of thyroid hormones. The thyroid is required for growth, energy, and metabolism. Kelp is especially useful for hypothyroid conditions (insufficient thyroid hormone production).

For its ability to restore normal metabolism and energy, some have marketed kelp as a metabolism stimulant to lose weight. Kelp helps individuals who have a dysfunctional thyroid gland lose weight and take off excess pounds in the hip area.

Kelp can act as an antibiotic. It assists the thyroid in releasing iodine into the bloodstream when pathogens are present. Iodine fights infection and helps prevent disease. Kelp also helps soothe an irritated throat and inflamed mucous membranes. It quiets coughs, dissolves firm masses (such as tumors), reduces edema, and is used for enlarged thyroid, lymph nodes, swollen and painful testes, all of which may be caused by malfunction of the thyroid gland.

Kelp activates endocrine glands of the body and helps regulate the thyroid and pituitary glands. (Among other things, the pituitary gland helps adjust the body's core temperature). Kelp aids in the function of digestive glands and other endocrine organs and stimulates the pancreas and adrenals.

Taken in normal doses, kelp is a good nutritional source during pregnancy, because it normalizes glands and hormones and has a high mineral content. Preliminary tests in Japan indicate kelp may help prevent certain fetus abnormalities.

Immune System

Japanese studies show a direct relationship between the ingestion of algin (found in kelp) and the prevention of breast cancer. Researchers conclude this is due to both a mechanical function (fiber content of the kelp) and a biochemical action

	(ability to enhance immune system function). It is believed alginates improve T-cell function in the immune system.
Cleansing	Kelp neutralizes wastes from the body fluids so they may be easily eliminated from the body. It also helps lower serum cholesterol and hypertension, relieving the heart and blood vessels.
Inflammation	Uric acid contributes to rheumatic pain. Kelp has elements that help contain and eliminate uric acid from the body. Kelp helps relieve rheumatism and rheumatoid arthritis when it is used both internally and as an external application upon inflamed joints.
	Acidity and lack of essential nutrients for nerves and their insulating sheaths lead to inflammation and neuritis. Iodine acts as a tranquilizer and interrupts the cycle of disease-pain-aggravation, more disease-pain, and so on.
Nervous System	Kelp provides nutritional support to the nervous system and heart and is important in herbal combinations for improving mental alertness.
Digestion	Another quality of alginic acid is that it swells upon contact with water. When it is taken orally, it forms a type of 'guard' at the top of the stomach and, for this reason, is used in several over-the-counter preparations for heartburn. Alginates give kelp its mild laxative properties as well.
Genitourinary Tract	Kelp is used by Asian herbalists to treat genitourinary tract problems of the kidney, bladder, prostate, and uterus. Clinical documentation shows taking kelp daily reduces enlarged prostates in older men and urination becomes painless.
Women	Bladderwrack helps women with abnormal menstrual cycles or menstrual-related disease histories. Repeated small doses can decrease breast milk in nursing mothers.
	In one Japanese study, it was observed taking bladderwrack appears to regulate the menstrual cycle by increasing the length of the cycle, stimulating ovulation, and lowering the estrogen-progesterone ratio in pre-menopausal women. Such changes may be beneficial to women at high risk of estrogen-dependent diseases or who are experiencing fertility problems.
	Results also suggest bladderwrack may alleviate hypermenorrhea (excessive menstruation) and dysmenorrhea (painful or difficult menstruation), which may provide some relief in the treatment of endometriosis.

Radiation and Pollution	Studies at the Gastrointestinal Research Laboratories of McGill University in Montreal found a factor called sodium alginate in kelp that binds with radioactive strontium-90 in the intestines and carries it out of the body. This factor aids in detoxification of the intestines. Sodium alginate also binds and cleanses the body of barium and cadmium. Barium sulfate is used as a radio-contrast agent for X-rays of the digestive system and is normally eliminated through digestion. Barium in higher doses begins to adversely affect the nervous system. Small amounts of cadmium are found in foods, but it is more readily absorbed through the lungs. Air-born cadmium exposure comes from tobacco smoke and air pollution around hazardous waste sites, metal refining factories, and cadmium product manufacturing plants (batteries, coatings, and plastics). Inhaling cadmium-laden dust quickly leads to respiratory tract and kidney problems, which may be fatal (due to renal failure). Kelp also helps to reduce the risk of poisoning from environmental pollution by providing fiber that increases digestive bulk, reduces cholesterol levels, and retards bile acid absorption.
Herb Parts Used	The whole plant.
Preparations and Remedies	Most kelp is harvested wild from the oceans. Norwegian kelp is considered by some to be a cleaner source of kelp, as it comes from the cold North Sea which is freer of pollution than other sources. The plants are dried on screens then powdered and put into capsules and other herbal preparations. Kelp is most often used in combination with other herbs.)
Poultices	*Slippery Elm Poultice:* (see SLIPPERY ELM preparations)
Safety	No health hazards or adverse side effects are known. If kelp is not needed, headaches may occur. Kelp is better tolerated when taken with other herbs.
Plant Profile	*Natural Habitat:* Kelp is a plant of the sea and is found along rocky seashores almost everywhere in the world. It is particularly harvested on the North Sea, Western Baltic, Atlantic, and Pacific coasts.

Description

Laminaria digitata (true kelp) have strap-like blades that grow three to four feet long and float upward toward the water's surface and sunlight.

Fucus vesiculosus (bladderwrack) have fronds that are thick and flexible but very tough. It has a dark, glossy brown-green color that is paler at the extremities and turns black when dried. The flattened, branching fronds grow up to six feet in length, have an obvious midrib, and are covered with spherical air bladders which tend to occur in pairs on either side of the mid-rib (in small plants, air bladders may be entirely absent). Forked and pointed reproductive structures occur at the tips of the fronds. There are separate male and female plants, and reproduction takes place once a year.

The air bladders keep the fronds in illuminated waters where they are able to photosynthesize. In exposed areas, it is beneficial for the water plant to lack bladders, as this minimizes the potential for severe damage and the risk of being detached and swept away.

Both plants of the sea have an extremely tough, expanded woody root fiber with a disc called a holdfast that attaches itself to rocks. These water plants live for up to three years. They smell strongly seaweed-like and have a nauseous saline taste.

Licorice

Latin Name: *Glycyrrhiza glabra*

Also known as: Licorice Root, Sweet Wood, Sweet Root

Scientific Classification

Family:	Fabaceae – pea family
Genus:	Glycyrrhiza – licorice
Species:	G. glabra – cultivated licorice
	G. glandulifera – Russian licorice

Influence on the Body	(PRINCIPAL ACTIONS are listed in CAPITAL LETTERS)
Addictions	DRUG WITHDRAWAL • tobacco addiction
Blood and Circulatory System	BLOOD CLEANSER • arteriosclerosis • POOR CIRCULATION • CIRCULATORY SYSTEM • heart • dropsy (edema due to heart insufficiency) • hypertensive (increases blood pressure)
Blood Sugar	DIABETES • raises blood sugar • HYPERGLYCEMIA • HYPOGLYCEMIA
Body System	TONIC • VITALITY • ENDURANCE • ENERGY • mild stimulant (strengthens metabolism and circulation) • fatigue • adaptogen (increases resistance to stress) • chills • dizziness • longevity • age spots • senility • inflamed mucous membranes • DEMULCENT (softens and soothes inflammation of mucous membranes) • catarrh (inflamed and congested mucous membranes) • abscesses
Digestive Tract	food poisoning • ulcers • duodenal (small intestine) ulcers • bowel • heals and lubricates intestinal tract • constipation • aperient (mild laxative without purging) • hemorrhoids
Ears	EAR INFECTIONS
Endocrine System	ADRENAL GLAND EXHAUSTION • GLANDULAR TONIC (increases energy and strength to the adrenal glands) • ADDISON'S DISEASE (caused by adrenal gland insufficiency) • Cushing's disease (hyperfunction of adrenal gland cortex) • natural cortisone • pancreas

Infections and Immune System	COLDS • antiviral • antipyretic (cools the body, reduces fevers) • herpes
Inflammation	anti-inflammatory • arthritis
Liver	liver • hepatitis • cirrhosis
Lungs and Respiratory System	COUGHS • expectorant (loosens and removes phlegm in the respiratory tract) • SOOTHES THROAT • asthma • bronchitis • mucous congestion • LUNG PROBLEMS • pneumonia • emphysema (enlarged air spaces in the lungs) • pectoral (healing to problems in the bronchio pulmonary area)
Mouth, Nose and Throat	sialagogue (promotes an increase flow of saliva) • SORE THROAT • VOICE • laryngitis • HOARSENESS • EXPELS PHLEGM
Reproductive System	SEXUAL STIMULANT • APHRODISIAC (stimulates sexual desire) • impotency • gonorrhea *Female:* FEMALE PROBLEMS • LOW ESTROGEN • menopause
Skin, Tissues and Hair	sores • emollient (softens and soothes skin when applied externally) • dermatitis
Urinary Tract	kidneys • bladder • diuretic (increases urine flow)
Other Uses	enhances properties of other herb combinations • sugar substitute • flavoring • covers taste of bitter herbs • coating for pills

Key Properties:

SUSTAINS ADRENAL FUNCTION	*stimulates and supports adrenal glands without depletion, raises blood sugar levels, boosts energy*
DEMULCENT	*softens and soothes inflammation of mucous membranes, loosens and removes phlegm*
SWEETNESS **natural cortisone hormonal properties**	*exhibits anti-inflammatory qualities*
Primarily affecting	ADRENAL GLANDS • MUCOUS MEMBRANES • LUNGS • STOMACH

History

Licorice use was first documented on Assyrian clay tablets (ca. 2500 BC) and Egyptian papyri. Ancient Arabs used licorice to treat coughs and relieve constipation. Indian Ayurvedic traditional medicine has a long history of using licorice as an expectorant, anti-inflammatory, and laxative.

Dioscorides, a first-century Greek physician, coined a name that was later developed into the genus name 'glycyrrhiza', derived from the Greek words 'glukos' for sweet and 'riza' for root. The Roman name 'gliquiricia' became 'liquiritia' and evolved further into the more common name licorice.

Theophrastus, an ancient Greek physician and botanist (ca. 371-286 BC), documented the use of licorice to assist with coughs and asthma.

Alexander the Great (ca. 356-323 BC) supplied his troops with rations that included licorice root. They could chew on the root in battle to alleviate thirst, increase stamina, and cleanse the eyes.

Licorice was prescribed by early physicians from the time of Hippocrates (ca. 460-370 BC) in cases of dropsy and to prevent thirst.

Since 25 AD, the Chinese have used the herb extensively to relieve and prevent coughs and as an expectorant. It also relieves spasms of the smooth (involuntary) muscles and exhibits a cortisone-like action. Licorice is included in most Chinese formulas to 'harmonize' the herbs.

Culpepper, the English botanist, herbalist, and physician (ca. 1616-1654) wrote of licorice, it 'helps the roughness of the windpipe, hoarseness, diseases in the kidneys and bladder, and ulcers in the bladder. It concocts raw humours in the stomach, helps difficulty of breathing, and is profitable for all salt humours.'

The German Commission E (first instituted in 1978) approved licorice root for inflammations of the upper respiratory tract and stomach ulcers.

My first memory of the wonderful healing abilities of licorice is when my father would eat it to relieve his stomach disorders. At the time, he didn't know it was healing his stomach. He just craved it. Later on, he noticed he didn't need his stomach medications any longer. This is just another testament to follow your body!

Attributes	Key Components: (including, but not limited to)
Nutrients	Vitamins B1 (thiamine) • B2 (riboflavin) • B3 (niacin) • B5 (pantothenic acid) • B6 (pyridoxine) • B9 (folic acid) • B12 (cobalamin) • Biotin • Choline • Inositol • PABA (Para-Amino Benzoic Acid) • E • Calcium • Chromium • Magnesium • Manganese • Zinc • Glycyrrhizin (has a sweet taste and cortisone-like activity) • Phytosterols (has some hormone activity) Glycyrrhizin is an active ingredient of licorice that has anti-inflammatory, cough-suppressant, antiviral, estrogen-like, and aldosterone-like qualities.
Adrenals	Studies have shown glycyrrhizin stimulates the excretion of cortisone and aldosterone without depleting the adrenal glands. Glycyrrhizin is similar in structure to cortisone (a hormone naturally released by the body as a reaction to stress which prepares the body for a fight or flight response). It helps the body handle stress, increases blood-sugar levels, elevates blood pressure, and gives a general feeling of well-being. Licorice is one of the best-known herbs used for hypoglycemia. Studies indicate licorice may help reduce body fat.
Digestion	Licorice is a useful demulcent and anti-inflammatory for treating irritated mucous membranes of the stomach and duodenum. When ulcers occur in these structures, licorice stimulates repair and regeneration of damaged tissues. Controlled clinical studies show glycyrrhizin acid and its derivatives accelerate the healing of gastric ulcers. In the 1950's, new research showed licorice-derived compounds can raise the concentration of prostaglandins in the digestive system that promote mucous secretion from the stomach and produce new cells in the stomach lining. A recent study from Iran used licorice-coated aspirin and found the licorice helped protect against ulcers irritated by aspirin use and reduced the size and number of ulcers. Licorice is a mild laxative that is safe and effective for delicate individuals with weak stomachs and children who are constipated and unable to take stronger laxatives. It softens, soothes, lubricates, and nourishes the intestinal tract.

Licorice is especially valuable for persons suffering with hemorrhoids, as softer stools diminish the discomfort accompanied by bowel movements. It is very effective for helping the body rid itself of hemorrhoids. Licorice is a corrective agent for stronger laxatives, modifying their action. It soothes and heals inflamed mucous membranes and catarrhal conditions of the bowel, kidneys, and bladder.

Sweet

Glycyrrhizin acid is 50 times sweeter than sugar cane and may safely be taken by diabetic patients. The dried roots may be chewed like candy. Glycyrrhizin has an agreeable taste, alleviates thirst, and soothes the throat.

Licorice is one of the few substances that is both naturally sweet and relieves thirst. Most sweets do the opposite. It is probably not the sweetness that affects thirst, but the 'bitter' which remains once the licorice juice is thoroughly chewed. The slightly bitter element stimulates the salivary glands and relieves thirst.

Respiratory Tract

Licorice relieves the discomfort of canker and mouth sores. The tea is used for laryngitis and will restore injured voice muscles, improving hoarseness and throat damage. Combined with other herbs, licorice is used for wheezing, shortness of breath, and pains of the chest and lungs.

Licorice is very soothing. It softens mucous membranes of the respiratory tract and cleanses them of catarrhal congestion. Licorice root reduces irritation of mucous surfaces, is useful for coughs and sore throats, and helps to loosen and bring up phlegm. It is often used in cough syrups and cough drops.

Immunity

Licorice stimulates production of interferons (glycoproteins) in response to the presence of viral infection. Interferons assist the immune response by inhibiting viral replication within host cells, activating the body's natural killer cells and macrophages, increasing antigen presentation to lymphocytes, and inducing resistance of host cells to viral infection.

Licorice is excellent for flu, colds, and lung congestion. For its antiviral activity and soothing qualities, it is often added to cough syrups and lozenges for both children and adults.

Liver

Glycyrrhizin acid is used in the treatment of viral liver inflammation. By inducing interferon activity, it works as an antiviral agent and helps protect the liver from diseases such as hepatitis and cirrhosis.

Inflammation	Licorice root exhibits substantial anti-inflammatory activity. The herb helps relieve arthritis by inducing the adrenal glands to release inflammation-soothing corticosteroids. Creams containing whole licorice (often combined with chamomile extract) are used for eczema, psoriasis, and herpes. One study suggests topical application of licorice extract may be effective in treating the itching and inflammation associated with dermatitis.
Women	Licorice contains phytosterols that facilitate estrogen production and help normalize ovulation in women experiencing infrequent menstruation.
	Studies indicate substances within licorice inhibit serotonin (a neurotransmitter) elimination and may be useful in the treatment of mild to moderate depression in women.
Circulation	Licorice affects the concentration of blood salts and minerals and strengthens the heart and circulatory system. Studies indicate dietary consumption of licorice root extract may help lower cholesterol and act as an antioxidant.
Commercial Uses	Licorice is added to candy, cakes, ice cream, and packaged desserts. Licorice candy sold in the United States is usually a synthetic-flavored licorice or combined with anise (a similar strong-flavored herb), but there are still a few brands that are based on true licorice. Much of the natural licorice imported to the United States today is used to flavor tobacco products.
	Licorice sticks consist of fresh or dried sections of licorice root that may be chewed. They are often used to help curb tobacco addiction by helping to discharge mucus from the upper respiratory tract and providing a tactile stimulus of having something to hold and chew.
	Because of its absorbent qualities, powdered licorice root is useful in pill making. It stiffens the pill mass and helps to prevent adhesion of pills to each other.
Herb Parts Used	Peeled or unpeeled dried roots, rhizome (underground stem), and root runners
Preparations and Remedies	Licorice root extract is used in cough drops, lozenges, nicotine lozenges, syrups, and laxatives. It is added to foods and other herbal combinations to sweeten and flavor them. The root is added to teas and may be purchased dried, sliced, or powdered.

In the powdered form, it is put into capsules, tablets, and tinctures for medicinal use.

DGL

Deglycyrrhizinated licorice (DGL) is a licorice preparation with the glycyrrhizin removed. However, it is not clear if DGL provides the same health benefits as whole licorice. I believe the Maker of licorice knew what He was doing!

Capsules

Allergies:
Take two capsules licorice root three times a day plus powdered, above-ground coral and Redmond clay to heal the stubborn hay fever problems. When the blood is clean and the adrenal glands are strong, there is less possibility of allergies or hay fever.

Powder

Mild Laxative:
Licorice powder taken internally will free and soften stools without griping, usually in 3-15 hours (3-6 hours if taken on an empty stomach). It is best given at bedtime. Take 1-2 teaspoonfuls of licorice powder daily for constipation, hemorrhoids, adrenal gland rejuvenation, blood sugar regulation, and (as needed) during pregnancy.

Extracts

Some people believe liquid extracts of licorice are incompatible with acid and should not be taken in citric juices.

Infusion

An infusion is made by boiling one ounce of the bruised root with a pint of water for a few minutes. The tea may be used for sore throats and in catarrhal conditions of the urinary and intestinal tracts.

In preparing an infusion for the purpose of sweetening or hiding the taste of other preparations, it should not be boiled over five minutes. When licorice is boiled any longer, its acrid, bitter-tasting resin is released into the infusion, and it is less palatable (though it still retains its healing qualities).

Yarrow Tea: (see YARROW preparations)
Liver / Jaundice Tonic: (see DANDELION preparations)

System Cleanse Tea: (see CHAPARRAL preparations)

Syrup

Laxative Syrup:
4 ounces Licorice root, cut or powdered
1 quart Distilled Water
8 ounces Honey

	Stir the herb into water while cold. Cover and soak overnight (or for at least 8 hours). Stir and bring to a slow boil. After boiling slowly for 20 minutes, strain and return liquid to a clean vessel. Bring to a boil again and stir in raw honey until dissolved. Remove from heat and allow it to cool, stirring occasionally. Take 1 tablespoonful or more, 3-4 times daily (regulate dosage according to bowel movements). Reduce child dose to 1-3 teaspoonfuls taken 2-3 times daily (according to need and size of child). *Syrup for Persistent and Irritated Cough:* 2 ounce cut Licorice root, or 1 ounce powdered 4 ounces ground Flaxseed 1 quart Water 1 tablespoon fresh lemon juice 1 tablespoon raw honey Simmer licorice and flaxseed in water until it reaches syrup consistency. Strain and add lemon juice and honey. Give freely warm or cold. Children may take up to four ounces a day for persistent and irritated coughs from chest colds. It will cause sweating and loosen the cough.
Ointment	*Skin Ointment:* Make an ointment for eczema, psoriasis, and redness of the skin by adding licorice extract to the goldenseal and myrrh salve (see GOLDENSEAL preparations) or adding to pure aloe vera gel.
Safety	No health hazards or adverse side effects are known. German health authorities recommend licorice not be used for more than four to six weeks at a time. German and French health agencies further suggest licorice not be used without the advice of a health care provider in cases of high blood pressure, potassium deficiency, or chronic liver inflammation and liver cirrhosis. Side effects are very rare when using whole licorice preparations (as compared to the isolated glycyrrhizin licorice products). Potassium-rich foods (like bananas and dried apricots) may be eaten while taking licorice to counter possible potassium loss.

Plant Profile

Natural Habitat:
Indigenous to Spain, Southern Italy, Greece, Asia Minor, Syria, Iraq, Russia, and Northern China, licorice is now widely cultivated throughout many parts of the world, including North America.

The plant grows best in sandy soil near streams and is rarely found in the wild more than 150 feet from a body of water. The plant succeeds better in a warm climate. Licorice cannot endure severe freezing. Cool weather interferes with the formation of its juices and renders it woody.

Description

Licorice is a perennial herb (tops of plant usually die back to the ground in the winter and grow again in the spring from a persistent rootstock) with woody stalks rising two to five feet in height, on which are set many long, narrow, green leaves on both sides with an odd leaf at the end. The plant can have many pale blue to light purple, pea-like flowers, one above another on the stalk. These turn into long, smooth, somewhat flat, tubular fruit containing one to six kidney-shaped, hard seeds.

The plant has a cylindrical taproot that runs to a considerable depth. It is grayish-brown externally and yellow inside and is succulent, tough, flexible, rapid in growth, and divides into three to five subsidiary roots and several horizontal woody stolons (underground stems). The roots and stolons are the most commonly used parts of the plant and may be harvested after three to four years of growth. The root has a peculiar earthy odor and a strong, characteristic, sweet taste.

Commercially, there are basically five grades, preferred in this order: Italian (best and sweetest), Spanish (or common licorice root), Syrian, Turkish, and Russian (the most bitter).

Growing Licorice

Planting:
Licorice prefers full sun and dry, alkaline, sandy soils. Plant in the fall or stratify seeds (chill in the refrigerator for 30 days) before sowing. Root cuttings may be planted in rows 4 feet apart (roots need space to spread). Thin or transplant seedlings 2-3 feet apart.

Harvesting

During the first two years, growth is slight. Plants do not rise above a foot the first season. The roots are not ready for harvest until the end of the third season but are sweeter still in the fourth season. Harvesting generally occurs in the autumn of the fourth

LICORICE — 229

year, preferably before the plant bears fruit, as it exhausts the sweetness of the sap. The same ground yields a crop every three or four years. After the fourth year, the texture of the root begins to take on a tough, coarse, and woody character.

Commercial harvesting is done by removing two to three feet of earth. This exposes the subterranean portion of the herb and allows the whole plant to be easily uprooted. Roots are severed, cleaned, washed, trimmed, sorted (older or 'hard' runners are sold, while the young 'soft' runners are reserved for replanting), cut, and marketed in bundles, bales, and bags.

When washed, fresh licorice root is externally a bright, yellowish brown. It is very flexible, easily cut with a knife, and has a light-yellow, juicy, internal substance. Both bark and wood are extremely tough, readily tearing into long, fibrous strings.

Lobelia

Latin Name: *Lobelia inflata*

Also known as: Indian Tobacco, Wild Tobacco, Asthma Weed, Pukeweed, Vomitwort, Bladderpod, Eyebright

Scientific Classification

Lobelia is a genus containing 350 species, many of them indigenous to America

Family:	Campanulaceae – bellflower family
Genus	Lobelia – lobelia
Species	L. inflata – Indian-tobacco
	Other lobelia species with medicinal qualities: Great Blue Lobelia (*L. siphilitica*) Pale-Spike Lobelia (*L. spicata*) Kalm's Lobelia (*L. kalmii*) Cardinal Flower (*L. cardinalis*)

Influence on the Body	**(PRINCIPAL ACTIONS are listed in CAPITAL LETTERS)**
Addictions	smoking • drugs • alcohol
Blood and Circulatory System	circulation • blood poisoning • BLOOD VESSELS • heart • heart palpitations • angina (chest pains)
Blood Sugar	Hypoglycemia
Body System	CATARRH • GENERAL CONGESTION • cleansing • mucous membranes • astringent (tightens, constricts and tones tissues) • HYPERACTIVITY • PAIN • analgesic (relieves pain) • PROMOTES SLEEP • INSOMNIA • sedative (calming, soothing, or tranquilizing) • relaxant (in larger doses) • stimulant (in small doses)
Bones and Teeth	TEETHING • TOOTHACHE • periostitis (inflammation or infection of the tissue covering bones)
Cancer	Tumors
Digestive Tract	digestive disorders • emetic (causes vomiting) • FOOD POISONING (as an emetic) • nervous dyspepsia (indigestion) • constipation • colic • small intestines • dysentery (large bowel inflammation and pain) • peritonitis (infection of the abdominal

	lining 'peritoneum') • cathartic • EXPELS WORMS
Ears	EARACHE • EAR INFECTIONS
Eyes	ophthalmia (eye inflammation)
First Aid	bruises • open wounds • cell rejuvenation • sprains • bites and stings • poison ivy • antivenomous • shock
Infections and Immune System	ALLERGIES • hay fever • COLDS • COUGHS • FEVERS • cold sweats • CHILDHOOD DISEASES • CONTAGIOUS DISEASES • CHICKEN POX • MUMPS • measles • ringworm • LOCK JAW (tetanus) • rheumatic fever • scarlet fever • diphtheria • WHOOPING COUGH • spinal meningitis • meningitis
Inflammation	ARTHRITIS • rheumatism • bursitis
Liver	liver • jaundice • HEPATITIS (heals and strengthens)
Lungs and Respiratory System	respiratory stimulant • esophagus • larynx • BRONCHITIS • bronchial spasms • bronchial asthma • ACUTE ASTHMA ATTACK • CROUP • EMPHYSEMA • LUNG PROBLEMS • PLEURISY • PNEUMONIA • EXPECTORANT (loosens and removes phlegm in the respiratory tract)
Mouth, Nose and Throat	CANKER SORES • hoarseness • laryngitis • tonsillitis
Muscles	MUSCLE SPASMS • cramps
Nervous System	CONVULSIONS • SPASMS • SEIZURES • EPILEPSY • palsy • St. Vitus' Dance • chorea (a nervous disease characterized by involuntary movements) • NERVE RELAXANT • neuralgia (sharp, stabbing pains due to deposits or congestion putting pressure on nerves) • HEADACHES • MIGRAINE HEADACHES • delirium • hysteria
Reproductive System	*Female:* MISCARRIAGE • emmenagogue (promotes menstrual flow)
Skin, Tissues and Hair	boils • felons (type of abscess) • eczema • skin infections • diaphoretic (promotes perspiration, increasing elimination through the skin) • scar tissue
Urinary Tract	urinary problems • diuretic (increases urine flow) • nephritis (kidney inflammation)

LOBELIA — 232

Key Properties:

ANTISPASMODIC NERVINE	*sedates and relaxes the body, relieves discomfort, improves nerve function*
EMETIC	*causes vomiting in large doses, expelling poisons and toxins out of the body*
RESPIRATORY STIMULANT and expectorant	*Relaxes and opens bronchioles, facilitates easier breathing, loosens and expels phlegm from the respiratory pathway*
Primarily affecting	NERVES • LUNGS • STOMACH • MUSCLES • CIRCULATION

History	Native Americans smoked lobelia leaves to stop asthma and bronchitis spasms and to ease breathing. Chewing the leaves soothed sore throats and coughs. Poultices were made from fresh leaves and roots to relieve body aches, soothe skin irritations, and heal sores. Lobelia was used to induce vomiting and treat infant colic.
	At least four other lobelia species were used medicinally by early Native Americans. Red Lobelia was used for syphilis and expelling worms. The Shoshones made a tea of lobelia for use as an emetic and physic. Native Americans introduced lobelia to European settlers.
	The herbalist Samuel Thomson (ca. 1769-1843) founded the alternative system of medicine that became known as 'Thomsonian Medicine.' It enjoyed wide popularity in the United States during the 19th century. Dr. Thomson championed lobelia use for emesis therapy (induced vomiting to purge toxins out of the stomach), as a muscle relaxant during childbirth, and as a poultice for healing abscesses. He believed lobelia was the most powerful herb that existed for removing disease and congestion, cleansing the body and promoting health.
	Dr. Thomson wrote of making a tincture using the ground-up, fresh herb and vinegar:
	> "This preparation is for the most violent attacks of disease, such as lockjaw, bite of mad dog, drowned persons, fits, spasms, and all cases of suspended animation, where the

vital spark is nearly extinct. It will not work in two cases: when the patient is dying, and when there is no disease. It clears all obstructions to the extremities and will be felt in the fingers and toes, producing a prickling feeling. It soon exhausts itself and, if not followed by some other medicine to hold the vital heat till nature is able to support itself by digesting food, it will not be sufficient to remove disease that has become seated..."

Dr. Thomson further recommended using cayenne tincture in conjunction with lobelia tincture 'to retain the internal vital heat of the system and cause a free perspiration.'

Lobelia was added to the pharmacopoeia of American herbalist physicians in the late 1700's. It was used for healing ulcers and treating dysentery, epilepsy, and respiratory diseases.

Our family's experience with this wonderful herb has been nothing short of amazing. I originally made this oil for my sore, pregnant belly. My husband would rub it on my tummy and it eased my discomfort. Remarkably enough, all of my old stretch marks seemed to disappear. We use what we call 'Lobelia oil' for just about everything. My fondest memories are when my children would ask me to rub 'Yobellia Oil' on their upset tummies, or when my husband would rub this oil on our nursing babies' feet to soothe them while I was away.

I remember when a friend carried his ailing wife into our home to see if I could help her get relief from severe discomfort in her swollen ankles. She couldn't even walk. I rubbed her feet and ankles with lobelia oil, and she was able to walk by the time she left our home. We have seen old and new scars dramatically lighten or disappear completely, tight muscles loosen up, and discomfort go away. We have also had lots of experience in helping lung issues to heal. Lobelia will always be in our family's cupboard.

Attributes	**Key Components: (including, but not limited to)**
Nutrients	Calcium • Cobalt • Copper • Iron • Potassium • Selenium • Sodium • Sulfur • other Trace Minerals • Lobeline (an alkaloid which is the main active ingredient in lobelia)

General	Many authorities consider lobelia to be the most important of all herbs. The proper use of lobelia can help alleviate an acute asthma attack and ease difficult breathing. It is useful in emergency cases of electrical shock, sunstroke, and heatstroke. It can force vomiting when the body is poisoned with narcotics, bad food, medicine, carbon monoxide, and infections. It has also been noted lobelia enhances pituitary function.
	In small doses, lobelia acts as a tonic and stimulant. In larger doses, it acts as a sedative relaxant. Large doses will also induce vomiting. It is a catalytic herb, energizing the body's ability to heal itself as needed. It resets the nervous system, opens up passages, and clears long-standing blockages.
	Lobelia's effect on the body can last for hours but, more likely, will fade out after 10-20 minutes. Using stimulant herbs such as cayenne or peppermint extends lobelia's effects.
	Copious amounts of water need to be taken with lobelia to aid the body in the elimination of drug-induced and metabolic toxic wastes.
Antispasmodic and Relaxant	Lobelia is a powerful nervine and antispasmodic. It can cause immediate relaxation and expansion of constricted parts of the respiratory system. This allows for the return of normal breathing and the flow of oxygen to exhausted tissues.
	Lobelia is considered the strongest relaxant in the herb kingdom. It has been successfully used to help relax the muscles in lockjaw. It is excellent for spasms, cramps, epilepsy, hysteria, chorea, tetanus, and convulsions.
	NOTE: Large doses will completely relax the entire body so even the smallest muscles cannot be used temporarily. In rare cases, people who are sensitive to lobelia's effects, or who are in a weak condition, may become over-relaxed and sleepy when using lobelia. This effect can be balanced by taking lobelia with cayenne.
	Keep lobelia tincture on hand for use in convulsions. It can be rubbed on the body, or drops may be put in the mouth, and the body will immediately absorb it and react to it.
	Rubbing a few drops of lobelia tincture or oil on the shoulders of a

restless child is an excellent way to help him/her calm down and go to sleep. Lobelia also helps relax the mother during delivery and speeds up the delivery of the placenta.

Heart and Circulation

Lobelia in small doses will relax the heart, lower a rapid pulse rate, and reduce palpitations of the heart. Lobelia is effective in removing obstruction and congestion within the body, especially the blood vessels. If blood flow through the vessels is depressed, lobelia works to correct the problem by strengthening muscular action of the vessel walls which propel blood forward.

Respiratory System

Lobelia is used internally in small doses for spasmodic lung and respiratory conditions. Lobelia first stimulates the nerves that go to the internal organs, then depresses and relaxes them. As lobelia depresses the nerve centers, the bronchial muscles relax, and the bronchioles dilate. This opens the bronchial tubes, esophagus, glottis (vocal cords), and larynx and allows for easier breathing.

Lobelia is used in this way for helping treat bronchitis, asthma, and croup. It is often added to cough medicines, as it loosens phlegm and can cause an impressive expulsion of thick, ropey mucus from sinuses and bronchi. Lobelia's stimulating effect on the respiratory system is quick, then it passes, diffusing throughout the body.

Nicotine Addiction

Lobelia has been used in lozenges, patches, chewing gums, and even smoked to relieve nicotine cravings. Research has shown lobeline has some of the same effects as nicotine in a milder, non-addictive form. It competes with nicotine for receptor sites in the body. Smokers may require more lobelia to get the same medicinal effects as non-smokers. Lobelia decreases the addictive need for tobacco, and its lobeline salts make nicotine taste bad when smoking normal cigarettes.

FDA Ruling:
In 1993, the U.S. Food and Drug Administration (FDA) prohibited the sale of lobeline-containing smoking products in the United States. The FDA reported such products lacked effectiveness in helping people quit or reduce smoking. However, other countries still use lobeline in smoking-reduction preparations.

Digestion

In the digestive tract, lobelia suppresses the appetite and increases peristaltic (intestinal) movement.

Emetic

In large doses, lobelia is an excellent emetic. Emesis is a therapy that induces vomiting. In many situations, it is better to cause vomiting to get the poison quickly up and out of the stomach. Digestion through the intestines could take days for some pathogens, allowing time to release its toxins into the blood (causing fevers and other symptoms) until finally expelled.

Emesis therapy is indicated when there is a feeling of nausea caused by bad food combinations, food or drug poisoning, and excessive mucus buildup in asthma, sinus congestion, or food allergies. Capsicum is often added to flush poisons from the stomach and bowels.

Much has been written regarding whether lobelia is poisonous, but experience suggests it is an antidote that purges poison from the body. It not only cleanses the stomach but exercises a beneficial influence over every part of the body.

Emesis therapy is for singular situations and not to be used on a regular basis. Habitual vomiting unbalances normal processes of the body and can be life threatening.

Infections and Fevers

Lobelia is not to be used continuously. The intent of use is to clean out, clean up, and keep clean the areas of congestion and infection.

Lobelia helps reduce fevers caused by infectious diseases. It induces perspiration and urine flow. Catnip and lobelia enemas are good for mumps as well as other infectious diseases.

External Uses

Lobelia tea may be used as a wash to help clear eyes in cases of ophthalmia or for infected or itchy skin rashes. Lobelia extract is good to rub on gums of a teething baby to relieve swelling, inflammation, and discomfort.

An extract of lobelia in extra-virgin olive oil is soothing and helpful when used topically. It can relax tight muscles, calm arthritic conditions, upset tummies, nausea, fussy babies, and soften and heal the skin (including acne and scar tissue). A poultice of lobelia soothes inflammations, rheumatism, ringworm, bruises, and insect bites. A natural soap poultice with slippery elm and lobelia added to it may be used to bring abscesses or boils to a

	head. Add lobelia to liniments for sore muscles, pains, and rheumatism.
Herb Parts Used	The whole plant (fresh or dried) and seeds are used medicinally. The root and inflated seed capsules are the most powerful. The seeds contain more lobeline than the rest of the plant.
Preparations and Remedies	Give lobelia in small quantities, as needed, to clean out waste material and relieve locked-up conditions of the body. When administered internally, it is used for acute, singular conditions, rather than for long-term use.
Powdered Formula	*Kidney Formula:* (see JUNIPER preparations) *Infection Formula:* (see GOLDENSEAL preparations)
Infusions	*Lobelia Tea:* 1 ounce Lobelia 1 pint boiling Water Steep for 10 minutes. Take lobelia tea in tablespoonful doses every hour or half-hour. A weak infusion given in teaspoonful doses every 10 minutes will thoroughly relax the muscular system.
Tincture	*Tincture of Lobelia:* 4 ounces Lobelia herb, stem, flowers, seeds or leaves 1 pint Raw Apple Cider Vinegar or Vodka (use alcohol for emergency first aid kits for external use). Macerate (soak to soften and release constituents) in a tightly capped bottle for 10-14 days. Shake every time you walk by, or at least once a day. Strain off the liquid and bottle it for use. *Neuralgia:* Using 10-40 drops of lobelia tincture in warm water (or in a good nervine tea) is a specific for neuralgia. *Massage:* Use tincture of lobelia to massage externally onto the afflicted area and take two or three drops internally at regular intervals until difficulty is resolved.

	Breathing Easy:
	2-5 drops (you may use up to 10 drops with caution) of lobelia tincture on the tongue will relax muscles in the throat and open bronchiole tubes.
	Baby Convulsions:
	Place a drop or two of the tincture on the tip of the finger and put it into the baby's mouth. This can help stop the problem immediately.
	Earache:
	Place a few drops of warm lobelia tincture or oil extract in the ear and plug it with cotton.
Fomentations	*Respiratory Fomentation:* (see MULLEIN preparation)
	Soothing Fomentation for Pains, Sprains, and Rheumatism:
	2 parts Ginger root
	1 part Slippery Elm
	1 part Cayenne
	1 part Lobelia
	Soak cloth with warm infusion and apply to affected area.
Poultices and Plasters	Lobelia tincture added to poultices and plasters sedates and relaxes the affected area and eases pain.
	Poultice for Boils and Abscesses:
	(see ECHINACEA preparations)
Salves	A salve or tincture of lobelia, along with other soothing barks and roots such as slippery elm bark, comfrey, and aloe, may be employed for inflammations, swellings, and discomfort (see COMFREY preparations for directions on how to make a salve formula).
Emesis Therapy	*Emesis (induced vomiting):*
	Take 1 teaspoon lobelia tincture every 10 minutes until vomiting is induced. Follow this therapy with several warm cups of peppermint or spearmint tea to soothe and relax the stomach.
	After vomiting (followed by a mint tea), fevers will usually reduce, and organ functions will return to normal. This therapy reduces

body energy and should not be used in weak, debilitated conditions, severe hypertension, or when hemorrhaging.

Emesis therapy is used in response to a toxic condition of the body and is not to be used on a regular basis.

Safety	Lobelia is powerful and effective in low doses. Getting to know the proper use of lobelia can be tricky, but it is well worth the trouble to have the knowledge and use of this valuable herb.

No health hazards or adverse side effects are known with proper dosages. Lobelia overdose is possible. To avoid the chance of overdose, internal preparations of lobelia are often mixed with other herbs and always taken with lots of water.

A dose of straight lobelia should usually be diluted in at least one full cup of water before ingestion. Lobelia may be used in tincture form directly under the tongue for emergencies. Large doses of lobelia may temporarily affect the heart muscle. Those suffering from a weak heart or heart disease should avoid emesis therapy.

Internal lobelia preparations should not be taken during pregnancy unless guided by a health-care provider that is familiar with this herb. Lobelia can help mothers-to-be avoid miscarriage and may be used during labor as a relaxant. Do not overuse, as large doses may cause nausea and vomiting.

Early physicians in the 1800's are said to have been jealous of Dr. Thomson's success and speedy results with his patients using lobelia. Even though there had never been a study proving it to be so, lobelia was labeled as a poison in official works of the day, such as the U.S. Pharmacopoeia and the American Dispensatory. |
| **Plant Profile** | *Natural Habitat:*
Indigenous to North America, lobelia grows wild in most sections of the United States. It is found in meadows, pastures, woods, and grassy places in Canada and the United States, and it is cultivated in Russia and India. |
| *Description* | This type of lobelia is not to be confused with the bright blue, low-growing ground cover that is popular in landscapes across America. |

The herb lobelia is an annual (must grow from seed every year) in warm latitudes and a biennial (must grow from seed at least every two years) in moderate and northern latitudes.

Lobelia has a fibrous root. The plant grows 1-3 feet with erect, angular, very hairy, and highly branched stems that have a milky sap. Lobelia has soft, pointed leaves (1-3 inches long) and loose terminal spikes of small and numerous pale-blue flowers (red, yellow, white, or blue in other species) from July to November.

Lobelia flowers give way to characteristic 'inflated' seedpods, two-celled puffy capsules (hence the species name 'inflata') housing numerous, small, brown-black-colored seeds.

Lobelia has a faint, irritating odor. When it is chewed, it doesn't have much flavor at first. It then produces a burning acrid taste, very closely resembling that of tobacco. It causes saliva to flow and produces an overall nauseating effect. However, lobelia is not related to tobacco and does not contain nicotine or other poisonous properties.

Growing Lobelia

Planting:
Lobelia plants prefer part to full sun, rich, acid soil, and plenty of water. Seeds are sown in spring or fall. Average germination time in warm soils is one to three weeks. Water very gently. In the wild, lobelia germinates in the fall, and the low-lying rosette (leaves) overwinters. The plant then flowers and goes to seed in the spring to early summer. When seed is planted and grown as a spring annual, it usually flowers early (once the soil warms) and gives very little yield.

Harvesting

The plant is best harvested in the green seedpod stage, usually from the end of July to the middle of October.

Storage

The plant should be dried in the shade and then preserved in covered containers, especially if reduced to powder.

Lobelia should never be stored in paper, as both the herb and the seeds contain a volatile oil that can be readily absorbed by the paper and lost. Potency of the herb deteriorates rapidly after drying, yet it is still very effective when dried and stored properly.

Milk Thistle

Latin Name: *Silybum marianum*

Also known as: Our Lady's Thistle, Marian Thistle, St. Mary's Thistle, Holy Thistle, Silybin

Scientific Classification
Only two species are currently classified in this genus

Family: Asteraceae – aster, daisy and sunflower family

Genus Silybum – milk thistle

Species S. marianum – blessed milk thistle

Influence on the Body	(PRINCIPAL ACTIONS are listed in CAPITAL LETTERS)
Blood and Circulatory System	heart problems • high blood pressure • varicose veins • hemorrhage
Blood Sugar	hypoglycemia • diabetes
Body System	Stimulant / tonic • depression • demulcent (softens and soothes inflammation of mucous membranes) • protects against chemotherapy
Digestive Tract	appetite stimulant • heartburn • indigestion • gas
Infections and Immune System	cholera • spleen congestion
Liver and Gallbladder	LIVER CONGESTION • LIVER DAMAGE • CIRRHOSIS (hardening of the liver) • alcoholism • fatty deposits • HEPATITIS • JAUNDICE • cholestasis (suppression of bile flow) • cholagogue (promotes the flow of bile) • gallbladder
Nervous System	convulsions • epilepsy • delirium • nervous conditions
Poisons	toxic poisons • snake bites • radiation
Reproductive System	*Female:* promotes lactation • galactagogue (enhances lactation of nursing mothers) • suppresses menstruation
Skin, Tissues and Hair	boils • skin diseases
Urinary Tract	KIDNEY CONGESTION

Key Properties:

HEPATIC	*supports and stimulates the liver, gallbladder, and spleen, increases the flow of bile*
Nervine	*improves nerve function*
stimulant / tonic	*increases internal heat, dispels chill, increases energy, strengthens metabolism and circulation*
Primarily affecting	LIVER • GALLBLADDER • KIDNEYS

History	According to tradition, the milk-white veins of the leaves of the plant came from the milk of the Virgin Mary, which fell upon the thistle plant and stained it forever more. Milk thistle thus became known as Our Lady's Thistle, St. Mary's Thistle, Holy Thistle, and other similar names.
	Pliny the Elder (23-79 AD), a Roman naturalist and philosopher, reported the juice of the plant mixed with honey was excellent for 'carrying off bile.' The Greek herbalist Dioscorides (ca. 40-90 AD) believed 'the seeds being drunk are a remedy for infants that have their sinews drawn together, and for those that be bitten of serpents.'
	It is recorded in old Saxon remedies 'this wort [plant], if hung upon a man's neck, it setteth snakes to flight.' By the Middle Ages, herbalists were using milk thistle to treat depression and other 'melancholy'. In 1597, Gerard, a prominent herbalist, wrote of this aspect. The word melancholy is taken from the Greek meaning 'black bile' and, in Gerard's day, it referred to any liver or biliary malady.
	Milk thistle was quite popular as a food, and almost all parts of it were eaten. The roots were eaten raw, boiled, and buttered, or parboiled and roasted. In spring, the young shoots were cut down to the root, then boiled and buttered. The spiny leaves on the flower head were eaten like globe artichoke, and the stems (after peeling) were soaked overnight to remove bitterness, then stewed. The leaves (trimmed of their spines) were boiled (which made a good spinach substitute) or added raw to salads.
	Nicholas Culpeper, English botanist, herbalist, physician, and astrologer (1616-1654), recommended the infusion of the fresh

root and seeds for jaundice, breaking and expelling stone, and dropsy when taken internally. In addition, the infusion was to be applied with cloths externally to the liver and the young leaves eaten in the spring as a blood cleanser. He also considered milk thistle to be efficient in preventing and curing the plague.

Today, milk thistle is used to protect and strengthen the liver. In 1986, Germany's Commission E approved an oral extract of milk thistle as a treatment for liver diseases.

Attributes	**Key Components:** (including, but not limited to)
Nutrients	Vitamin E Bitter • Mucilage • Silymarin Complex including the group of flavonoids: Silybinin • Silidianin • Silicristin Silymarin is the active component in milk thistle found principally on the inner seed coat.
Functions of the Liver	Milk thistle protects and supports the liver. By so doing, it has the overall effect of preserving health and well-being of the entire body. The liver is a vital organ which is responsible for a wide range of functions in the body and is necessary for survival. Among other tasks, the liver acts to: • Help filter, cleanse, and detoxify the blood (it is the toxic waste disposal plant of the body) • Break down toxic substances and most medicinal products • Synthesize and degrade proteins • Produce and excrete bile (assists in the digestion of fats) • Metabolize fats • Produce albumin (part of blood serum), coagulation factors, fetal red blood cells, and insulin-like growth factors • Break down insulin, other hormones, and hemoglobin • Store glucose, Vitamins A, D, B12, iron, and copper • Help filter out antigens

Liver, Spleen and Gallbladder

Milk thistle helps eliminate obstructions and detoxify the liver and spleen.

Milk thistle helps repair and rejuvenate liver cells damaged by alcohol and other toxic substances. Reversal of acute and chronic liver problems has been observed, including viral hepatitis, alcohol (and chemically induced fatty liver disorders), cirrhosis, cholestasis, and hepatic organ (liver) damage. It also helps rebuild the gallbladder.

Multiple studies from Europe suggest benefits of oral milk thistle for cirrhosis. In experiments that follow subjects for up to five years, milk thistle has improved liver function and decreased the number of cirrhotic patient deaths.

Researchers have shown silymarin stimulates liver regeneration by stimulating ribosomal RNA (Ribonucleic acid) activity, which helps carry out and control protein synthesis in liver cells.

After just one week of therapy with oral silymarin, decreased serum transaminases (elevated levels can be an indicator of liver damage) and decreased bilirubin values (higher bilirubin levels occur in certain diseases) were observed.

Workers who had been exposed to vapors from toxic chemicals (toluene and/or xylene) for 5-20 years were given either a standardized milk thistle extract (80 percent silymarin) or placebo for 30 days. Workers taking milk thistle extract showed significant improvement in liver function tests over the placebo group.

Milk thistle protects liver cells and stabilizes liver-cell membranes. Silymarin induces an alteration of liver cell membranes that prevents toxins from penetrating into the interior of the cells. Silymarin appears to displace toxins trying to bind to the liver. This has been observed and recorded with liver-toxic medications (such as acetaminophen, Dilantin, alcohol, psychotropic drugs, and phenothiazines), amanita mushroom poisoning, common dry-cleaning fluid (carbon tetrachloride poisoning), and cadmium poisoning.

Milk thistle is especially indicated for people living in or working around environmental toxicity, industrial pollution, radiation, hydrocarbon fumes, and bad water.

Antioxidant	Milk thistle is a potent antioxidant which inhibits free radical oxidation. It stimulates the liver to produce superoxide dismutase (SOD), an antioxidant enzyme.

In a study to determine the efficacy of silymarin in preventing liver damage in patients taking long-term psychotropic drugs (known to cause liver damage from oxidation of lipids), patients taking silymarin had less hepatic damage than patients taking the placebo. |
| *Digestion* | Traditionally, a tea made from the whole plant is used to improve appetite, allay indigestion, and restore liver function. |
| *Other Organs* | Milk thistle has also been shown to protect the kidneys, brain, and other tissues from chemical toxins. It strengthens memory because of its effect on circulation. Cleansing the blood of toxins directly affects the healing of skin. Milk thistle has been found to be beneficial to those with psoriasis and other skin conditions. |
| *Blood Sugar* | Medical research suggests milk thistle may improve diabetes. Studies have shown a decrease in blood-sugar levels and an improvement in cholesterol and serum-triglyceride levels in people with Type 2 diabetes.

In a randomized, placebo-controlled trial, glycemic control was significantly improved, indicated by lower blood glucose, glycosylated hemoglobin, and improved insulin resistance.

Diabetic patients taking silymarin should carefully monitor their blood glucose when fasting, as they may require a reduction in medications. |
| *Immunity* | Milk thistle blocks allergic reactions, eradicates infection, and soothes inflamed tissues. It is mucilaginous (a slippery substance that protects and soothes mucous membranes and inflamed tissues) in nature and aids the immune response by increasing the production of T-lymphocytes and interferons (soluble proteins). |
| *Cancer* | Early reports indicate silymarin and silibinin in milk thistle reduce the growth of breast, cervical, and prostate cancer cells. There is one report of a patient with liver cancer who improved following treatment with milk thistle. |

Herb Parts Used	Seeds harvested when mature and dried, roots, sprouts, and fresh, young leaves (divested of the spines)
Preparations and Remedies	*Fresh:* For a wonderful tonic, the stalks and young leaves are palatable and nutritious. Young shoots should be cut in the spring, close to the root with part of the stalk. They are generally eaten fresh in a salad, cooked as greens, or included in hearty soups. Milk thistle is a bitter and, therefore, good for digestion.
Sprouted Seeds	Sprouted seeds are quite good in salads and provide a gentle stimulant to the liver and bile.
Dried Seeds	Dried seeds are ground and taken plain, mixed into yogurt, sprinkled on cereal, or put into herbal preparations.
Infusions	Water extracts are not very useful, unless the seed is ground and the whole plant consumed. *Milk Thistle Tea:* Steep 2-3 teaspoons of dried, ground seeds in 1 cup of hot water for 10-15 minutes. Do not strain. Consume the whole plant and all the water from the tea.
Encapsulated	*Liver Formula:* 8 parts Milk Thistle 8 parts Barberry root 2 parts Wild Yam root 1 part Cramp bark 1 part Fennel seed 1 part Catnip leaves 1 part Peppermint leaves Combine herbs in quantities indicated and encapsulate. This formula nutritionally supports the body by assisting, repairing, and rebuilding the liver; thus, cleansing the bloodstream more effectively. It is not recommended this formula be made into an extract. Milk thistle is not water soluble, and the active ingredients must be extracted into an alcoholic liquid. Alcohol is hard on the liver and would be counterproductive.

Safety	No health hazards or adverse side effects are known.
Plant Profile	*Natural Habitat:* Milk thistle is native to the Mediterranean regions of Europe, North Africa, and the Middle East. It has been naturalized in North America and Australia and is widely cultivated.
Description	The stout thistle grows on an erect stem that branches at the top and reaches a height of four to six feet. It has wide, waxy, green-toothed leaves with white blotches that exude a milky white fluid when crushed. The solitary flower head at the end of the stem is pink to purple and surrounded with thistle spines.
Growing Milk Thistle	The small, hard-skinned fruit is first white, then turns nearly black, spotted, and shiny with hairy tufts at maturity. Milk thistle's active ingredients are more abundant in the mature, darker seeds.
Planting	Milk thistle thrives in dry, well-drained, or even stony soils in fields and roadside ditches. The plant self-sows freely and spreads quickly. It matures in less than a year. Many farmers consider it to be a nuisance weed. The best way to grow milk thistle for seed production is to sow it directly in the garden in the summer. Leave plenty of room for these plants to grow (a healthy one can easily be 4 feet across and up to 6 feet tall). The first germination is about 30 percent (fairly typical for wild plant seeds that contain plenty of inhibitors). These first plants will develop strong rosettes, which then overwinter and go to flower the following spring, producing the thorny capitula filled with liver-protective seeds by midsummer. Over the next year or two, the majority of seeds will eventually germinate.
Harvesting	For medicinal use, collect the seeds when ripe, as the purple flower dies back. Put seed heads in a container and stir daily with a stick (not by hand) to dry evenly.
Storage	Whole seeds are naturally protected against degradation, but when ground, the seed flour easily goes rancid. Seeds are best stored whole and only ground as needed.

Mullein

Latin Name: *Verbascum thapsus*

Also known as: Mullein Dock, Lungwort, Cow's Lungwort, Bullock's Lungwort, Flannel Flower, Flannel Leaf, Velvet Leaf, Velvet Dock, Feltwort, Bunny Ears, Begger's Blanket, Shepherd's Club, Aaron's Rod, Jacob's Staff, Candlewick, Torch Weed

Scientific Classification

There are over 360 species of Verbascum. Other species commonly used in herbal traditions include V. phlomoides (orange mullein), V. nigrum (black mullein) and V. densiflorum (large-flowered mullein), which are also found in North America

Family: Scrophulariaceae – figwort family

Genus Verbascum – mullein

Species V. thapsus – common mullein

Influence on the Body	(PRINCIPAL ACTIONS are listed in CAPITAL LETTERS)
Blood and Circulatory System	dropsy (edema due to heart insufficiency) • HEMORRHAGE
Body System	MUCOUS MEMBRANES • DEMULCENT (softens and soothes inflammation of mucous membranes) • CATARRH (mucous membrane inflammation and congestion) • PAIN RELIEVER • ANODYNE (relieves pain and reduces nerve excitability) • SWOLLEN JOINTS (use as a fomentation) • cramps • spasms • INSOMNIA
Cancer	tumors • malignant throat cancer
Digestive Tract	colic • ulcers • constipation • DIARRHEA • BLEEDING BOWELS • DYSENTERY (bowel inflammation) • hemorrhoid discomfort (use herb as a fomentation) • anthelmintic (kills parasites and worms)
Ears	EARACHES • EAR INFECTIONS
Eyes	sore eyes
First Aid	sprains • vulnerary (promotes healing of wounds by protecting against infection and stimulating cellular growth)
Infections and Immune System	hay fever • colds • flu • antiseptic • antibacterial • LYMPHATIC CONGESTION • SWOLLEN GLANDS • herpes simplex • mumps • childhood diseases

Inflammation	rheumatism • bursitis • immuno-suppressant
Lungs and Respiratory System	RESPIRATORY • RESPIRATORY ALLERGIES • asthma • breathing problems • BRONCHITIS • COUGHS • EXPECTORANT (loosens & removes phlegm in the respiratory tract) • ANTITUSSIVE (inhibits the cough reflex) • CROUP • EMPHYSEMA (enlarged air spaces in the lungs, making breathing difficult) • LUNG PROBLEMS • BLEEDING LUNGS (hemorrhage) • PLEURISY (painful inflammation of chest cavity lining) • pneumonia • PULMONARY DISEASES • CONSUMPTION (TUBERCULOSIS) • THICKENING OF LUNG TISSUE
Mouth, Nose and Throat	toothache • nasal congestion • nosebleed • SINUS PROBLEMS • SINUSITIS • sore throat • hoarseness • gargle • tonsillitis
Nervous System	NERVOUSNESS • antispasmodic
Reproductive System	*Male:* swollen testicles *Female:* mastitis (breast inflammation, use as a fomentation)
Skin, Tissues and Hair	boils • bruises • skin disorders • emollient (softens and soothes skin and mucous membranes) • SORES • poison ivy • rashes • infant rashes • diaper rash • warts
Urinary Tract	nephritis (kidney inflammation) • dysuria (impaired ability to pass urine, painful voiding) • astringent (tightens and constricts tissues, reducing swelling) • diuretic (increases urine flow)

Key Properties:

RESPIRATORY TRACT	*soothes mucous membranes, loosens phlegm, heals pulmonary organs*
ANODYNE	*relieves pain, reduces swelling of glands and joints, soothes inflammation*
ARRESTS BLEEDING	*heals blood vessels, particularly noted in lungs and bowels*
Primarily affecting	RESPIRATORY TRACT • GLANDS • LYMPH
History	The plant's scientific name 'Verbascum' is a corruption of the Latin words 'barbascum', 'barba' meaning beard. The name 'mullein' comes from the Latin word 'mollis' for soft. The flowers impart a yellow color to boiling water, which was used by Roman women to dye their hair golden.

Asian Indians used the stalk for cramps, fevers, and migraine headaches. The power of driving away evil spirits was ascribed to mullein both in Europe and Asia. It has the reputation among the natives in India as a sure safeguard against evil spirits and magic. In their medicine, it was primarily used to treat diarrhea, respiratory diseases, and hemorrhoids.

Throughout the Middle Ages, the plant had many uses. The dried leaves are readily flammable, and the down on the leaves and stem make excellent tinder. Before the introduction of cotton, the dried, downy hairs were used as lamp wicks. When dried and dipped in oil, whole stalks were burned like torches.

Both men and livestock were given mullein to chew for respiratory congestion and breathing difficulties. Herbalists made mullein poultices of the fresh, bruised leaves for rashes, slow-healing wounds, ulcers, and tumors. A mullein flower tea wash was made for burns, sores, and ringworm. Taken internally, mullein is a mild diuretic and was used to treat kidney infections and digestive upsets. Mullein tea, brewed from either the leaves or the flowers, was used as a remedy for coughs and colds.

Prominent English herbalist John Gerard (1545-1612) wrote of mullein, 'The leaves are worn under the feet in a manner of a shoe sole or sock and assist to bring down in young maidens their desired sickness being so kept under their feet that they do not fall away.' He considered mullein to be an admirable bactericide, stating, 'Figs do not putrefy at all that are wrapped in the leaves of mullein.'

Nicholas Culpeper, English botanist, herbalist, physician, and astrologer (1616-1654) stated, 'The powder of the dried flowers is an especial remedy for those that are troubled with the belly-ache or the pains of colic.'

Native Americans smoked the dried leaves to relieve lung congestion. During the Civil War (1861-1865), the Confederates turned to mullein to treat respiratory problems when their conventional medical supplies ran out.

Germany's Commission E has approved mullein flowers to be used as an expectorant for inflammation of the upper respiratory tract.

Attributes	Key Components: (including, but not limited to)
Nutrients	Vitamins A • B1 (thiamine) • B2 (riboflavin) • B3 (niacin) • B5 (pantothenic acid) • B6 (pyridoxine) • B9 (folic acid) • B12 (cobalamin) • Biotin • Choline • Inositol • PABA (Para-Amino Benzoic Acid) • D • Iron • Magnesium • Potassium • Sulfur Verbascoside • Mucilage

Mullein has a high mineral content of iron, magnesium, potassium, and sulfur.

Verbascoside, the active ingredient isolated in mullein, shows antiseptic, antitumor, antibacterial, and immuno-suppressant activities.

The leaves are high in mucilage (soft and slippery sugar molecules) that protects and soothes mucous membranes and inflamed tissues. |
| *General* | Mullein is one of the most important known plants for its ability to reduce swelling in the glandular system and heal serous (blood) vessels and mucous membranes. It has numerous medicinal uses but is principally employed in the treatment of lung disease, coughs, consumption, and hemorrhage of the respiratory organs. |
| *Lungs and Respiratory Tract* | Mullein has a special affinity for the respiratory organs and is valuable for all pulmonary complaints. It strengthens sinuses and allows for free breathing. Mullein provides mucilaginous protection to mucous surfaces, inhibiting the absorption of allergens through mucous membranes. As an antispasmodic and astringent herb, it helps reduce swollen membranes and relieve painful seizing in the respiratory system.

The plant helps to alleviate chest ailments by clearing the lungs of excess phlegm and reducing bronchial and lymphatic congestion. Mullein quiets coughs and mucous membranes. As a bacteriostatic, it has been used to treat tuberculosis for centuries. Science confirms mullein's antiviral activity against herpes simplex and influenza viruses.

Taken internally, mullein is also good for lung hemorrhaging and shortness of breath. It stops the escape of fluids from ruptured vessels and rids the body of toxins. |

Urinary Tract	Mullein is used in kidney formulas to soothe inflammation, increase the flow of urine, and strengthen the renal system.
Pain	Mullein helps relieve pain and calm inflamed and irritated nerves. It is very effective for swollen joints. The herb has mild narcotic properties (blunts the senses, reduces pain, and may induce sleep), without being poisonous or harmful. The seeds of some mullein species, when thrown into the water, are said to be strong enough to intoxicate fish and have been used by poachers for that purpose.
Ear	Mullein oil is considered one of the best remedies for earaches and ear infections.
Digestion	Mullein heals the mucous membranes lining the bowels. A mullein infusion is generally given to relieve diarrhea. When bleeding of the bowels is present, a stronger decoction prepared with milk is recommended. Mullein is also used for relief of hemorrhoidal pain and swelling.
Herb Parts Used	Leaves, flowers, fruit, and root
Preparations and Remedies	Do not use dried flowers that have turned brown. The leaves become dark green when they are dried.
Powdered	The combination of three parts mullein and one part lobelia is used for glandular problems including thyroid, swollen lymph glands, breasts, male testicles, etc.
Infusions	**Mullein infusions must be strained to remove the fine, downy hairs of the herb. Hairs may cause intolerable itching in the mouth and throat.** Use an extract, tea infusion, or inhale the smoke of the burning herb for bronchial problems. Inhaled steam is also useful for bronchial and lung conditions. *Mullein Tea:* 1 ounce Mullein leaves, cut 1/2 pint Distilled Water

Pour boiling water over leaves. Cover and steep for 15 minutes. Strain through muslin (to filter out the hairs), sweeten with honey to taste, or add 1 ounce glycerin to preserve. Cool, bottle, and store in a cool place. Take 2-3 ounces (or more) 3-4 times a day, as warranted. Mullein tea is useful for coughs, colds, asthma, and respiratory diseases.

For sinusitis, snuff a teaspoon of tea up each nostril several times a day (but not enough to irritate the condition).

Drink an infusion made with flowers to induce sleep, relieve pain or, in large doses, as a laxative.

Yarrow – Mullein Tea: (see YARROW preparations)

Decoctions

The taste of a mullein decoction is bland and mucilaginous and roughly four times the strength of a normal infusion. It is more astringent and soothing. When working with advanced conditions, use the stronger decoction of leaves and flowers alone or in combination with comfrey root and garlic juice.

Strong Decoction:
4 ounces (equal parts) cut Mullein leaf and flowers
3 pints Distilled Water
4 ounces Glycerin

Place the herb in a pan and cover with distilled water. Bring to a boil and simmer slowly for 15 minutes. Strain, press, return the liquid to a clean pot, and reduce it to 1 pint and add the glycerin while hot. Allow to cool, bottle, and keep refrigerated.

Take 1 tablespoon 3-4 times daily (may be taken in much larger doses). A child's dose is 1 teaspoon 3-4 times daily.

For diarrhea, dysentery, and bleeding of the bowels:
Boil one ounce of mullein herb in one pint of raw milk for a few minutes, strain, and take in half-cup doses after each bowel elimination. Milk from an animal source is used like a glue to adhere the mullein to the lining of the bowel. Mullein tea may also be used as an enema for double application.

Fomentations

Breathe Easy Mullein and Lobelia Fomentation:
2 ounces Mullein
1/2 ounce Lobelia herb powder
1 teaspoon Cayenne

2 quarts Raw Apple Cider Vinegar

Simmer ingredients in vinegar, closely covered, for 15 minutes. Take from heat and strain.
Use fomentation (towel soaked in infusion or decoction) and place as warm as can be tolerated over the lungs or other affected areas. Use for bronchitis, croup, cough, rheumatism, stiff joints, mumps, glandular swellings, and dropsy.

For Burns:
Apply juice of mullein leaves mixed with apple cider vinegar.

Poultice

Apply as a poultice for swollen glands, stiff neck, and mumps. Apply bruised leaves for diaper rash.

Oil

Mullein Oil:
2 ounces Mullein flowers dried
Sufficient Extra-Virgin Olive Oil

Place mullein flowers into a jar or wide-mouthed bottle and cover with olive oil up to an inch above the flowers. Stopper and shake well. Place in a warm place or expose to the sun for 7-14 days, shaking well every day.

Note: When using fresh mullein flowers, instead of using a lid, cover the top of the bottle with several layers of cheesecloth secured by an elastic band to allow moisture to escape.

When maceration (soaking to soften and release constituents) is complete, carefully pour off the oil from the flower sediment, press oil through cheesecloth or unbleached muslin, and store in a dark glass bottle in the refrigerator.

Put two to six drops of the warmed oil in the ear overnight two to three times daily until healed. Let it absorb for a few minutes, then cover with a clean cotton ball (if needed). Rub oil on any area that is swollen or irritated. Mullein oil makes a good ointment for bruises and frostbite.

Vermicide and Parasiticide:
Take one teaspoonful mullein oil internally 3-4 times daily.

For Hemorrhoids:
Apply mullein ointment topically and take the tea internally. If hemorrhoids are inflamed, apply fomentation (or wash) of a hot tea (or decoction) made from the leaves.

Safety	Mullein leaves and flowers are on the U.S. Federal Drug Administration's GRAS (generally recognized as safe) list. Mullein hairs may irritate the skin or, if swallowed, the mouth and throat.
Plant Profile	*Natural Habitat:* Mullein is widespread in Europe, temperate Asia, and North America. It grows on banks, roadsides, waste ground, and slovenly kept fields. It prefers gravel, sandy, or chalky soils.
Description	Mullein is a biennial (grows for at least 2 years before dying) that produces a rosette of large (6-15 inches long), fuzzy, gray-green leaves the first year, and it adds an attractive spike that grows 1-4 feet in height with light yellow flowers the second year. The straight, stout, unbranched stalk and large thick leaves are velvety and flannel-like with branched, downy hairs. The leaves are arranged such that the smaller leaves above drop the rain upon the larger ones below, directing the water to the roots. Flowers appear the second year, here and there along the spike, in July and August. Each flower has five golden-yellow, rounded petals with a large number of tiny white hairs. These hairs are full of sap and attract bees and flies. The nectar is readily accessible, though the supply is not very great. The fruit is a capsule or pod. While the herb has a bitter taste, the odor of the flowers is faint and rather pleasant.
Growing Mullein	Mullein grows freely in certain low mountain locations, and it may easily be propagated in most medicinal gardens. Be sure that the soil is not too rich. Mullein seems to thrive in the poorest of soils. Germination takes about 10 days.

Peppermint

Latin Name: *Mentha pipertita*

Also known as: Balm Mint, Curled Mint, Brandy Mint, Lamb Mint, Lammint, American Peppermint, Northern Mint, White Peppermint, and Black Peppermint

Scientific Classification

The genus Mentha is composed of at least 25 species that tend to freely hybridize and integrate. Besides peppermint and spearmint (M. spicata), which are considered official, other distinct species demonstrating similar therapeutic properties are water mint (M. aquatica), field mint (M. arvensis), and European horsemint (M. longifolia).

Family: Lamiaceae – mint family

Genus Mentha – mint

Species M. x piperita – peppermint

Influence on the Body	(PRINCIPAL ACTIONS are listed in CAPITAL LETTERS)
Addictions	Smoking
Blood and Circulatory System	mild alterative (purifies and cleanses the blood) • HEART • HEART PALPITATIONS
Body System	stimulant • tonic • pale countenance • FAINTING • SHOCK • astringent (increases the tone and firmness of tissues) • insomnia • NIGHTMARES
Digestive Tract	AROMATIC (contains volatile oils which aid digestion and relieve gas) • IMPROVES APPETITE • HEARTBURN • DIGESTIVE AID • GASTRIC STIMULANT • STOMACHIC (strengthens stomach function) • DYSPEPSIA (indigestion) • GAS • CARMINATIVE (relieves intestinal gas, promotes peristaltic movement) • COLIC • ANTINAUSEA • ANTI-EMETIC (helps prevent vomiting) • motion sickness • seasickness • VOMITING • STOMACH SPASMS • stomach cramps • griping • DIARRHEA • constipation • COLITIS • diverticulitis • ulcers • DYSENTERY
Ears	Earache
Infections and Immune System	CHILLS • COUGHS • COLDS • antibacterial • antiviral • herpes simplex • antimicrobial • antiseptic • FEVERS • FEBRIFUGE (reduces fever) • FLU • childhood diseases • measles • cholera

Inflammation	inflammation • rheumatism • gout
Liver	liver • cholagogue (promotes the flow of bile) • gallbladder
Lungs and Respiratory System	BRONCHITIS • hiccup
Mouth, Nose and Throat	toothaches • mouth sores • mouthwash • sore throats • gargle
Muscles	muscle spasms • lumbago (back pain)
Nervous System	NERVINE (soothes and strengthens nerves) • neuralgia (sharp, stabbing pains due to deposits or congestion putting pressure on nerves) • analgesic (relieves pain) • anodyne (relieves pain and lessens the excitability of nerves) • dizziness • HEADACHE • nervous headache • migraine • convulsions • antispasmodic • depression • hysteria • calmative (gently calms nerves) • sedative
Reproductive System	*Female:* morning sickness • menstruation pain • menstrual cramps • menstrual obstructions • emmenagogue (promotes menstrual flow)
Skin, Tissues and Hair	boils • itching • shingles • diaphoretic (promotes perspiration, increasing elimination through the skin) • the oil is rubefacient (increases blood flow to the skin and local reddening)
Other Uses	MINT FLAVORING AGENT • MENTHOL

Key Properties:

DIGESTIVE AID	*has a refreshing, uplifting scent, improves appetite, settles the stomach, relieves gas and intestinal spasms, strengthens and soothes the digestive system*
NERVINE	*Stimulates and strengthens the nervous system, revives sensibility, gently calms nerves, spasms, convulsions, cramps, and relieves pain*
STIMULANT	*Warms, induces perspiration, cools to the touch, improves circulation, cleanses the blood*
Primarily affecting	*STOMACH • INTESTINES • NERVES • MUSCLES • CIRCULATION*

History

'Peppermint', the herb's common name, comes from the species name 'piperita' meaning peppery. Pliny, a Roman naturalist of the first century, tells us that the Greeks and Romans crowned themselves with peppermint at their feasts and adorned their tables with its sprays. Their cooks flavored both sauces and wines with its essence.

Two species of mint were used by ancient Greek physicians, but some writers doubt whether either was the modern peppermint plant we know today. There is evidence M. piperita was cultivated by the Egyptians. It is mentioned also in Chinese medical literature as early as 659 AD and in the Icelandic Pharmacopoeias of the 13th century.

References to 'mint' appear in medieval texts and, through the centuries, it became a symbol for purity and hospitality. Tables and floors were scrubbed with the refreshing essence.

The peppermint species we know today was recognized as a distinct species in the 1696, 2nd edition of *Synopsis Methodica Stirpium Britannicorum* by John Ray (English naturalist 1627-1705). It was found growing in England as a natural hybrid of spearmint and water mint. Peppermint's medicinal properties were soon recognized, and it was admitted into the London Pharmacopoeia in 1721 under M. piperitis sapore.

Colonists carried peppermint to the New World and used it for digestive complaints such as heartburn, nausea, colic, and gas. It was also used to cure hiccups, induce sleep, relieve headaches, and as a general stimulant to the body. Native Americans used peppermint for bowel complaints, toning the digestive tract, healing colds, and controlling fevers.

Peppermint leaf is approved in Germany for use in muscle spasms of the gastrointestinal tract as well as for spasms of the gallbladder and bile ducts.

The Japanese have long recognized the value of extracted menthol and, over 200 years ago, carried it about with them in little silver boxes hanging from their girdles. The distillation of peppermint oil forms a considerable industry in Japan. Most of the menthol is taken out of their essential oil for other uses. By cooling the oil, the menthol separates and crystalizes out, leaving a cheaper (though marketable) by-product of dementholised oil.

The cheapest variety of peppermint essential oil available in commerce is the partially dementholised oil imported from Japan. Adulteration of American peppermint oil with dementholised Japanese oil is frequently practiced. Other essential oil adulterations exist, mixing peppermint with other herbs before distillation, using synthetic oils, etc.

These cheaper oils are used most often for their mint-like scent and flavor, but do not contain the same therapeutic properties as pure peppermint essential oil.

Attributes	Key Components: (including, but not limited to)
Nutrients	Vitamins A • C • Copper • Iron • Magnesium • Potassium • Sulfur • other Trace Minerals Menthol (30-48 percent of the essential oil is menthol) Menthol is the chief constituent of peppermint oil. It is antibacterial, antiviral, and antispasmodic.
Opposing Properties	Peppermint has seemingly opposing properties that affect the system, according to what resonates with the body's needs. The herb can be calming or energizing; sedative or stimulating; warming or cooling, all depending on how the body puts it to use. Peppermint has warming, stimulating, digestive, antispasmodic, and decongestant properties. Peppermint and elder tea is a traditional treatment for flu, pneumonia, and high-fever diseases. Both the herb and the essential oil are very versatile when combined with other herb and oil formulas, adding a freshness to them and boosting the combination's therapeutic actions.
Digestion	Peppermint is one of the oldest and most popular remedies for simple colic and minor bloat in children and adults. It may be used in pregnancy to soothe the stomach, relieve nausea, and alleviate vomiting. It is excellent for calming a queasy stomach caused by motion sickness, sea sickness, morning sickness, or illness. Peppermint oil temporarily quiets hunger pangs in the stomach, but they will return if the stomach is not satisfied. Peppermint stimulates digestion, increases bile flow, and strengthens and tones the stomach.

Menthol relaxes the lower sphincter muscle of the esophagus, aiding digestion and easing gas, burping, and bloating after eating. It helps to prevent the gripping effect caused by disease or strong laxatives and is a favorite remedy for soothing the intestinal tract. Peppermint is excellent for diarrhea, ulcers, and colitis. Peppermint tea enemas are very useful for colonic problems.

In 2007, Italian investigators reported 75 percent of the patients in their study who took peppermint oil capsules for 4 weeks had a major reduction in irritable bowel syndrome (IBS) symptoms. Another study involving 146 individuals with IBS found peppermint provided significant relief from abdominal cramps. Research shows coated capsules permit peppermint oil to reach the colon without breaking down in the stomach. Because of this, it is believed by some to be more effective in healing IBS and lower bowel afflictions.

Nervous System

Peppermint is good for the nerves. It is one of the great stimulant herbs. Using a strong peppermint tea is excellent for chills and a pale countenance. Peppermint can assist the body in raising internal heat. It strengthens the nerves and heart muscle and acts as a marvelous antispasmodic. The oil inhibits smooth muscle cramping and is good for helping alleviate infant convulsions.

Conversely, peppermint can act as a mild, soothing sedative for nervous and restless individuals of all ages and can promote relaxation and sleep.

Peppermint is used in plasters for neuralgia, rheumatism, chronic gout, and lumbago. Peppermint oil can be used instead of aspirin for neuralgic headaches by rubbing it on the temples or areas of discomfort (remember to keep the oil out of the eyes).

Infections

Peppermint inhibits the growth of bacteria and fungus and is excellent for fevers and flu. It also relieves symptoms of allergy and asthma. Drinking hot peppermint tea induces perspiration, which purges toxins and cools down the body. Using peppermint in a bath cools the body and helps soothe itching skin.

Cleansing

Peppermint increases respiration, the oxygen supply in the blood, and cleanses the blood. As a nerve stimulant, it strengthens and tones the entire body.

Commercial Uses	The oil is used for its well-known, refreshing, minty taste in toothpaste, dental creams, mouthwash, cough drops, candies, chewing gum, and baked goods. Menthol is an active ingredient in Vicks VapoRub (used for chest congestion) and in local anesthetics such as Solarcaine and Bengay. Unfortunately, most of the menthol used commercially is synthetically produced, rather than extracted from peppermint, thereby missing out on most of the long-term healing properties that could be obtained if the natural oil is used.
Herb Parts Used	Leaves, stem, essential oil
Preparations and Remedies	Peppermint is most often used as a tea, powdered and included in herb combinations, or distilled into an essential oil. The oil is often adulterated or artificially made, but these products do not effectively duplicate peppermint's true aroma or the medicinal effects of real peppermint oil.
Powdered Formula *Infusions*	*Liver Formula:* (see MILK THISTLE preparations) **Do not boil peppermint leaves, as the medicinal principles are extremely volatile and will be lost.** Peppermint leaves make a delicious, mild tea. The infusion is a wonderful beverage and can be taken hot in the winter and cold in the summer. Do not underestimate the powerful healing effects of peppermint tea. It seems mild, yet it is very effective in so many areas of health and rejuvenation. *Peppermint Tea:* Pour boiling water over the leaves (1 teaspoon herb to 1 cup water). Cover and keep in a warm place for 10 minutes. Strain, sweeten, and drink hot or cold. Drink a hot, strong peppermint tea for fainting or dizzy spells. It can also soothe the gastrointestinal area irritated by foods and unripe fruits. A strong cup of peppermint tea and 10 minutes of relaxation can often prevent the need for aspirin. *Alkaline Formula Tea:* (see DANDELION preparations)

Enemas	*Cold and Flu Tea:* (see YARROW preparations) Use peppermint tea as an excellent enema for cholera, colon problems, convulsions, and stomach spasms, even for children.
Poultices	For gastrointestinal complaints, the fresh leaves may be bruised and applied to the stomach and the tea taken internally.
Compress	*Cooling Compress*: ½ cup Peppermint leaves 1 quart Distilled Water Ice cubes Pour boiling water over peppermint leaves, cover and let steep until cool, and then strain. After the mixture has cooled down, put in the freezer or add ice cubes to make the infusion really cold. Soak a cloth in the tea and wring it out so it does not drip, yet still retains enough liquid to stay cold. Apply the cloth to the body. When the cloth warms, re-soak and re-apply. Repeat this procedure three to five times, adding ice cubes, if necessary, to keep the liquid cold. When finished, dry the area thoroughly. Use this compress to cool fevers and reduce swelling. This preparation can help stimulate the production of both white and red blood cells and reduce pulse rate and fevers, especially when applied to the feet.
Peppermint Essential Oil	Essential oils are concentrated and powerful. A few drops are all that are needed for therapeutic effects. Keep away from eyes and mucous membranes. If contact burning occurs, dilute with a carrier oil like coconut oil or extra virgin olive oil.
Inhalant	Boil 2 quarts water, remove from heat, and add 5-10 drops peppermint oil. Quickly enclose the pot and head with a heavy blanket or towel to capture the steam, and inhale deeply through the mouth and nostrils. Menthol inhalation can help open the sinuses and relieve bronchial cough, colds, and flu symptoms. It is also an excellent facial steam bath. *Alternative:* Inhale peppermint oil directly from the container to reduce jet lag and vitalize the mind.

Gargle	Use one drop of peppermint oil to one cup of water for a stimulating and antiseptic gargle for canker sores, bad breath, bleeding gums, or pyorrhea.
Rub	For toothache or tender gums, rub the afflicted area directly with one drop of peppermint oil.
	Apply essential oil externally on affected areas for rheumatism, neuralgia, and sore muscles. Rub the back of the neck with one drop of peppermint oil neat (directly on the skin) or diluted in one teaspoon of olive oil.
Soak	To refresh sore feet, add 5 drops of peppermint oil to a large bowl of cold water. Bathe the feet and ankles for 10 minutes.
Sponge Bath	*For Fevers:* Menthol coolness helps to control body temperature. Peppermint essential oil blended in a carrier oil (such as almond or olive oil) and applied on the bottoms of an overheated, feverish child or adult's feet can gently reduce and regulate body temperature. An application of peppermint oil also helps reduce hot flashes.
	As an alternative, sponge the body with cool water to which has been added one drop each of eucalyptus, peppermint, and lavender oils.
Drops	*Digestive Aid:* To aid digestion and relieve an upset stomach, place one drop peppermint oil in a half cup of water and slowly sip.
	Caution: **Use only pure peppermint essential oil for internal applications. Synthetic or adulterated oils may cause illness when ingested.**
	Rodent Repellent Place several drops of peppermint oil on cotton balls and place them in problem locations to repel mice.
Safety	No health hazards or adverse side effects are known.
	Essential oils are potent. Only a small amount is needed. They should never be put into the eyes nor directly contact mucous membranes. If contact burning occurs, soothe the area with a carrier oil such as almond or olive oil. Be careful to purchase only pure essential oils when using them for therapeutic purposes.

Plant Profile

Natural Habitat:
The plant is indigenous to Europe and is now widely cultivated throughout all regions of the world, including North America.

Description

Peppermint is a hybrid plant of spearmint (*M. spicata*) and water mint (*M. aquatica*). The well-known scent of 'mint' is the aroma of peppermint. Menthol, a principal component of peppermint oil, gives the 'cool' sensation felt on the skin and upon inhalation. Peppermint is the most pungent of all the mints. The entire plant has a characteristic odor due to the volatile oil present in all of its parts.

Peppermint is an herbaceous perennial plant (dies back in winter and grows back from a persistent rootstock each year) which reaches one to three feet tall. It has smooth, square, purple stems (not greenish as in spearmint) and dark green (sometimes tinged with purple), opposing leaves that are toothed on the margins. The rhizomes (underground root or stem) are wide-spreading and fleshy with bare, fibrous roots.

It is easy to confuse spearmint with peppermint. Spearmint grows wild along ditch banks and has dull leaves, whereas peppermint has shiny leaves and requires special growing conditions.

Peppermint typically grows in moist habitats, including sides of streams and drainage ditches. Flowers appear in July and August and are pale violet or whitish on terminal spikes. They are usually sterile, producing no seeds. Peppermint principally reproduces vegetatively through its spreading rhizomes.

A crop that yields a high percentage of essential oil exhausts the soil. After cropping with peppermint for four years, the land must be put to some other purpose for at least seven years. In some areas, plantations are renewed annually to strengthen their yield.

Growing Peppermint

Peppermint generally thrives in shade and spreads quickly by underground rhizomes. When growing peppermint, it is advisable to plant prepared cuttings in a container, otherwise it can rapidly take over the whole garden. Place a saucer beneath the pot to prevent the roots from creeping into the ground. Peppermint needs a good water supply and is ideal for planting in part-sun-to-shaded areas.

PEPPERMINT — 265

Planting

Today, peppermint is cultivated through vegetative propagation. Seeds require especially favorable conditions. Only a small percentage will thrive. Root starts or cuttings grow rapidly in a glass of water. Transplant rooted starts in pots with well-soaked heavy soil. Be careful to keep different mints apart, as they cross hybridize easily. The plant prefers cool and moist conditions.

Harvesting

The leaves and flowering tops are the usable portion of the plant. For drying, collect herbs just before the plant blooms, during dry weather (August through September). If harvesting for oil, collect just after the flowers have opened for best potency. However, the plant may be used fresh at any time.

Wild peppermint is less suitable for commercial use. Cultivated plants have been selected for higher yield and better oil content. Peppermint seeds sold at many stores will generally not germinate into true peppermint but, more likely, into a poor-scented spearmint plant. True peppermint rarely produces seeds of its own. I recommend you find a reliable source of certified seeds and roots such as Horizon Herbs out of Oregon.

Drying

Just before blooming, cut the stalks and hang upside down in bunches to dry. Hang the cut plant inside paper bags (slotted on the sides for ventilation) and store the herbs in airtight containers once they are sufficiently dried.

Freezing

Peppermint leaves may be frozen. Harvest the herb at its peak and wash gently but thoroughly, then pat dry. Herbs may be chopped by hand or in the food processor until the pieces are the right size to use for teas and other recipes. Pack and seal in freezer bags, first squeezing out the air until herbs are in a flat layer. Label the bags immediately, as many herbs look alike. When ready to use, simply break off what is needed and return the rest to the freezer.

Red Clover

Latin Name: *Trifolium pratense*

Also known as: Purple Clover, Wild Clover, Meadow Clover, Clover Grass, Cow Grass, Trefoil

Scientific Classification
True clover plants number about 250 species,
80 or more are listed as indigenous to North America

Family: Fabaceae – pea family

Genus Trifolium – clover

Species T. pratense – red clover

Influence on the Body	(PRINCIPAL ACTIONS are listed in CAPITAL LETTERS)
Blood and Circulatory System	BLOOD CLEANSER • BLOOD PURIFIER • depurative (cleanses blood by promoting eliminative functions)
Body System	insomnia • sedative • mild stimulant • deobstruent (removes obstructions)
Cancer	ANTICANCER • CANCER • TUMORS • LEUKEMIA
Cleansing	TOXINS • cleansing
Digestive Tract	nutritive • rickets (a Vitamin D deficiency) • appetite suppressant • digestive • antiemetic (helps prevent vomiting) • constipation • laxative • rectal irritation
Eyes	Eyewash
First Aid	fresh wounds • burns
Infections and Immune System	colds • coughs • flu • lymphatic congestion • mild antibiotic • antiviral • antifungal • athlete's foot (use as a fomentation) • antimicrobial • childhood diseases • scarlet fever • whooping cough • AIDS • leprosy
Inflammation	anti-inflammatory • gout • rheumatism • rheumatoid arthritis
Liver	gallbladder • LIVER CONGESTION
Lungs and Respiratory System	expectorant (loosens and removes phlegm in the respiratory tract) • BRONCHITIS • inflamed lungs • tuberculous

Muscles	muscle cramps • SPASMS
Nervous System	nerves • NERVOUS CONDITIONS • St. Vitus Dance (a nervous disease characterized by involuntary movements) • antispasmodic
Poisons	poisonous bites • stings
Reproductive System	Syphilis *Male:* prostate health *Female:* female tonic • strengthens ovaries • dysmenorrhea (painful or difficult menstruation) • vaginal irritation • improves lactation • mastitis (breast infection)
Skin, Tissues and Hair	ACNE • BOILS • SKIN DISORDERS • sores • skin ulcers • PSORIASIS • scrofuloderma (tuberculosis infection of the skin)
Urinary Tract	diuretic (increases urine flow) • urinary problems • BLADDER PROBLEMS • kidney problems
Other Uses	fodder for cattle • ground cover crop • nectar source for clover honey

Key Properties:

ALTERATIVE	*cleanses and purifies the blood, improves circulation, and gradually detoxifies the blood vessels, spleen, liver, kidneys, bowels, and lungs, improves digestion, respiration, heart and skin health*
ANTICANCER	*traditionally used for cancerous tumors, skin ulcerations, and ridding the body of cancerous wastes*
hormone activity	*has estrogenic properties that promote hormone balance and counteract bone loss in women*
Nutritive	*roots pull nutrients from deep within the earth, providing vitamins and minerals that sustain and restore weakened body systems*
Primarily affecting	*BLOOD • LIVER • LYMPH • NERVES • LUNGS*
History	The genus name 'Trifolium' is derived from the Latin 'tres' meaning three and 'folium' for leaf. The species 'pratense' is Latin for 'growing in meadows.'

RED CLOVER — 268

Ancient Celtic Druids saw the three-leafed clover as a symbol of earth, sea, and heaven; Middle-Age Christians as a symbol of the Trinity.

Chinese physicians and Russian folk healers used red clover to treat cancer and respiratory problems.

Native Americans used red clover for food and as a remedy for burns and sore eyes. In the 19th century, it became popular among herbalists as an alterative blood purifier.

For over 100 years in America and Europe, red clover has been used not only as a diuretic and expectorant but also to treat gout, treat and prevent cancer, and heal whooping cough.

Attributes	Key Components: (including, but not limited to)
Nutrients	Vitamins A • B1 (thiamine) • B2 (riboflavin) • B3 (niacin) • B5 (pantothenic acid) • B6 (pyridoxine) • B9 (folic acid) • B12 (cobalamin) • Biotin • Choline • Inositol • PABA (Para-Amino Benzoic Acid) • C • Bioflavonoids • Calcium • Cobalt • Copper • Iron • Magnesium • Manganese • Molybdenum • Selenium • other Trace Minerals Dietary Isoflavones: Formononetin, Daidzein, Genistein, and Biochanin A (as estrogen regulators) • Coumarins (thins blood) The molybdenum (an essential trace element in nutrition) in red clover tops accelerates the discharge of nitrogenous wastes, aids in cleansing the system of impurities, and helps retard the spread of infection.
Nutritive	As with alfalfa, red clover sends roots far into the ground. This makes it possible to draw upon an abundance of vital nutrients, nitrogen, vitamins, and minerals. Clover is a dependable source of nutrients for relieving general weakness, shortness of breath, and all forms of degenerative diseases. Red Clover is important for individuals suffering from anemia. Molybdenum and iron together can more rapidly produce hemoglobin than iron alone. Molybdenum and iron also help form protective antibodies against rattlesnake, scorpion, and other poisonous bites and stings.

Cleansing

Red Clover is a blood-thinning and cleansing alternative. It is especially effective when combined with other blood purifiers such as yellow dock, chaparral, dandelion root, buckthorn bark, or burdock root. Red Clover helps ease arthritic pain by increasing urine flow and ridding the system of uric acid (considered by some as a main cause of arthritis).

Red Clover flower infusions are recommended to efficiently remove metabolic waste products, eliminate toxins from the liver and bowels, stimulate immune function, and inhibit the attachment and metastasis (spread of disease from one part of the body to another) of abnormal cells.

Red Clover is one of the best mucus clearing sources in nature and is often used for bronchitis and pulmonary congestion. It has expectorant properties. Taken as a warm infusion, red clover helps cleanse and soothe bronchial nerves, relieves dry coughs and wheezing, and heals laryngitis, weak chests, bronchitis, and whooping cough.

Red Clover's antibiotic properties fight several bacteria, including tubercular bacilli. The tea is used as a gargle for infections and glandular swelling of the throat.

To promote the skin's healing process, use red clover in an herbal tea wash or as an external salve for boils, sores, eczema, psoriasis, acne, and other kinds of dermatitis. Clover is used by Russian healers as a strong natural antiseptic and in poultices for burns and abscesses. The fresh leaf juice and a dried leaf tea are used as an eye wash.

Drinking the tea helps cleanse the blood, liver, and skin. Red Clover's cleansing properties can counteract scrofuloderma and other skin diseases.

Circulation

Isoflavones found in red clover have numerous potential benefits. They help promote cardiovascular health and maintain normal blood pressure, cholesterol levels, and youthfulness.

An initial study in Australia reported red clover extract produced a 23 percent increase in elasticity of arteries compared to the placebo. Additional trials suggest red clover has beneficial effects on lipid levels in men and women, including the following: a significant increase in high-density lipoprotein (HDL) cholesterol in post-menopausal women, a significant decrease in triglyceride levels among women, and a lowered low-density lipoprotein (LDL) cholesterol in men.

Digestion

Red Clover stimulates the liver, activates the gallbladder, and improves digestion. It has a slight laxative effect on the digestive system and is good for stomach problems and intestinal elimination.

Nervous System

Red Clover is a tonic for nerves and can help strengthen the systems of delicate children. It is beneficial in wasting diseases such as rickets (a Vitamin D deficiency disease) and lack of vitality. A warm infusion of red clover is soothing and relaxing to nerves and the entire body. Red Clover calms nervous energy and exhaustion and has antispasmodic effects. It is an effective sedative.

Cancer

Red Clover is a powerful remedy for cancerous growth anywhere in the body. In combination with chaparral and other herbs, red clover is used to break up growths and tumors. Red Clover has been used effectively for both esophageal and breast cancer.

Fomentations and poultices of red clover have been used for cancerous skin growths. Dr. Harry Hoxsey, N.D. (1901-1974) started the first cancer clinic in Mexico, using red clover in his treatments.

Rich in phytoestrogenic compounds like genistein, red clover is an important component of well-respected formulas for assisting the body in its fight with cancer and helping to prevent the disease.

Red Clover extracts have also shown potential for promoting male prostate health. Population studies suggest a high dietary intake of isoflavones reduces the risk of prostate cancer and supports general prostate health. A review of phyto-therapies (plant-therapies) for men with benign prostatic hyperplasia (BPH) concluded isoflavones, particularly from red clover extract, are potential therapies for prostate health in men with non-cancerous prostate growth associated with advancing age.

Women

The isoflavones found in red clover have hormone activity and help maintain normal estrogen levels. Red Clover has been used to restore fertility, alleviate bleeding of dysmenorrhea, and support the maintenance of healthy bones, skin, and arteries.

	Studies suggest red clover isoflavones slow the rate of bone loss and may even build bone in post-menopausal women. One study showed decreased bone loss over 12 months compared to placebo, and the study concluded red clover isoflavones may have a protective effect on the lumbar spine in women. Another trial demonstrated a significant increase in bone mass after 6 months of use. The mineral molybdenum affects mammary glands, which helps improve lactation in nursing mothers.
Other Uses	Clover has been cultivated as a ground-cover crop, a forage crop, and for making hay for centuries. Red Clover is recognized for its importance in soil conservation and crop rotation due to clover's ability to fix nitrogen in the soil.
Herb Parts Used	Flowering tops
Preparations and Remedies	Red Clover leaves are eaten as nutritious salad greens, and the flowers are dried for use in teas. Leaves and flowers may be dried and powdered for encapsulation and inclusion in herb formulas and preparations.
Infusions	*Blood Cleansing Tea:* Make a strong tea by simmering 1 tablespoon of the herb for each cup of water, for 15-20 minutes. Drink 1 cup, 2 or 3 times daily. Drink the infusion freely for soothing nerves and for bronchial, spasmodic, and whooping cough ailments. *System Cleanse Tea:* (see CHAPARRAL preparations)
Gargle	Make a strong tea as a gargle for a sore and inflamed throat. Gargle four to five times a day, swallowing a fresh mouthful after each cleansing.
Enema or Douche	Use a strong tea for rectal and vaginal irritations, making sure to hold in the solution for several minutes before releasing.
Fomentation	Use a strong tea as a wash or fomentation (towel soaked in infusion and placed on affected area) for athlete's foot, arthritic pain, psoriasis, eczema, deep burns, rashes, and hardened breasts of nursing mothers.

Poultice	Chop the fresh herb, combine with a little water, and mash or blend to make a poultice. Apply directly to lesions.
Ointments	Apply red clover ointment to scaly skin as needed.
Safety	Red Clover is on the U.S. Federal Drug Administration's GRAS (generally recognized as safe) list. Red Clover has blood-thinning components that may affect blood-thinning medications.
Plant Profile	*Natural Habitat:* Red Clover is indigenous to Europe, Central Asia, Northern Africa, and naturalized in many other parts of the world. It is commonly found in pastures, lawns, roadsides, and meadows throughout the United States and Canada. In the United States, Red Clover is the state flower of Vermont.
Description	The herb is a stout clover with hairy, erect (or reclining), branching stems reaching 6-24 inches. The stem supports generous numbers of terminal, purplish-pink, sweet-scented, and rounded blossom heads that appear from April to November. The leaves grow on alternate sides of the stems in three-leaflet branches. Each fine-tooth-edged leaf has a whitish crescent 'V' along the center.
Growing Red Clover	Red Clover is a biennial (germinates, flowers, sets seed, and dies within a two-year cycle) that flowers in the second year. In warm winter climates, it may be sown in the fall, for an overwintering cover, or in cold winter areas, it is best sown in the spring or summer. The plant is powerfully effective for loosening poor, rocky, or clay soils and for fixing atmospheric nitrogen in its roots. It feeds crop plants after being turned under into the soil.
Planting	To sow seeds, scatter or drill them shallowly in early spring. Thin plants to one foot apart. Red Clover may be grown as a living mulch or a green-fertilizing crop. The flowers attract beneficial insects, and the nitrogen-fixing bacteria on the roots work to enhance soil fertility.
Harvesting and Storage	Gather the flowers while in perfect bloom. Dry them on paper in the shade and store in airtight containers.

Red Raspberry

Latin Name: *Rubus idaeus*

Also known as: Garden Raspberry, Hindberry, Hindbur

Scientific Classification

Rubus idaeus is the cultivated variety. Rubus strigosus is the wild variety.

Family:	Rosaceae – rose family
Genus	Rubus – blackberry
Species	R. idaeus – American red raspberry

Influence on the Body	(PRINCIPAL ACTIONS are listed in CAPITAL LETTERS)
Blood and Circulatory System	HEART • mild alterative (purifies the blood, cleanses, and induces efficient removal of waste products)
Blood Sugar	Diabetes
Body System	stimulant • tonic • MUCOUS MEMBRANES • astringent (tightens, constricts, and tones tissues, reduces swelling and mucous discharge)
Digestive Tract	stomachic (strengthens stomach function) • ulcers • DIGESTIVE DISORDERS • indigestion • antacid (corrects acid conditions in the stomach, blood, and bowels) • NAUSEA • ANTI-EMETIC (relieves stomach, helps prevent vomiting) • VOMITING • GAS • GASTRITIS • BOWEL PROBLEMS • colic (severe abdominal pain) • constipation • laxative • DIARRHEA • dysentery (bowel inflammation) • hemorrhoids
Eyes	eyewash • ophthalmia (eye inflammation)
First Aid	wounds • fractures
Infections and Immune System	COLDS • coughs • FEVERS • refrigerant (cools, reduces fever) • diaphoretic (promotes perspiration, increases elimination through the skin) • FLU • cholera (serious infectious disease) • measles
Inflammation	Rheumatism

Nervous System	nervous conditions • ANTISPASMODIC
Reproductive System	gonorrhea *Male:* prostate gland *Female:* FEMALE ORGANS • MENSTRUAL IRREGULARITIES • emmenagogue (promotes menstrual flow) • leukorrhea (vaginal discharge) • vaginitis (vaginal inflammation) • douche • strengthens and tones UTERUS • MORNING SICKNESS • PREGNANCY • MISCARRIAGE preventative • anti-abortive • LABOR PAINS • oxytocic (stimulates contractions accelerating childbirth) • PAINLESS CHILDBIRTH • AFTER-BIRTH PAINS • hemostatic (stops bleeding) • breastfeeding discomfort • LACTATION • galactagogue (enhances lactation of nursing mothers)
Urinary Tract	urinary problems • cystitis (urinary bladder inflammation)

Key Properties:

FEMALE HERB	*normalizes menstrual flow, strengthens uterus and female organs, helps prevent miscarriage, regulates birth contractions, eases labor and childbirth, helps stop hemorrhaging*
ASTRINGENT	*has anti-inflammatory and toning effects on mucous membranes, cleanses and firms tissues of the mouth, throat, stomach, intestines, and urinary tract*
digestive aid	*relieves nausea, gas, and diarrhea, soothes mucous membranes of the digestive tract*
Primarily affecting	*FEMALE ORGANS • MUCOUS MEMBRANES • GENITO-URINARY SYSTEM • STOMACH*

History	Red Raspberry has been used for many centuries by women for morning sickness and to strengthen the walls of the uterus and female organs. Native Americans used the herb as a healing astringent by making an infusion of the root bark and applying it to sore eyes. The fresh fruit of red raspberry was used for dissolving tartar on the teeth.

Attributes	Key Components: (including, but not limited to)
Nutrients	Vitamins A • B1 (thiamine) • B3 (niacin) C • D • E • Calcium (good source) • Iron (good source) • Magnesium • Manganese (good source) • Phosphorus • Potassium • Selenium • Sodium • Sulfur Fruit Sugars • Pectin • Tannins
	Raspberry leaves are a rich source of calcium, iron, and manganese. Red Raspberry leaves have at least twice the manganese content of any other herb. Raspberries rank near the top of all fruits for antioxidant strength.
Hormones for Men and Women	The benefits of red raspberry leaves are well known. They have been used by herbalists and midwives for hundreds of years to balance hormones. The herb is a specific for reproductive health in both men and women of all ages. Raspberry leaves contain raw materials that help the body produce its own estrogen.
	Drinking raspberry leaf tea helps relieve painful menstruation and regulates menstrual flow. If menstruation is too heavy, it will lighten without abruptly stopping.
Pregnancy and Childbirth	Red Raspberry helps to strengthen the walls of the uterus and supports the entire female reproductive system. Raspberry leaf tea is commonly used to relieve morning sickness and may be taken throughout pregnancy.
	Red Raspberry helps reduce the chance of miscarriage and premature birth. It helps the body coordinate uterine contractions. It decreases contractions in the second trimester of pregnancy, reduces false labor pains prior to birth, and assists labor by stimulating contractions at the time of delivery. Herbalists and midwives recommend taking raspberry leaf tea freely throughout pregnancy to render childbirth less laborious.
	Regular use of the tea will fortify uterine tissues to the extent that it helps prevent tearing of the cervix during birth. Red Raspberry helps prevent hemorrhaging during and after labor, and it can reduce afterbirth pains. It is not a conventional painkiller, so red raspberry can safely cross the placental membrane without depressing the respiratory and circulatory centers in the brain of the developing fetus.
	Observational studies were conducted wherein midwives monitored the efficacy and safety of raspberry leaf tablets (2.4gm

daily) taken from 32 weeks pregnancy until the commencement of labor. Analysis of the findings suggested labor was shortened by an average of 10 minutes. An unexpected finding was the women in the raspberry leaf group were less likely to require an artificial rupture of membranes, a caesarean section, forceps, or vacuum birth than the women in the control group. No adverse side effects were identified for mother or baby while taking the herb.

If the women had taken red raspberry leaf from the beginning of their pregnancy in a liquid form such as tea or tincture, I believe the outcome would have been much more dramatic.

Raspberry leaf tea helps prepare the breasts for nursing by cleansing and purifying the blood. Its high iron content enriches the early colostrum found in mother's milk and increases overall milk supply.

Mucous Membranes

Raspberry leaves have been used to clean and heal cankerous conditions of mucous membranes throughout the body. Tannins found in red raspberry tighten tissues and have an anti-inflammatory effect on mucous membranes and skin abrasions. Tannin-rich raspberry leaves are used as a wound treatment, mouthwash, gargle, and internal tea for the digestive tract.

Raspberry tea is mild and pleasant to the taste. It is soothing for stomach aches and bowel problems in children and adults. Red Raspberry's astringent qualities help control the bowels and is a long-established remedy for dysentery and diarrhea, especially in colicky infants. For flu and diarrhea in children, drink the tea and use as an enema (if needed). Raspberry leaf is an excellent herb for children to use for colds and fevers.

Red Raspberry helps relieve urethral irritation and is soothing to the kidneys, urinary tract, and ducts. The herbal tea makes an effective eyewash for swollen and inflamed eyes.

Herb Parts Used	Leaves and fruit
Preparations and Remedies	Red Raspberry is a mild, pleasant, stimulating, astringent tonic.
Infusions	*Red Raspberry Leaf Tea:*

RED RASPBERRY — 277

Pour 1 cup of boiling water over 1 or 2 teaspoons of the dried leaf. Steep for 10 minutes, strain, and sweeten to taste.

During pregnancy, drink two to three cups daily. Use for morning sickness, to neutralize acid, aid digestion, and strengthen the uterus for childbearing.

Use a strong infusion as a gargle for cankers, sore throat, thrush, and spongy gums.

For hemorrhoids, drink plenty of red raspberry leaf tea daily. Make a decoction with equal parts witch hazel and red raspberry. Apply to the affected area with a clean cloth or cotton ball (which may be left on overnight for added benefit).

A cold infusion of raspberry leaves is a reliable remedy for extreme laxity of the bowels. It is also useful in stomach complaints of children.

Lactation Tea: (see BLESSED THISTLE preparations)

Ginger Tea: (see GINGER preparations)

Yarrow Tea: (see YARROW preparations)

Stomach Tea:
A strong tea made from slippery elm and red raspberry is excellent to help cleanse the stomach and soothe irritation and relieve gas.

Enema and Douche

Use tea for an enema preparation and as a douche to soothe irritated membranes, as needed.

Douche:
Mix together equal parts of the following:
Goldenseal • Red Raspberry • Echinacea • Slippery Elm

Wash

Make a strong infusion using one ounce of the herbs to one pint of boiling distilled water. Cool and strain. Add one teaspoon of raw apple cider vinegar (if desired). Douche in the morning and evening. Use for problems with the uterus, infections, candida, and vaginitis.

The infusion is a valuable wash for sores, wounds, skin ulcers, and raw surfaces.

Eye Wash: (see GOLDENSEAL preparations)

Ointment

Yarrow Ointment: (see YARROW preparations)

Safety	No health hazards or adverse side effects are known. Red Raspberry leaf tea has been used safely for centuries by children, adults, pregnant women, nursing mothers, and the elderly.

I hear of more and more women being told red raspberry leaves are dangerous during pregnancy. Considering the vast amount of historical data we now have, I find this to be simply absurd. Once again, I question the motives behind these suggestions. |
| **Plant Profile**

Description

Growing Red Raspberry | *Natural Habitat:*
Indigenous to Europe and Asia, red raspberry is widely cultivated in temperate climates and grows abundantly in North America.

Red Raspberry is a perennial plant with a biennial growth habit (meaning it dies down in winter and revives each spring from the root, not flowering until the second year). It grows in hedges, thickets, and neglected fields. The stalks are generally erect (growing three to six feet), freely branched, covered with small, straight, slender thorns, and have pale green leaves that are double serrated on the edges.

Small, white, or rose-colored flowers bloom from May through July in simple clusters, followed by fruit. The fruit is not a true berry, but an aggregate of a number of red, hairy drupelets containing small seeds. The red juice is sweet, acidulous, and pleasant to the taste. The odor is characteristic and aromatic.

Red Raspberry hedges are generally propagated by suckers (secondary shoots from the base of the plant). Place the plants about two feet apart in rows, allowing four or five feet between each row. If planted too closely, the fruit does not fully develop. It is wise to replant every three or four years, as the fruit on old plants is apt to deteriorate.

In October, cut down all the old wood that has produced fruit in the summer and shorten the young shoots to about two feet in length. Dig spaces between rows and dress with a little manure. Beyond weeding during the summer, no further care is needed. |

Saw Palmetto

Latin Name: *Serenoa repens*

Also known as: Sawtooth Palm, Windmill Palm, Shrub Palmetto, Dwarf Palmetto, Sabal

Scientific Classification
Serenoa repens is the only species in the genus Serenoa.

Family: Arecaceae – palm family
Genus Serenoa – serenoa
Species S. repens – saw palmetto

Influence on the Body	(PRINCIPAL ACTIONS are listed in CAPITAL LETTERS)
Addictions	Alcoholism
Blood Sugar	Diabetes
Body System	stimulant • tonic • GLANDS • anti catarrhal (eliminates mucous conditions) • anti-inflammatory • astringent (tightens, constricts, and tones tissues, reduces swelling and mucous discharge) • general debility
Digestive Tract	nutritive • DIGESTIVE AID • parasiticide
Infections and Immunity	colds • antiseptic • whooping cough
Liver	gallbladder problems
Lungs and Respiratory System	mucous discharge (head area) • sore throat • bronchitis • asthma • lung congestion • expectorant (loosens and removes phlegm from the respiratory tract)
Nervous System	nervine • nerves • neuralgia (sharp, stabbing pains due to deposits or congestion putting pressure on nerves) • antispasmodic • sedative
Reproductive System	HORMONE REGULATION • REPRODUCTIVE ORGANS • INFERTILITY • SEXUAL STIMULANT • frigidity • libido • mild aphrodisiac *Male:* MALE HORMONE IMBALANCE • PROSTATE GLAND ENLARGEMENT • BPH (benign prostatic hyperplasia) • PROSTATITIS (prostate inflammation) • IMPOTENCY *Female:* BREAST ENLARGEMENT • anti galactagogue (limits milk secretions)

Urinary Tract	diuretic • urinary tract infections • cystitis (bladder inflammation) • bladder • kidney diseases • Bright's disease (kidney inflammation)
Weight	PROMOTES WEIGHT GAIN when undernourished • obesity

Key Properties:

GLANDULAR TONIC	*supports glandular system, builds and restores tone to weakened body systems*
HORMONAL REGULATOR	*enhances reproductive system balance in both men and women, promotes prostate health and healing*
MUCOUS MEMBRANES	*increases urine flow, reduces mucous conditions, soothes inflammation in the lungs, urinary tract, reproductive organs, and glands*
Primarily affecting	GLANDS • HORMONES • GENITO-URINARY SYSTEM • MUCOUS MEMBRANES
History	Saw Palmetto is an old American tonic known to early Mayans. Native Americans, in the region that is now Florida, used saw palmetto not only as a food source to increase strength and weight, treat digestive problems, dysentery, genitourinary inflammation, urinary problems, and women's breast disorders, but also as an aphrodisiac.
	Early American settlers also used the fruits to promote reproductive function, as a sedative, and as a tonic to improve general health. However, one settler wrote of its taste as unpalatable, describing it as being similar to eating 'rotten cheese steeped in tobacco juice.'
	The genus name 'Serenoa' was named for Sereno Watson (1826-1892), a Harvard botanist. Scientists noticed animals that fed on saw palmetto berries grew sleek and fat. Observational human studies found eating the berry improved digestion and increased strength and weight. It was recommended in wasting diseases and for reproductive glandular weaknesses such as atrophy of the testes and prostate problems.
	In 1879, Dr. J. B. Read wrote of saw palmetto in the *American Journal of Pharmacy*:
	> 'By its peculiar soothing power on the mucous membranes it induces sleep, relieves the most troublesome coughs, promotes expectoration, improves digestion, and increases fat, flesh, and strength. Its sedative and diuretic properties are remarkable.'

In the 1900's, doctors in Europe and America, took up saw palmetto as a treatment for male prostate enlargement and urinary tract infections in both men and women. Its use fell out of favor with American physicians as other pharmaceutical medications were created for treatment. Meanwhile, saw palmetto research and treatment increased in European countries.

French researchers in the 1960's discovered by concentrating the oils of the saw palmetto berry, they could maximize the herb's effectiveness. German health authorities approved saw palmetto preparations containing the fat-soluble components for conditions associated with benign prostatic hyperplasia (BPH).

Saw Palmetto remains an acceptable medical treatment for BPH in New Zealand, France, Germany, Austria, Italy, Spain, and other European countries. Some countries use saw palmetto as the standard that prostate medications must meet to be considered effective.

In the 1990's, along with the general increased interest in using herbs in America, the virtues of saw palmetto had a resurgence of popularity. It has since been one of the top-selling herbs in the United States.

Attributes	**Key Components:** (including, but not limited to)
Nutrients	Vitamin A Fatty Acids • Volatile Oil • Sterols The fruit is rich in fatty acids and sterols which appear to give saw palmetto its therapeutic properties
Hormone System	Saw Palmetto supports the glandular hormonal system and helps to regulate hormone balance. It is recommended in wasting diseases because of its nutritive and healing effects on all the glandular tissues. In cases of under-nutrition, saw palmetto can directly enhance body weight in those that are malnourished. It can also stimulate the glands, thus assisting the body to improve the appetite, and aid digestion and assimilation. Saw Palmetto is often used in herbal combinations to provide nutrients and heal hormonal glands and organs that are unbalanced or diseased. It is specifically used in normalizing

blood-sugar levels of diabetics, decreasing ovarian irritability, increasing the size of under-developed breasts, improving the secreting ability of the mammary glands, and restoring sexual desire.

The reproductive organs are greatly benefited by the use of saw palmetto. It assists the thyroid gland in regulating normal sexual and physical development and function. It promotes increased blood flow and nourishment to the sexual organs. Saw palmetto is used in diseases of both male and female reproductive systems. In general, saw palmetto improves health, disposition, and tranquility.

Prostate Health

Numerous studies with several thousands of participants have been conducted to determine the effectiveness and method of action of saw palmetto therapy on men with benign prostatic hyperplasia (BPH) and related conditions.

BPH is a non-cancerous prostate enlargement. Abnormal prostatic growth is believed to begin as early as age 30, with 50 percent of men showing histological evidence of BPH by age 50, and 75 percent by age 80. When the prostate gland is sufficiently large, it begins to constrict the urethral canal. This leads to symptoms of painful urination, increased frequency, urinary retention and hesitancy, and increased risk of urinary tract infections. Although prostate specific antigens, or PSA levels, may be elevated (an indicator of possible malignant cancer) in individuals with BPH because of increased organ growth and inflammation (due to urinary tract infections), BPH alone is not considered to be a pre-cancerous condition.

Dihydroxy-testosterone (DHT) is a powerful hormone (three times as potent as testosterone) derived from testosterone by enzyme action of 'testosterone-alpha-reductase.' Like testosterone, DHT is responsible for many male characteristics (such as a deepened voice, facial hair, sex drive, and muscle growth). However, unbalanced hormones with increased levels of DHT cause cells to multiply excessively, leading to the prostate enlargement. DHT is also a primary contributing factor to male-pattern baldness.

As a side note, increased levels of DHT in women result in the development of certain male characteristics, including facial hair and deepened voice. A high level of DHT is one factor that contributes to hair loss in women.

Urinary System

Saw Palmetto's known method of action on BPH is two-fold. In order to assist the body to restore hormone balance, (1) it can inhibit the enzyme responsible for converting testosterone into DHT, and (2) it has the ability to help the body balance estrogen and progesterone hormone production.

A major study of 1,098 patients compared the effects of saw palmetto extract to conventional drug therapy. The study concluded both treatments relieved symptoms in two-thirds of their patients. It was also noted adverse side effects when using conventional medications included impotency and decreased libido. Fortunately, these side effects did not occur with the use of saw palmetto.

Saw Palmetto helps the body to balance male sex hormones, restore normal function, and increase sexual desire and potency. Many clinical trials corroborate the ability of saw palmetto extract to improve the signs and symptoms of BPH. Saw Palmetto not only inhibits further enlargement, it also helps reduce existing inflammation, swelling, and pain of the prostate gland.

Preliminary medical literature has recently reported reduced occurrence of prostate cancer with the use of active components in saw palmetto. In addition, saw palmetto's anti-inflammatory action reduces the occurrence and severity of androgenic alopecia (hair loss due primarily to hormone imbalance).

Saw Palmetto calms uterine irritability and inflammation, increases the bladder's ability to contract and expel its contents, increases urine flow, tones the urethra, removes uterine blockage, and heals infection and rupture. A double-blind French clinical trial published in 1984 involving 110 BPH patients reported saw palmetto reduced the number of times patients had to urinate at night by more than 45 percent and increased urinary flow by more than 50 percent. Painful or difficult urination was significantly reduced in the treatment group, as compared to the placebo group. Reported benefits required 4-6 weeks of treatment to develop.

Saw Palmetto is a natural urinary antiseptic that helps prevent infection. Positive clinical results have been shown in women who use saw palmetto for repeated bladder infections.

Mucous Membranes	Saw Palmetto soothes inflamed mucous membranes. It reduces excessive mucus in the head, nose, throat, air passages, and in cases of chronic bronchitis and lung asthma. Saw Palmetto is quieting to the nerves and has a sedative effect on the body.
Herb Parts Used	Ripe berries
Preparations and Remedies	Saw Palmetto berries may be eaten fresh, though many find the taste disagreeable. The fruit may be dried and powdered for herbal preparations. Studies have shown the rich oils must be present for saw palmetto to be effective. Special care must be taken to retain the active, therapeutic components when saw palmetto is harvested, stored, dried, and processed for encapsulation in herbal formulas.
Safety	Saw Palmetto is generally considered safe and side-effect free. There are no known drug interactions. Saw Palmetto is not recommended for use when pregnant, due to its effect on hormone levels.
Plant Profile *Description*	*Natural Habitat:* Saw Palmetto is native to North America. It grows wild along the coastal regions of the southern states of the United States, from South Carolina to Florida and west to Texas. Most saw palmetto is wild-harvested in Florida. Saw Palmetto is a fan palm consisting of 20 or more leaf blades radiating from a central point. The plant grows as a shrub (2-7 feet) or as a small tree (20-25 feet). The thick, tough stems and leaf blades are lined with sharp, saw-like teeth that can easily tear skin and clothes. Each blade ends in two sharp points. The stout evergreen shrub is supported by a large, underground trunk. Whitish-green flowers with three to five petals appear May through July. Deep purple to almost black ovate berries (about one inch long) follow in branched clusters. Each berry contains one large seed. The fruit ripens in the high humidity and heat of August and September, and is usually ready to harvest October

through November. The fruit has a rather rancid smell (The fruit isn't bad. It really just smells that way!) and is soapy and unpleasant to the taste.

Growing Saw Palmetto

Saw Palmetto thrives in dappled shade and moist, well-drained soils. It is propagated by seed or by separation of suckers (secondary shoots from the base of the plant).

Harvesting

Fruits are harvested when ripe and dried for use in herbal preparations.

Slippery Elm

Latin Name: *Ulmus rubra*

Also known as: Indian Elm, Red Elm, Rock Elm, Moose Elm, Elm Bark, Sweet Elm, Winged Elm, Gray Elm

Scientific Classification

There are about 20 species belonging to the elm family. Slippery (or Red) Elm is smaller than the rest of the elm family. California Slippery Elm (Fremontia californica) is not botanically allied to Ulmus rubra, but its bark is said to have the same properties and may be used for similar medicinal purposes.

Family: Ulmaceae – elm family

Genus Ulmus – elm

Species U. rubra – slippery elm
U. fulva – synonymous classification: the species name U. rubra was made and published just prior to U. fulva and is technically more correct. Herbalists have used both nomenclature systems.

Influence on the Body	(PRINCIPAL ACTIONS are listed in CAPITAL LETTERS)
Addictions	Smoking
Blood and Circulatory System	Hemorrhage
Blood Sugar	Diabetes
Body System	odorous perspiration • mucous membranes • DEMULCENT (softens and soothes inflammation of mucous membranes) • removes mucus • mild astringent (tightens and constricts tissues, reduces swelling)
Cancer	cancer • tumors
Digestive Tract	NUTRITIVE TONIC (supplies nutrients, aids in building and toning, and increases energy and strength throughout the body) • hiatal hernia • nutrition (good source of nutrients and sustenance) • weak and debilitated nutrition • DIGESTIVE DISORDERS • gas • stomach problems • stomach acidity • ULCERS • COLITIS • COLON • DIARRHEA • CONSTIPATION • dysentery (bowel inflammation) • diverticulitis (bowel wall 'out-pouch' inflammation) • hemorrhoids • expels worms • appendicitis

Endocrine System	adrenal glands
Eyes	eyes • purulent ophthalmia (eye inflammation with discharge)
First Aid	BURNS • sores • fractures • wounds • gangrenous wounds • vulnerary (promotes healing of wounds by protecting from infection and stimulating cellular growth) • poison ivy rash
Infections and Immune System	hay fever • fevers • flu • herpes • CATARRHAL INFECTIONS • COUGHS • whooping cough (also known as pertussis, a contagious disease characterized by severe coughing and 'whooping' sound when breathing in)
Inflammation	internal inflammation • gout • arthritis • painful joints
Liver	Jaundice
Lungs and Respiratory System	PECTORAL (healing to problems in the bronchopulmonary area) • ASTHMA • BRONCHITIS • LUNGS • phlegm • expectorant (loosens and removes phlegm in the respiratory tract) • croup (inflammation of larynx, accompanied by cough, difficult breathing and fever) • pneumonia • tuberculosis • lung hemorrhaging • pleurisy (painful inflammation of chest cavity lining) • diphtheria (contagious disease characterized by difficult breathing)
Mouth, Nose and Throat	hoarseness • sore throat • tonsillitis
Pain	pain • lumbago (back pain)
Reproductive System	libido • venereal disease • syphilis *Female:* ovaries • uterus • cramps • female problems • vaginal discharge • douche • leucorrhea (vaginal discharge due to infection)
Skin, Tissues and Hair	EMOLLIENT (softens and soothes skin externally, and mucous membranes when taken internally) • ABSCESSES • boils • warts • ulcerous sores • chafed skin • rashes • DIAPER RASH • eczema • skin diseases
Urinary Tract	urinary tract infections • kidney disorders • water retention • diuretic (increases urine flow) • cystitis (bladder inflammation) • bladder problems

Key Properties:

MUCILAGE DEMULCENT and EMOLLIENT	*protects, soothes, softens, and heals inflamed mucous membranes, particularly of the skin and digestive, respiratory, and urinary systems.*

NUTRITIVE	*supplies nourishment, soothes digestion, assists nutrient assimilation, restores strength and tone to the body*
mild astringent	*increases tissue tone and firmness, reduces mucous discharge from the nose, intestines, and draining sores, etc*
Primarily affecting	*MUCOUS MEMBRANES • STOMACH • RESPIRATORY TRACT • URINARY TRACT*

History

The species name 'rubra' means red and refers to the rust color of the tree's buds before the leaves appear in the spring.

Native Americans ate the nourishing inner bark and made a soothing laxative tea. They called it 'oohooska,' meaning 'it slips.' The Osage found the inner bark made an effective poultice for healing wounds and extracting thorns and gunshot. Among the Cree tribe, a poultice of the bark was a toothache remedy.

Early American settlers learned to soak the bark in water and apply it to wounds as a natural bandage. Slippery Elm was used by colonists to make pudding, thicken jelly, preserve grease, and as a survival food on long trips.

George Washington's army endured the bitter winter at Valley Forge (1777-78) by eating porridge made from the inner bark of the slippery elm tree. Army doctors used it as a primary treatment for gunshot wounds. Later, when food was scarce during the War of 1812, British soldiers fed their horses slippery elm bark.

Skin washes and teas were made using dried elm leaves. The inner bark was used to waterproof canoes, baskets, and places of living. Physicians In the 19th century recommended slippery elm bark be taken as a nourishing broth for children, the elderly, wasting diseases, and convalescing invalids who had difficulty digesting food.

The bark was recommended as a reliable remedy for gastrointestinal disorders (stomach aches, ulcers, gastritis, colitis, diarrhea, dysentery, and intestinal worms), respiratory afflictions (sore throats, coughs, pneumonia, consumption, and pleurisy), injuries, and skin ailments.

Slippery Elm throat lozenges made by the Henry Thayer Company have kept the herb on drugstore shelves for over a century. Thayer's Slippery Elm Lozenges first appeared sometime in the late 1800's. Slippery Elm bark continues to be used today, much in the same way as in the past.

Attributes	Key Components: (including, but not limited to)
Nutrients	<u>Bioflavonoids</u> • Vitamins <u>E</u> • <u>K</u> • <u>Calcium</u> (good source) • <u>Copper</u> • <u>Iron</u> • <u>Phosphorous</u> • <u>Potassium</u> • <u>Selenium</u> • <u>Sodium</u> • <u>Zinc</u> <u>Linoleic acid</u> • <u>Mucilage</u> (soft and slippery sugar molecules) When the inner bark of the slippery elm gets wet, gummy substances surrounding its fibers swell and produce a slippery, gel-like compound called mucilage.
Nutritive	Slippery Elm is recognized as a mild-flavored, wholesome, and nutritious food that is safe enough for babies and recovering convalescents. It is an excellent sustaining food possessing as much nutrition as oatmeal, though it is much easier to digest. Slippery Elm helps to nourish the adrenal glands, which gently stimulate and energize the entire body. Slippery Elm helps the body break down dairy products, and is indicated whenever there is difficulty in digesting or holding down foods. The gruel made with slippery elm bark is a valuable remedy in cases of malnutrition, weakness, stomach inflammation, pulmonary complaints, lung hemorrhage, etc.
Mucous Membranes	Slippery Elm has a wonderfully soothing, healing, and strengthening action on inflamed mucous membranes and irritated tissues. Its abundant mucilage naturally coats, softens hardened tissues, draws out impurities, absorbs poisons, and buffers inflammation. Names of disorders ending in '-itis' indicate an inflamed and irritated condition. Slippery Elm is used for its abilities to rapidly heal and relieve discomfort in conditions such as bronchitis, colitis, cystitis, arthritis, tendinitis, prostatitis, and conjunctivitis.
Digestive Tract	This versatile herb provides nutrition and a soothing coat to the digestive tract. Slippery Elm is a great friend to the stomach, small intestine, and colon. It has the ability to protect sore throats, help neutralize stomach acidity, absorb foul gases, heal damaged tissues, speed digestion, and enhance beneficial bacteria growth. Slippery Elm acts as a deterrent to many toxic substances through its ability to absorb and pass toxins harmlessly out of the

body. It lubricates the bowel, allowing for smooth and softer eliminations. Parasites literally slide out of the digestive tract of a person taking a large dose of the tea.

Slippery Elm works as a 'contact healer', as well as by way of digestion. For sore throats and hiatal hernias, slippery elm is best consumed either in tea form or by stirring the powder in water, juice, or applesauce. Once swallowed, slippery elm is able to directly contact the surfaces above the stomach and begin its healing action.

Taking a heaping teaspoon of slippery elm powder every two to five hours can soothe the worst digestive inflammation of nervous diarrhea or soften and lubricate areas of constipation. It may be taken by mouth or used as an enema to normalize stools and soothe, protect, and heal the entire intestinal tract inner lining.

Slippery Elm bark powder is a good addition to douches and enemas when inflammation and burning are present. When it is used this way, it needs to be diluted with enough water, so as not to plug the orifice as it swells. Slippery Elm is also an excellent remedy for irritated kidneys and the mucous membranes of the urinary and respiratory tract.

Lungs and Respiratory Tract

Slippery Elm tea and lozenges are great for coughs, sore throats, bronchitis, lung diseases, and lung hemorrhaging.

Skin

Slippery Elm acts on the skin and tissues to relieve painful inflammation, draw out impurities, soothe, smooth, soften, speed healing, and strengthen tissues.

Slippery Elm bark may be applied as a poultice or a fomentation to inflamed surfaces, rashes, chafed skin, ulcerous sores, wounds, burns, boils, skin diseases, and even purulent ophthalmia. It also makes a wonderful topical application for deeper inflammations such as gout, arthritis, and painful joints.

Antioxidant

Antioxidants found in slippery elm bolster the immune system and reduce inflammation. Slippery Elm is one of four ingredients in Essiac Tea, which is used for stimulating the immune system and helping the body fight cancer (see recipe in BURDOCK preparations section).

Other Uses

Slippery Elm's mucilage gives it the ability to bind together herbal preparations such as suppositories, boluses, and lozenges.

SLIPPERY ELM — 291

	Poultices made with leaves of other herbs are frequently combined with slippery elm to give the combination cohesiveness.
Herb Parts Used	Inner bark, fresh or dried
Preparations and Remedies *Powder*	*Fresh:* The inner bark may be chewed and the fluid swallowed for irritation of the throat. The powder should be gray or fawn colored. If powder is dark or reddish, good results may not be obtained. It has a bland flavor that hints of burnt caramel candy. Most babies willingly eat slippery elm mixtures. It may be added to juices or apple sauce. Lukewarm liquid activates the mucilage immediately. *Tooth Powder:* A pinch of the powder placed in the tooth where decay has started is said to reduce discomfort and delay further decay.
Infusions	Slippery Elm is mucilaginous and expands when mixed with water. It should be taken with lots of water. The powder mixes easily with plenty of liquid. You may also use a blender, wire whip, fork, or shake it in a bottle vigorously until well blended. *Mild:* Pour one cup of hot water over one teaspoon of powdered bark and steep for one hour or overnight. Infusions may be simmered, strained, and then consumed, giving a thick syrup consistency. *Medium:* Pour one cup of hot water over one tablespoon of powdered bark. *Strong:* Pour one cup of hot water over two to four (or more) tablespoons of the powdered bark, stirring constantly. It will make a thick, slimy, healing, brown sludge. *Essiac Tea:* (see BURDOCK preparations) *Red Raspberry Tea:* (see RED RASPBERRY preparations) *Urinary Tract Infection Tea:* (see UVA URSI preparations)
Wash / Fomentations	*Athlete's Foot Soak:* (see CHAPARRAL preparations) *Soothing Fomentation:* (see LOBELIA preparations)

Slippery Elm Gruel

Mix one teaspoon of slippery elm powder and one teaspoon of honey or maple syrup into one pint of hot water, stirring to eliminate lumps. Flavor with lemon rind, cinnamon, cloves, nutmeg, or other spices.

Alternative:
Ginger is a good addition because it significantly increases the focus and action of slippery elm. Use one-fourth or a half-part of ginger for each one part of slippery elm. Individuals who cannot keep anything down are often able to tolerate slippery elm gruel when it is taken a teaspoonful at a time.

Extended Internal Use:
It may be necessary to use the soothing, healing effects of slippery elm bark for an extended period of time in cases of prolonged, severe colitis or surgery. Some practitioners recommend a day's break be taken once a week from continuous slippery elm use (or mix slippery elm with other herbs such as ginger) to ensure against a non-stop coating of the intestines.

Enema

Use mild infusion as an enema for diarrhea and nausea.

Enema/Douche: (see RED RASPBERRY preparations)

Bolus

Bolus: (vaginal or rectal suppository)
Hold inside for a day, wash out with douche, and repeat if necessary. A bolus is an excellent treatment for uterine problems, cancer and tumors of the womb, all growths in the female organs, fallen womb, leucorrhea, or inflammation and congestion of any part of the vagina or womb.

Poultices

Soak the inner bark in water (warm water works the quickest) until a gel substance forms and apply directly to the area of concern. Always clean and flush open wounds with an anti-infection tincture before applying a poultice. Use slippery elm alone, or mix with other herbs such as:

    Goldenseal root, to disinfect
    Cayenne (in small amounts), to stop bleeding
    Plantain
    Echinacea, for bites, stings, and blood poisoning
    Aloe vera gel, to promote healing
    Tea tree oil
    Kelp
    Powdered Myrrh gum

Black Walnut inner hulls
(the inner goo just inside the outer shell)

Make slippery elm inner bark at least a third of the poultice mixture. Blend all the herbs by hand or in a blender. Add enough hot water to make a gummy consistency and apply to the affected area.

In simple inflammations, the poultice may be applied directly onto the affliction. If the area has hair, smear the face of the poultice with olive oil or fold it within a piece of clean, unbleached muslin before applying.

For abscesses and open wounds, poultice ingredients should be placed between cloths. Always use clean muslin (cotton) and change often if drainage occurs. When covering a deep wound or cut, the poultice may stay in place for three or four days. Adding a layer or two of cotton gauze over the poultice and pressing will make a secure cast.

While acting as a binding agent, slippery elm will help draw out poisons, soothe the skin, and reduce inflammation. It is excellent for abscesses, burns, skin inflammation, congestion, eruptions, enlarged prostate, swollen glands of the neck and groin, severe rheumatic problems, gout, and other joint problems. Slippery Elm inner bark works so well, once it dries, it may take some effort to remove it.

Boils and Abscess Poultice: (see ECHINACEA preparations)

Poultice for Burns: (see FLAXSEED preparations).

Cough Syrups

Slippery Elm makes a great cough syrup when used either alone or as a base for other herbs. It helps to soften and expel mucus and relieve inflammation.

Slippery Elm Cough Syrup:
Make the syrup fresh when it is needed, or it may be stored in the refrigerator for a few weeks. After that time, it is best to start with a fresh batch to ensure potency.

In a saucepan, mix a quarter cup of slippery elm powder with one cup of water. Simmer and stir gently for twenty minutes. Let cool and add two tablespoons each of raw honey and fresh squeezed lemon juice (raw apple cider vinegar can be used if lemon is not available). It is difficult and unnecessary to strain out the used herb powder.

Option 1: Substitute part of the slippery elm for other herbs such as comfrey, chopped raw onion, ginger, or clove. Cayenne may be used in small quantities as well.

Option 2: Add a few drops of an essential oil to supplement the healing action and taste of the syrup. Peppermint oil is refreshing, and clove oil would be a fine choice for its antiseptic and pain-numbing qualities.

For children up to about six years old, most syrups should be taken one teaspoon at a time, every two hours, or as needed. For older children and adults, one tablespoon per dose may be taken as needed.

Salve

Lobelia Salve: (see LOBELIA preparations)

Safety

No health hazards or adverse side effects are known.

Slippery Elm is approved by the Federal Drug Administration as an over-the-counter ingredient in throat lozenges.

Plant Profile

Natural Habitat:
Elm trees are native to the Appalachian Mountains of eastern North America and in Asia. They grow in the moist (though not waterlogged) woods of eastern Canada and the United States.

Description

Slippery Elm grows 50-60 feet high with a trunk 1-4 feet in diameter. The reddish-brown bark is very rough and scaly and has deep, perpendicular furrows. Young branches are red-brown to orange and more or less downy. The twigs are rough, grayish, and hairy. The under layers are ruddy brown, and the innermost layer, next to the wood, is buff white, aromatic, and very mucilaginous. It is this inner layer that is used medicinally. Small flowers appear (before the leaves) in clusters at the extremities of young shoots in March and April.

Its large leaves (four to eight inches long, two to three inches broad) are sandpaper-rough on both sides. They have a deep, olive-green color above and a lighter, sometimes rusty, color beneath. Leaf color darkens in the fall. The leaves have double-serrated margins, and are noticeably asymmetrical at the base.

The fruit ripens in early summer every two to four years. It encircles a single, flat brown seed. The thin, green, membranous capsule makes a flat circular wing that flies away on the spring wind. In the wild, only a few seeds are fertile.

Slippery Elm Growth

Slippery Elm grows in moist soils in full or partial sun. It seems to be less susceptible than other species to Dutch Elm Disease, which devastated other elm populations when it spread to the United States in the 1930's.

Harvesting

In the spring, the herb is collected from wild trees. To be effective, the tree must be at least ten years old. It should be gray in color, not red. The rough outer bark is removed, and the inner bark retained and dried. The wood does not have commercial value; therefore, it is left. When harvested commercially, the tree is fully stripped and consequently dies.

So much bark was harvested at one time, slippery elm became a threatened species. In an 1837 study conducted for the state of Massachusetts, George B. Emerson wrote, 'In many places I have found it dead or dying, from having been stripped of its bark... It is much to be regretted that the slippery elm has become so rare.'

Responsible harvesting and repopulation are essential to maintaining an adequate supply of herbs. It would have indeed been a shame to have lost the benefits of this marvelous plant.

St. John's Wort

Latin Name: *Hypericum perforatum*

Also known as: St. Johns Wort, Johns-Wort, St. John's Grass, Goatweed, Klamath Weed, Tipton Weed, Hardhay, Amber

Scientific Classification

There are 300 species in the Hypericum genus found worldwide.
None of the others live up to true St. John's Wort in terms of medicinal qualities.

Family: Clusiaceae – mangosteen family

Genus: Hypericum – St. John's Wort

Species: H. perforatum – common St. John's Wort

Influence on the Body	(PRINCIPAL ACTIONS are listed in CAPITAL LETTERS)
Blood and Circulatory System	heart • blood cleanser • anemia • internal bleeding • hemorrhage • reduces capillary fragility
Body System	insomnia • chronic fatigue syndrome (debilitating fatigue of six months or more) • ANTI CATARRH (eliminates inflammation and congestion of mucous membranes)
Cancer	CANCER • ANTI TUMOR
Digestive Tract	aromatic (contains volatile oils which aid digestion) • appetite • stomachache • stomach spasm • ULCERS • colic (severe abdominal pain) • diarrhea • dysentery (bowel inflammation) • WORMS
First Aid	bruises • burns • scrapes • wounds • septic (infected) wounds • leg ulcers • vulnerary (promotes healing of wounds by protecting against infection and stimulating cellular growth)
Infections and Immune System	anti-bacterial • antiviral • herpes • human immunodeficiency virus (HIV) • acquired immunodeficiency syndrome (AIDS)
Inflammation	anti-inflammatory • gout • arthritis • rheumatism • cellulitis (inflammation of connective tissues just beneath skin surface) • lymphangitis (inflammation of lymph vessels)
Liver	gallbladder • jaundice • hepatitis (inflammation of the liver)

Lungs and Respiratory System	BRONCHITIS • LUNG CONGESTION • coughs • expectorant (loosens and removes phlegm from the respiratory tract)
Muscles	myalgia (muscular pain) • strains • pulled muscles or ligaments
Nervous System	NERVINE (improves nerve function) • nervous conditions • nervous tension • headaches • neurasthenia (lack of energy) • ANTI DEPRESSANT • melancholy • sedative (calming, exerts soothing, tranquilizing effect) • anxiety • hysteria • palsy • antispasmodic • spasms • lower back spasms • sciatica • neuralgia (pain due to congestion or impingement of nerves) • BEDWETTING • peripheral neuropathy (nerve function disorders outside the spinal cord, with symptoms such as numbness, weakness, burning pain, or loss of reflexes) • multiple sclerosis (disease of the myelin sheath of the nerves marked by numbness, weakness, loss of muscle coordination, and problems with vision, speech, and bladder control) • nerve damage
Poisons	insect bites
Reproductive System	*Female:* swollen breasts • REGULATES MENSTRUATION • PAINFUL MENSTRUATION • UTERINE CRAMPS • AFTER-BIRTH PAINS • menopause
Skin, Tissues and Hair	boils • external skin problems • shingles • varicose ulcers
Urinary Tract	URINARY DISORDERS • SUPPRESSED URINATION • astringent (tightens and constricts tissues, reduces discharge and swelling) • water retention • diuretic (increases urine flow)

Key Properties:

NERVINE	*regulates the nervous system, relieves pain, quiets nerves and spasms, repairs damaged nerves, mildly sedative*
ANTI-DEPRESSANT	*regulates balance of many neurotransmitters, calms anxiety, elevates mood*
ANTI-CATARRHAL	*relieves congestion and soothes inflammation of mucous membranes of the lungs, digestive tract, and genitourinary systems*
alterative	*purifies and cleanses the blood of impurities and wastes*
Primarily affecting	NERVOUS SYSTEM • MUCOUS MEMBRANES • BLOOD • UTERUS
History	Its scientific name 'Hypericum' is derived from the Greek words 'hyper' and 'eikon,' meaning 'to overcome an apparition,' relating

to ancient belief in its ability to ward off evil spirits. The species name 'perforatum' is derived from the translucent dots that can be seen when the leaf is held up to the sun, making it look perforated.

First century Greek physicians Galen and Dioscorides both recommended St. John's Wort as a wound healing herb, a diuretic, and a treatment for menstrual disorders.

'Wort' is the Old English word for plant and, according to legend, St. John's Wort carries St. John the Baptist's name because of its use as a healing balm on battle wounds incurred during the crusades (1095-1099). The plant also tends to flower around the feast of St. John on June 24th. It exudes a red color when bruised, seen as symbolic of his blood.

It was later believed during medieval times on St. John's Eve, if an unwed woman gathered St. John's Wort that yet had the dew on the leaves, she would find a husband, or if gathered by a barren wife, it would secure conception.

In the 16th century, Paracelsus (1493-1541), a Renaissance physician, botanist, alchemist, and astrologer, used the plant externally for treating wounds and painful contusions (bruises).

During the Middle Ages, St. John's Wort was popular for casting out demons (possibly an archaic description of treating emotional disorders). In the 1800's, the herb was classified as a nervine and was used internally for mild depression, anxiety, hysteria, and insomnia. St. John's Wort was also recommended for pulmonary complaints, jaundice, diarrhea, dysentery, bleeding, worms, bladder ailments, and children's bedwetting.

The fresh flowers were infused in teas, tinctures, and oils for treatment (especially indicated when nerve damage was present) of external ulcers, wounds, sores, cuts, and bruises.

Native Americans dried the plant and used it as a meal. They were also known to eat the fresh leaves for a soothing effect. The Cherokee used the plant to treat bloody diarrhea, intestinal complaints, fever, and suppressed menstruation. The crushed plant was sniffed to treat nosebleed, and it was rubbed on venereal sores. Roots of the plant were chewed and swallowed or made into a poultice for snakebites. The Montagnais tribe used a plant decoction to treat coughs. The Iroquois used the plant to treat fevers and the root to enhance fertility.

In 1793, St. John's Wort was collected in Pennsylvania, where it was first recorded as a specimen in the United States. American eclectic physicians were doctors who practiced with a philosophy of 'alignment with nature' at the turn of the 20th century. They promoted the use of St. John's Wort for the healing of wounds and lacerations that involved nerve damage. Eclectics also used it as a diuretic, astringent, nervine, and mild sedative.

St. John's Wort became more popular as a treatment for depression in the early 1900's. As pharmaceutical antidepressants became available, German researchers began looking to herbs for similar properties. Today, St. John's Wort is one of the best-documented herbal treatments for depression, with scientific research and testing approaching that of many prescription drugs.

Attributes	
Nutrients	**Key Components: (including, but not limited to)** Choline (an essential nutrient, usually grouped with the Vitamin B complex) • Hypericin (a red pigment that exudes from the flower petals when crushed) • Hyperforin (a bitter found in the leaves that stimulates digestive juices and improves appetite) • Pseudo-hypericin • Pectin • Tannins • Flavonoids • Alkaloids The action of the principle active ingredients of St. John's Wort is not precisely known. There seems to be a synergistic effect as the components work together. Hypericin appears to have antidepressant and antiviral properties. Studies show hypericin and pseudo-hypericin have potent antiretroviral activity, without serious side effects. Hyperforin has antidepressant, antibiotic, and anticarcinogenic qualities.
Nervine and Anti-inflammatory	St. John's Wort has a deep-seated nervine effect. It helps restore damaged nerve tissue, can relieve nerve pain, calms the system, and has a mild sedative effect. St. John's Wort is also used to improve the quality of life for individuals suffering from chronic diseases, including arthritis, multiple sclerosis, neurasthenia, and chronic fatigue syndrome.

Externally, the herb is invaluable for reducing inflammation and the pain of scrapes, bruises, strains, burns, and other trauma. St. John's Wort may be applied as a liniment salve or poultice over the spine for relief of nerve disorders that are related to the spine, sciatica, neuralgia, and rheumatic pains. St. John's Wort is specific for deep, low pain of the coccyx (vertebrae at the base of the spine).

St. John's Wort relieves chronic nerve pains such as peripheral neuropathy. The herb is very useful for treating athletic injuries with nerve damage and/or pulled muscles and ligaments.

Wounds

St. John's Wort is especially useful in cases of dirty, septic wounds. It has been proven effective in cases of putrid leg ulcers that resist healing. The herb cleanses out infection without destroying healthy tissue. It helps reduce the inflammation in septic sores, boils, cellulitis, and lymphangitis.

In Germany, St. John's Wort is approved as an external preparation for the treatment of sharp or abrasive wounds, myalgias (muscles pains), and first-degree burns.

Antidepressant

St. John's Wort is prescribed in Germany for mild to moderate depression more often than prescription medications. Typical symptoms of depression include poor stress tolerance, difficulty concentrating, depressed mood, anxiety, nervous tension, irritability, lack of energy, sleep problems, and appetite disturbance.

St. John's Wort can be used to help alleviate chronic insomnia and anxiety when they are related to depression. It may be effective in relieving seasonal affective disorder (SAD) as well.

Controlled clinical trials of St. John's Wort conclude it is significantly more effective than placebo and is found to be generally as effective (with fewer adverse side-effects) as standard antidepressant medications. Recent scientific findings support the use of St. John's Wort as a safe and effective treatment of major depression. [1]

A 1993 German study compared St. John's Wort to placebo. An incredible 80 percent of the participants had significant improvement based on a standardized set of questions regarding depression, compared to only 26 percent of the placebo group.

A placebo controlled, double-blind study of 105 patients

diagnosed with mild to moderate depression was conducted more recently. Patients who took St. John's Wort felt significant improvement in depressive mood indicators (feelings of sadness, hopelessness, helplessness, uselessness, fear, and difficult or disturbed sleep) with no significant side effects being observed.

Cumulative research indicates St. John's Wort is effective in at least 55 percent of the cases studied. As with other antidepressants, the full benefit takes approximately 4-6 weeks to develop, sometimes taking up to 3 months for complete effect.

How It Is Believed To Work:
The latest research suggests St. John's Wort blocks the reabsorption (re-uptake) of the neurotransmitter serotonin. This leaves more serotonin available in the brain. Increased serotonin levels enhance neurotransmission (sending of nerve impulses). This process categorizes St. John's Wort as a selective serotonin re-uptake inhibitor (SSRI).

Research has found abnormalities in neurotransmitter activity affect mood and behavior. Both hypericin and hyperforin (found in the blossoms and leaves of St. John's Wort) have qualities that regulate brain levels of important compounds such as:

Serotonin – regulates mood, appetite, muscle contraction, sleep, and some cognitive functions, including memory and learning

Melatonin – affects the regulation of the circadian rhythms, including sleep cycles

Dopamine – affects heart rate, blood pressure, cognition, attention, learning, motivation and reward, voluntary movement, sleep, mood, and feelings of pleasure

Norepinephrine – a stress hormone
Monoamine-oxidases – affects levels of certain neurotransmitters and their by-products

Interleukins – signals proteins used primarily in the immune system.

Overall, the effect of St. John's Wort on neurotransmission is to help reduce symptoms of depression, uplift mood, and calm anxiety, distress, mental burnout, and nervous depression.

Blood Flow

St. John's Wort is an excellent blood cleanser and purifier. It is

	valuable for treating internal bleeding and helps reduce capillary fragility. The herb contains an alkaloid that is a heart and artery stimulant. Hypericin increases blood flow to stressed tissues.
Antimicrobial	Modern clinical research supports St. John's Wort's use as an antibacterial, antifungal, antiviral, and anti-inflammatory compound. Hypericin is used for viral infections such as hepatitis, HIV, and herpes simplex.
Congestion	St. John's Wort is used for persistent mucous catarrh (congestion and inflammation) in the lungs, bowels, and urinary tract. It helps relieve phlegm build-up and obstructions in the chest, and is used as an expectorant to loosen and expel accumulated mucus. It has been very effective in relieving bronchitis, and contributes to the healing of all pulmonary complaints.
Digestive Tract	The herb tea is effective for digestive disorders. It has been used to treat stomachache, stomach spasms, dysentery, colic, and diarrhea. The tea, with a small amount of aloe powder, helps cleanse the liver. Whole flakes of morbid matter can wash away in the urine.
Urinary Tract (UT)	St. John's Wort increases the flow of urine and has a toning, tightening, astringent quality on distressed tissues. It strengthens urinary tract (UT) organs and helps the body in cases of urinary suppression and chronic UT and bladder disorders.
Women	St. John's Wort is specific for chronic uterine disorders and enhances uterine tone. Along with proper diet, it can control uterine cramping and help ease irregular and painful menstruation. It helps alleviate afterbirth pain and is often used when there are menopausal changes triggering irritability and anxiety.
Cancer	Hypericin has shown potent antitumor activity, helping the body reduce and control tumor growth.
Herb Parts Used	The herb tops and flowers are used medicinally. The leaf contains active flavonoids, which augment the activity of the hypericin found in the flowers and buds.
Preparations and Remedies	*Fresh:* Rub crushed petals on cold sores and fever blisters.
Infusions	*St. John's Wort Tea:*

Pour 1 cup of boiling water over 2 teaspoons of fresh, flowering tops. Steep for 10 minutes and strain. Drink 1 cup, 2-3 times a day for colds or flu. The tea is also a good blood purifier and can be used for boils, diarrhea, dysentery, jaundice, uterine cramping, uterine pain, suppressed urine, bedwetting, insomnia, and other nervous conditions.

Remedy for bedwetting:
A half teaspoon each of leaves and flowers steeped in four to eight ounces of boiling water for one hour. Take every night before going to bed.

Oil

Hypericum Oil:
It is best to use flowers and herbs fresh, as hypericin may degrade when dried. The fresh herb should be thoroughly cut, bruised, or mashed prior to combining with extra-virgin olive oil. Including the flower stems serves the function of allowing the olive oil to flow around the mashed flowers and leaves, which otherwise tend to clump.

Combine one part (by volume) of the fresh herb and flowers to three parts (by volume) of extra-virgin olive oil. As it pulls out the reddish resin of hypericum from the blossoms, the oil will turn blood red in color.

Alternative:
Take about one cupful of the fresh flowers and add a sufficient quantity of extra virgin olive oil to just cover the flowers.

Solar maceration (soaking an herb in oil and exposing it to sunlight for a few hours the first three days to soften and release constituents) of the oily mixture improves extraction of certain properties, although maceration in the dark is also effective. Maceration must be continued for two full weeks. Shaking the container each day will enhance the extraction process. After two weeks, the infused oil should be pressed, strained, and stored in a closed container in a cool, dark location for up to one year.

Salves

Apply the infused oil topically to hasten the healing of burns, wounds, swellings, bruises, sprains, swollen breasts, hard tumors, ulcers, varicose ulcers, hemorrhoids, and rheumatic ailments.

Hypericum oil may also be taken internally for indigestion and gastric ulcers. Take one teaspoon, two to three times daily.

The oil may be further processed into a salve or cream, which retain the same effects. Apply liberally throughout the day to hemorrhoids and slow-healing wounds.

Safety

In the extensive German experience with St. John's Wort being prescribed as a treatment for depression, there have been no published reports of serious adverse consequences from taking the herb with normal dosages.

Concurrent use of St. John's Wort preparations with prescription drugs should be discussed with your health care professional. It may alter the effectiveness of certain medications, including drugs taken for depression, heart transplants, HIV, blood thinners, and some anesthetics.

St. John's Wort can be very effective in helping wean off chemical medications used to treat depression. If needed, find a health care provider who can assist you.

It is recommended by some to not take St. John's Wort 21 days before surgery.

It is reported overdose of the herb may cause photosensitivity, generally characterized by an increased optical sensitivity to sunlight (and radiation from tanning salons) and an increased tendency for the skin to burn. To my knowledge, there have been no studies on humans using the whole plant. The only studies used to substantiate this caution have been done with cattle.

Areas treated with St. John's Wort infused oil should be kept covered from the sun, due to an increased risk of burning or blistering. A rare side effect of permanent darkening of skin pigmentation may result from solar exposure after applying the oil.

Plant Profile

Natural Habitat:

St. John's Wort is indigenous to all of Europe, Western Asia, and Northern Africa. It was introduced to Eastern Asia, Australia, New Zealand, North and South America, and is cultivated elsewhere.

The herb grows wild in unused ground, woods, hedges, roadsides, and meadows. St. John's Wort has been reduced to one percent of its original population in the Pacific United States by ranchers who consider it a bothersome weed. The plant is particularly aggressive in range lands with dry summers.

Description

St. John's Wort is an upright perennial (grows back in the spring from a persistent rootstock), with many branched stalks that grow to about two feet high. The plant has a hard and woody root, which abides in the ground for many years, shooting up new growth every year.

St. John's Wort has numerous, small, lemon-scented flowers and each bright-yellow petal has black glandular dots on the outer rim. The five-petaled flowers have long, feathery stamens clustered at the center. One way to identify St. John's Wort is to pinch the leaves or blossoms. They will turn red due to the release of hypericin (and stains the fingers blue-violet).

After flowering June through September, small, round heads form which contain tiny blackish seeds smelling like resin. The fruit is a three-celled capsule. The seeds ripen in August.

Slender, oblong leaves grow in opposite pairs. The deep green leaves appear perforated when held up to the light. These 'holes' are actually transparent oil glands. The entire plant smells faintly of turpentine or balsam. Its taste is bitter, resinous, and somewhat astringent.

Growing St. John's Wort

St. John's Wort loves sunny, warm locations but will grow in partial shade. The plant likes well-drained soil and is perfectly cold hardy. It does not grow well in waterlogged soil but does tolerate dryness, making additional irrigation unnecessary in most cases. St. John's Wort readily self-sows once it is established.

Planting

The growth rate of the seeds is typically 30 percent the first year. A considerable amount of the remaining hard seeds will reside for years in the soil and finally germinate at a later date. Direct seeding of such small seeds is tricky. Green-house propagation of seedlings works somewhat better with this plant.

Between March and May, sow verified St. John's Wort seeds thinly in a small box or seedling tray filled with potting soil. Cover the seeds with a thin layer of soil. Mist thoroughly with water and keep seeds moist. They will germinate in approximately 14-30 days.

After the seedlings have reached a height of 1-2 inches, transplant them in clusters of 3 into small pots filled with growing soil. Place the potted plants in sunny locations during the summer and make sure they receive sufficient water.

Harvesting

In early fall, set the plants out about 12 inches apart in well-drained soil. Cover the base of the plants with a light mulch after the first frost. They will bloom the next summer.

Harvest the plant between June and August, traditionally around June 24th (St. John's Day), near the time of the summer solstice. Never dig up wild plants because it could harm the balance of the natural habitat.

Take care while harvesting and handling the fresh herb, as the hypericin oil is readily absorbed through the skin. Using gloves is recommended. While harvesting in the hot sun, be careful not to wipe the delicate tissues around the eyes or brow with hypericin-laden hands. These areas are particularly sensitive. After handling large quantities of fresh St. John's Wort, make sure all exposed skin surfaces are thoroughly washed with soap and water.

Cut back the stems of cultivated plants to just above ground level and hang them in a dark place with the flower heads down. Though it is possible to harvest the upper plant from June through August, it contains the highest active constituents at the end of June, just after flowering.

St. John's Wort should be dried quickly (in warm weather or in a drying room), in order to preserve its oils. Gather seeds (a thimbleful of seeds should suffice) in the fall. Store seeds in a dark, dry place during the winter to sow in March.

Uva Ursi

Latin Name: *Arctostaphylos uva ursi*

Also known as: Bearberry (bearberry is also a common name for another herb, Cascara), Bear's Grape, Kinnikinnick (Indian name), Mountain Cranberry, Mealberry, Fox Berry, Rockberry, Arberry, Mountain Box, Barren Myrtle, Coralillo.

Note: Sometimes uva ursi is confused with the common plant name 'arbutus.' It is called arbutus-uva ursi in at least one early herbal reference, but it differs from the true arbutus plant.

Scientific Classification
Bearberries are three species of dwarf shrubs in the genus Arctostaphylos.

Family: Ericaceae – heath family

Genus Arctostaphylos – manzanita

Species A. uva ursi – common bearberry

Influence on the Body	(PRINCIPAL ACTIONS are listed in CAPITAL LETTERS)
Blood and Circulatory System	alterative (purifies the blood, cleanses, and induces efficient removal of waste products) • anemia • strengthens heart muscle • cardiac dropsy (swelling of tissues around the heart)
Blood Sugar	DIABETES • pancreas
Body System	mucous membranes • astringent (tightens, constricts, and tones tissues, reduces swelling and mucous discharge)
Digestive Tract	improves appetite • aromatic (contains volatile oils which aid digestion) • digestive disorders • dysentery (bowel inflammation) • diarrhea • hemorrhoids • emetic (causes vomiting in large doses) • purgative (in large doses causes watery evacuation of intestinal contents)
Inflammation	arthritis • rheumatism
Infections and Immune System	fevers • disinfectant • antibiotic • SPLEEN • herpes
Liver	liver • gallstones
Lungs and Respiration	lung congestion • bronchitis
Reproductive System	GONORRHEA • venereal diseases • syphilis *Male:* prostate gland weakness

	Female: female problems • excessive menstruation • UTERINE ULCERATION • prolapsed uterus • vagina • vaginal discharge • leucorrhea (vaginal discharge due to infection) • parturient (in large doses stimulates uterine contractions which induce and assist labor)
Skin, Tissues and Hair	Shingles
Urinary Tract	lower back pain • RENAL ULCERATIONS • renal sedative (exerts calming, soothing or tranquilizing effect on the kidneys) • urinary antiseptic • KIDNEY INFECTIONS • NEPHRITIS (kidney inflammation) • BRIGHT'S DISEASE (chronic kidney inflammation) • kidney stones • gravel • urolithiasis (process of forming stones in the urinary tract) • anti lithic (prevents or relieves calculi stones) • lithotriptic (dissolves and discharges urinary and gallbladder stones) • uric acid • urinary disorders • water retention • DIURETIC (increases urine flow) • BLADDER INFECTIONS • CYSTITIS (bladder inflammation) • BLADDER CATARRH (congestion and inflammation of the mucous membranes in the bladder) • dysuria (impaired ability to pass urine, painful voiding) • bladder incontinence (involuntary voiding) • bedwetting • strangury (difficult, painful urination, with passage of only a small amount at a time) • CHRONIC URETHRITIS (inflammation of urethra) • pyelitis (infection of the pelvic outlet of the kidney)
Weight	obesity • weight loss

Key Properties:

HEALS AND SUPPORTS URINARY TRACT HEALTH	*the body uses the herb's healing qualities to strengthen, repair, cleanse, and tone the entire urinary tract system*
ASTRINGENT	*increases the tone and firmness of tissues, reduces discharges of the urinary tract, lungs, intestines, and draining sores*
alterative **DIURETIC**	*increases urine flow, purifies, and cleanses the urinary system*
antiseptic and anti-inflammatory	*kills bacteria, soothes, and reduces congestion of mucous membranes*
Primarily affecting	*KIDNEYS • GENITO-URINARY SYSTEMS*
History	Uva ursi, from the Latin 'uva', meaning grape (berry of the vine) and 'ursi', meaning bear, is also known as Bear's Grape and

Bearberry. The fruit of the plant is edible and said to be enjoyed by bears, a few species of songbirds, and other game animals.

Venetian merchant and explorer Marco Polo (1254–1324) reported Chinese physicians were using this herb as a diuretic and to treat kidney and urinary problems. Kublai Khan (1215-1294), who welcomed Marco Polo to China, had learned of uva ursi during his invasion of China.

According to *Physicians of Myddfai*, a 13th century Welsh herbal text, uva ursi was used as a powerful astringent.

Early colonists found Native Americans mixed the leaves of uva ursi with tobacco to create a smoking combination they called 'kinnikinnick', meaning mixture. They used kinnikinnick in religious ceremonies (as a smoldering smudge or smoked in a sacred pipe) to carry the smoker's prayers to the Great Spirit.

Native Americans used uva ursi in a wide variety of healing applications. In addition to smoking the leaves for sacred purposes, the smoke from the leaves was used for earaches, and the leaves were chewed to suppress thirst.

A leaf tea was made and used for sore gums, canker sores and as a mouth wash. The tea was also used as a diuretic tonic, antiseptic, and astringent to heal urinary tract ailments such as urethritis, kidney stones, and cystitis. The Cheyenne used the tea to treat back sprains and chronic back pain. Other tribes drank it to treat venereal disease.

The entire plant was utilized to make an infusion to wash hair in cases of dandruff and scalp disorders and to clean and heal skin sores.

Leaves and stems were ground up, made into a poultice paste, and applied to sores, cuts, burns, boils, and pimples to accelerate healing. Moistened leaves were rubbed on the back for pain relief.

Berries were eaten raw or cooked and considered quite nutritious. They were eaten in large quantities as a laxative. The leaves and fruit mixed with fat were given to children for diarrhea and used as a salve for rashes, boils, burns, and skin sores.

Until the development of sulfa drugs in the 1940's, uva ursi's principal active component, arbutin, was frequently prescribed for urinary infections. In Germany, bearberry is approved as a urinary antiseptic.

Attributes	
Nutrients	**Key Components: (including, but not limited to)**
	• <u>Allantoin</u> (accelerates healing) • <u>Arbutin</u> (glycoside found in the leaves) • <u>Tannins</u> (found in leaves and berries, has astringent qualities)
	Uva ursi's diuretic action comes from arbutin, which is largely absorbed into the system (unchanged by digestion) and excreted by the kidneys. It has an antiseptic effect on the urinary mucous membranes. The leaves have a high tannic acid composition (six to eight percent).
Urinary Tract	Uva ursi has a specific healing action upon the genitourinary organs, especially in cases of gravel or ulceration of kidney or bladder membranes. The herb helps balance the pH of highly acidic urine and acts as a solvent to uretic calculi deposits.
	It is effective in kidney disorders, including mucous buildup with pus and blood. Uva ursi soothes inflammation and decreases excessive mucous discharge. It has no equal for addressing chronic inflammation of the bladder and kidneys, as it strengthens and tones the mucous membranes of the urinary passages.
	Uva ursi has antiseptic and antibiotic properties for infections and diseases that occur in the kidneys and bladder. The herb has effectively healed urinary infections that were unresponsive to pharmaceutical antibiotics. Uva ursi has been shown to work in various types of bladder and kidney diseases, including pyelitis, nephritis, cystitis, urethritis, and others.
	As a diuretic, uva ursi increases the flow of urine, helping the body to discharge residual stone material, mucus, and infections. It is important to not force cleansing through over-dosage. This may dislodge mucus and wastes so quickly they block or damage organ structures. It is best to gradually cleanse overtaxed, eliminative organs.
	Uva ursi is a powerful astringent herb that stimulates kidney activity. It has sedative and tonic qualities, which affect weakened kidneys, bladder walls, and the sphincter muscle of the bladder (helping prevent leaking). It is used to alleviate bedwetting and in the treatment of involuntary loss of bladder control.

	Uva ursi is a kidney healing herb. It works well in combination with other mucilaginous, diuretic herbs in urinary tract formulas.
Blood Sugar	Uva ursi helps the body cleanse and purify the blood. It washes out excessive sugar in the blood and assists the body in controlling diabetes.
Inflammation	The leaves of uva ursi contain more than a dozen anti-inflammatory and antiseptic compounds that help rid the body of arthritis and inflammation.
Infections	Research confirms uva ursi is a strong antimicrobial agent against many organisms including Staphylococcus and E. Coli. Two studies evaluated the antibacterial potency of the urine of people who were taking uva ursi and found activity against most major bacteria that infect the urinary tract.
Tonic	Uva ursi has invigorating and body-strengthening properties. It cleanses and reinforces the spleen and is a tonic for a weakened liver and other glands. It is considered to be a digestive stimulant.
Reproductive System	Due to the proximity of the prostate to the urinary tract in males, uva ursi has also been found to be effective in prostate remedies. It is reported to aid in treating certain sexually transmitted diseases.
Women	Uva ursi is used for womb problems and is very good as a post-partum remedy to help prevent infections. An uva ursi bath helps soothe the discomfort of inflammation, skin infections, hemorrhoids, and after-childbirth trauma. It is also used as a douche for vaginal infections and other problems of the pelvic region. Ingesting uva ursi in large doses stimulates the uterus to contract, helping to assist labor and hasten childbirth.
Herb Parts Used	Leaves
Preparations and Remedies	Leaves are dried and cut or powdered to be made into teas, tinctures, and other herbal preparations.
Powdered Formula	*Kidney Formula:* (see JUNIPER preparations)
Infusions	*Uva Ursi Tea:* 1 tablespoon Uva Ursi leaves, cut

1 cup Water

Boil the water and immediately pour over the leaves. Cover and steep for ten minutes. Strain, cool, bottle, and keep in a cool place. Drink two ounces, three to four times a day before meals.

Take the tea internally for urinary infections and disorders. Use the tea as a wash for hemorrhoids or as a douche for uterine ulceration or infection.

Tea for Urinary Tract Infections:
1 part Plantain
1 part Slippery Elm
1/2 part Ginger
2 parts Goldenseal
1 part Uva Ursi
1 part Juniper Berry

Mix herbs together. Make a tea using 1 tablespoon of herb mix per cup of boiling water, steep for 10 minutes, and strain. Drink a half cup of tea every 1-2 hours.

Kidney / Lower Back Tea:
4 parts Uva Ursi
4 parts Juniper Berry
1 part Dandelion root
1 part Marshmallow
1 part Parsley
1 part Ginger
1 part Plantain

Simmer 2 tablespoons of herb mixture for 10 minutes in pure water with lid on tight. Remove from heat, leave cover on, and steep for 20 minutes. Strain and drink 1-2 cups, as needed, for lower back discomfort. The herb nutrients used to support the kidneys travel to the lower back and strengthen and assist in healing the entire area.

Herbal Bath

Uva ursi put in a stocking and added to a hot tub of water makes a healing bath.
Alternative:
Boil 2 ounces of uva ursi for 5 minutes in a gallon of water. Let cool and add to bath water. Soak for 30 minutes morning and night. The herbs help relieve symptoms of herpes and shingles.

Safety

No health hazards or adverse side effects are known.

The herb has a large amount of tannins, which could cause an upset stomach when taken in large quantities. Begin with smaller amounts of uva ursi and increase gradually. You may notice the herb often turns urine a dark green. Do not be alarmed. This is normal. Some recommend uva ursi not be given to children under the age of two.

In large quantities, the herb stimulates the uterus to contract and acts as a vasoconstrictor (cuts down circulation) to the uterus. Pregnant women should not take large amounts of Uva ursi.

Plant Profile	*Natural Habitat:* Uva ursi grows abundantly in cool, temperate regions of the northern hemisphere including North America, Europe, and Asia. The low-growing evergreen shrub is found in pine woods and sterile, sandy, and gravelly soils.
Description	This extremely-winter-hardy, slow-growing shrub will typically grow to 6-12 inches high and 3-6 feet wide. Over time, and in the proper environment, bearberry can spread (by stem rooting) to cover a larger area (up to 15 feet in diameter and up to 20 inches in height). Uva ursi features reddish-gray branches with numerous, lustrous, dark-green leaves, which turn reddish-brown in the winter. As the plant spreads, it forms a dark-green carpet ground cover. The small leathery leaves are a shining deep green on the upper surface, and paler beneath. The leaves have no distinctive odor but have a very astringent and somewhat bitter taste. At the ends of the branches, 3-15 small, waxy-looking, white (or pink), bell-shaped flowers droop in closely crowded clusters. These flowers appear June through September (showing as early as April in some areas). Bright-red berries do not ripen until winter. They are extremely sour, but are readily eaten by birds. The quarter to half inch fruit is smooth and glossy, with a tough skin enclosing a mealy pulp and up to seven kidney-shaped seeds.
Growing Uva Ursi	As well as being a valuable herb, uva ursi is an excellent, although slow-growing, ground cover. The plant can provide erosion protection for slopes and hillsides, and has been adopted by landscapers for use as a drought-tolerant, glossy-leaved evergreen.
Planting	Bearberry grows best in cool surroundings and acid, rocky, well-

drained soils. It should not be fertilized. The plant prefers full sun, or light shade, and does well in pots. Propagation by seed is difficult. It is generally sown in the fall, spring, or summer by cuttings or layerings.

Harvesting

Most of the leaves in commerce are wild harvested by hand. They should be collected on fine September or October mornings, after the dew has dried. Select only green leaves and reject any leaves that are stained or broken.

Drying

Drying may be done in half-shade, out of doors, in warm, sunny weather. Leaves dried in the shade retain their color better than those dried in direct sun. Spread leaves in a single layer (preferably not touching) on frames covered with wire or garden netting, ensuring air circulation, and turn as needed. If there is any risk of dampness from dew or showers, take indoors to a dry room or shed. Leaves may also be dried by exposure to gentle heat.

Storage

Once the leaves are dried, they should be packed quickly away in closed containers (leaves re-absorb moisture from the air). Store in a cool, dry, dark location.

Valerian

Latin Name: *Valeriana officinalis*

Also known as: English Valerian, Cat's Valerian, All-Heal, Setwall, Setewale, Garden Heliotrope, Capon's Tail, Vandal Root, Amantilla, Phu

Scientific Classification

There are over 200 species in the Valeriana genus found worldwide. Valerian officinalis is sometimes classified into four sub-species because of a variety of plant characteristics, including whether it flourishes in damp or dry locations. All four variations have similar herbal qualities and are considered one herb in this text.

Family: Valerianaceae – valerian family

Genus Valeriana – valerian

Species V. officinalis – garden valerian

Influence on the Body	(PRINCIPAL ACTIONS are listed in CAPITAL LETTERS)
Addictions	alcoholism • hangover • drug addiction • smoking
Blood and Circulatory System	HIGH BLOOD PRESSURE • HYPERTENSION • HEART PALPITATIONS • dyspnea (shortness of breath)
Blood Sugar	hypoglycemia • diabetes
Body System	Nerve-healing stimulant (increases circulation and healing of nerves) • SEDATIVE (exerts a soothing or tranquilizing effect) • hypnotic (induces sleep) • fatigue • insomnia • restlessness • cramps • spasms • twitching spasms • stress • shock
Digestive Tract	aromatic (contains volatile oils which aid digestion and relieve gas) • heartburn • digestive disorders • stomach problems • gas • carminative (brings warmth and circulation, relieves intestinal gas discomfort, and promotes peristaltic movement) • ulcerated stomach • ulcers • intestines • colic (severe abdominal pain) • constipation • cathartic (strong laxative causing rapid evacuation) • parasiticide (kills parasites and worms) • expels worms
Infections and Immune System	colds • coughs • antibacterial • fevers • diaphoretic (promotes perspiration) • scarlet fever • contagious diseases • measles • whooping cough • cholera (serious infectious disease with symptoms of vomiting, diarrhea, dehydration, and high fever) • typhoid (disease principally caused by infected water or food,

	with symptoms of high fever, ulcers, diarrhea, headache, and hemorrhages)
Inflammation	arthritis pain
Liver	liver protective
Lungs and Respiration	BRONCHIAL SPASMS
Muscles	MUSCLE SPASMS • lumbago (back pain)
Nervous System	nervine (improves nerve function) • nerve tonic (feeds and cushions nerves) • nerve weakness • NERVOUS CONDITIONS • NERVOUS SLEEPLESSNESS • despondency • delirium • NERVOUS BREAKDOWN • HYSTERIA • HYPOCHONDRIA • PAIN RELIEF • neuralgia (sharp, stabbing pains) • headaches • migraine headaches • vertigo • head congestion • ANTISPASMODIC • CONVULSIONS • epilepsy (brain disorder accompanied by periodic convulsions and loss of consciousness) • palsy • St. Vitus Dance (nerve disease characterized by irregular and involuntary movements) • paralysis
Reproductive System	*Female:* dysmenorrhea (painful or difficult menstruation) • promotes menstruation • menopause • menopausal headaches • menstrual cramps • uterine spasticity • AFTER-BIRTH PAINS
Skin, Tissues and Hair	acne • skin eruptions
Urinary Tract	diuretic/antidiuretic (helps body regulate urine flow) • bladder • bladder gravel • lithotriptic (dissolves urinary stones)

Key Properties:

NERVINE TONIC	feeds and tones the nerves, supports nerve function, helps rebuild nerve vitality, has a gentle, stimulating, healing action, especially cushions and heals nerve endings, eases pain and calms spasms, is indicated for nervous debility, weakness, overstimulation, and irritation
SEDATIVE	calms frayed nerves and nervous energy, very soothing and quieting to the nervous system, relaxes the body, induces quality sleep, without 'hangover' feeling upon awakening
Stimulating ANTISPASMODIC	supports, warms, and heals the nerves, calms spastic nerve firing
Primarily affecting	NERVES

VALERIAN— 317

History	Early Greek physician Hippocrates (ca. 460-370 BC) recommended valerian use primarily for digestive problems, nausea, liver complaints, and urinary tract disorders. Valerian root has been used both as a sedative and for anxiety since pre-Christian times. It is cited in virtually every pharmacopoeia in the world.
	Discorides, a Greek physician (ca. 40-90 AD), recorded, 'The dry root is put into counterpoysons and medicines preservative against the pestilence.' Galen (ca. 129-217 AD), a prominent Roman physician, recommended valerian for insomnia and epilepsy. Fabio Colonna (born in 1567), an Italian nobleman, suffered from epilepsy. He came upon Galen's reference regarding the use of valerian for this affliction and took it. Colonna thereafter claimed it completely restored his health. Use of valerian to relieve spasms and induce sleep evolved in the 17th and 18th centuries.
	The common name 'all-heal' arose from the popular medieval belief it could cure almost anything (including the plague). The genus name 'Valeriana' comes from the Latin 'valere,' meaning 'to be in good health.'
	Valerian root has been used for many centuries to calm all kinds of nervous disorders. It was supposedly taken as often as coffee by ladies in Germany, resulting in their lack of nervous irritability. During World War II, it was used in England to relieve the stress resulting from air raids.
	Modern scientific studies on valerian in humans began in the 1970's, leading to its approval as a mild sedative and sleep aid by Germany's Commission E in 1985. Today, valerian is approved in the United States for use in flavoring foods and beverages such as root beer.
	Dogs, cats, and rats find the odd smell of the root irresistible. It is reputed to be the magical attractant carried by the Pied Piper of Hamelin in the children's story of the same name.
	As a child, my mother took valerian so she could get off prescription Valium.
Attributes *Nutrients*	**Key Components: (including, but not limited to)** Calcium • Copper • Magnesium • Potassium • other Trace Minerals

VALERIAN— 318

Volatile Oil (including Valerenic Acid) • Starches • Albumin • Iridoids (also known as valepotriates)

Valerian is one of the best herbal sources of calcium and magnesium.

Valerian's volatile oil has a pale, greenish color which becomes yellow and viscid with exposure. The oil contains esters similar to those found in rosemary. It develops the 'dirty sock / rotten cheese' odor during the drying process, when these esters undergo a chemical decomposition to iso-valerianic acid.

Valerian has more than 150 different chemical components, but it is not yet clear which ones are responsible for the herb's activities.

Nerve Health

Valerian supports nerve health and function. It particularly serves to cushion and heal frayed and stripped nerve endings. It naturally reduces tension and anxiety. Significant results have been obtained in cases of emotional (or mental) hysteria and hypochondria.

Nature's tranquilizer valerian, calms and cushions the nerves, leaves no 'hangover' stupor upon waking, does not require increased dosage over time, is not habitual nor addictive, and improves quality of sleep.

Valerian improves coordination, tones nerves, and raises serotonin levels. It is especially active when an individual is in pain or under emotional stress. Valerian both excites and depresses the central nervous system (CNS). Before the sedative effect can be felt, components in valerian's essential oil must be broken down by body enzymes into valeramic acid (the calming element).

In a double-blind study of 48 participants, individuals in the valerian treated group reported less anxiety when placed under situations of 'social stress.'

Sedative

Valerian is the first remedy herbalists consider for calming the nervous system and promoting healthy sleep. It is a clinically-proven sedative and sleep inducer. Its use is indicated when sleep disorders are a result of nervous tension, anxiety, exhaustion, headache, or hysteria.

Valerian affects the cerebrospinal system. It is employed as a calming sedative of the primary nerve centers for afflictions such as St. Vitus Dance, nervous unrest, neuralgia pain, epileptic fits, hysteria, and wakefulness. Valerian is very relaxing to the whole system without narcotic effect. It helps lower anxiety and aggression and promotes sleep when taken at night.

As one of the safest, best, and most gentle herbal sleeping remedies, valerian enhances the natural body process of slipping into sleep and helps to reduce stress. For individuals who do not need as much sleep as they once did, it also mellows while lying awake in bed, ensuring a restful and relaxing experience. Conventional sleeping pills can have a marked impact on REM (rapid eye movement) sleep, but valerian does not interfere with this process.

Valerian's method of action is attributed to a number of its components, with no single ingredient considered to be the only active element. Knowledge of how valerian functions is still limited, but science has revealed more than one process.

Sleep cycles go through a sleep-wake rhythm throughout the night. The rhythm is related to natural changes in adenosine levels within the central nervous system (CNS). Studies have shown administration of adenosine induces sleep. Valerian exhibits adenosine activity.

Valerian contains constituents that bind to adenosine receptors. This enables some of the valerian compounds to act partially like adenosine in the brain, yet they do not stimulate the receptor as fully as adenosine itself. The authors of these studies concluded a valerian/hops combination extract functions as a sleep aid by suppressing wakefulness through the central nervous system (CNS) adenosine process. Also, they found the onset of its action to be relatively fast.

Whatever the process, results of studies have shown use of valerian can produce an improvement in sleep quality. When valerian root function was studied in healthy young people, they experienced an easier and quicker descent into sleep.

In two randomized, blind, and placebo-controlled crossover trials, valerian (400-450 mg before bedtime) resulted in significantly improved sleep quality and decreased sleep latency with no residual sedation in the morning. Habituation or addictions have not been noted.

Muscle Relaxant	Much research has demonstrated valerian root has safe relaxing properties that work to slow down the central nervous system (CNS), calm nerves, relax muscles, and relieve muscle spasms. It can be used safely for muscle cramping, bronchial spasms, uterine cramps, and intestinal colic. Valerian will decrease both spontaneous and caffeine-stimulated muscular activity, significantly reduce aggressiveness, and alter a number of processes in the brain and nervous system. It has also been used since ancient times in the treatment of epilepsy.
Heart	Valerian is used for circulatory problems and suggested in cases of heart palpitation. Several of the alkaloids present in valerian have blood pressure lowering qualities. It slows the action of the heart, while increasing the strength of its beats. Valerian is used worldwide as a relaxing agent for lowering hypertension and easing stress-related heart conditions.
Women	Valerian produces an exhilarating sensation and is especially useful for women of all ages who have emotional swings during their menstrual cycles. The tea or tincture will help reduce menstrual cramps and relieve menopause-induced headaches.
Digestion	Valerian stimulates glandular secretions of the stomach and increases intestinal peristalsis (contractions that propel contents onward). It helps to heal stomach ulcers and is powerful in preventing digestive fermentation and gas. Valerian has long been used as an antispasmodic to relieve stomach cramps and stress.
Addictions	Valerian root works counter to the hypnotic effects of alcohol and drugs. It has been used to assist the rehabilitation of many addicts. It serves as a substitute for some chemical medications, helping the addict sleep easier, and allowing relaxation and 'mellowing out.'
Herb Parts Used	The roots and rhizomes (underground stems) are used medicinally.
Preparations and Remedies	Roots and rhizomes may be dried and cut or powdered to put in infusions, capsules, extracts, and other herbal preparations. **Never boil the root, as much of its therapeutic value is in the volatile oil that will evaporate in the steam.**

Infusions	Make an infusion with 1 tablespoon of the cut and sifted root for every cup of water. Steep the valerian for 30 minutes in a closed pot. Drink about half a cup once or twice daily to calm nerves and relieve insomnia, headaches, stress, and menstrual tension and discomfort.
	When taken hot, valerian will promote menstruation in women who are having difficulty. Drink hot valerian with cayenne pepper for heart palpitations.
	Give small doses of valerian infusion two to three times daily for both infantile convulsions and restlessness of children with measles and scarlet fever. A sound sleep will generally result.
External Wash	Drink and externally apply valerian root tea for acne and irritated skin.
Soothing Bath	An infusion of a half cup of the root may be used in a bath to relieve nervous exhaustion.
Vapor Inhalation	Children can inhale vapors to quiet tension and encourage restful sleep.
Valerian Essential Oil	Diffuse or apply the essential oil topically (especially in a soothing massage) to calm, relax, ground, and balance emotions. It is also a sleep aid.
Safety	No health hazards or adverse side effects are known. Valerian is on the U.S. Federal Drug Administration's GRAS (generally recognized as safe) list and has been approved for use as a food.
	Valerian should not be taken with other central nervous system (CNS) sedatives, before driving, or in other situations when alertness is required.
	Over-dosage is highly unlikely, even with very large doses. For situations of extreme stress, where a sedative or muscle relaxant effect is needed quickly, a single dose may be repeated two or three times at short intervals.
	Essential oils are potent. Only a small amount is needed. They should never be put into the eyes nor directly contact mucous membranes. If contact burning occurs, soothe the area with a carrier oil such as almond or olive oil. Be careful to purchase only pure essential oils when using them for therapeutic purposes.

Plant Profile

Description

Natural Habitat:
The valerian plant is found in Europe and the temperate regions of Asia and the United States. It grows in damp places such as low-lying woods and meadows, along banks of rivers and lakes, and, generally, in marshy, swampy areas. However, some varieties flourish equally well in dry places.

Valerian is a large, handsome, perennial plant (after tops die down in the winter, it grows back from a persistent rootstock in the spring) that grows two to four feet high. The coarse, green, opposing, fern-like leaves (one to two and a half inches long) give off a sharp scent. They form rosettes from which the tall stems grow.

The pale green stem is thick, round, grooved, and hollow. It is branched at the top, with large terminal clusters of small, lacy white or pale pink flowers that appear June through August. The flowers are agreeably fragrant. The fruit is a capsule containing one oblong compressed seed, easily carried away with the wind.

The roots tend to merge into a short, conical shaped root stalk with an erect rhizome. They develop for several years before a flowering stem is sent up. Slender, underground, horizontal branches terminate in buds, which produce fresh plants where they take root. Only one stem arises from the root, which attains a height of three or four feet. The root crown often shows above ground at the stem base. Old roots become hollow and pithy.

The mature root is dark yellowish-brown externally and whitish within. Slender and brittle rootlets of the same color are numerous. The odor of the fresh root is pleasantly aromatic, but the smell becomes strong and less agreeable as it dries. The taste is sweet at first and then bitter.

The smell of the growing valerian plant is highly attractive to cats, rats, and dogs. If the leaves or roots are bruised, some cats may roll around the plant and tear it to pieces. Valerian was once planted in outer borders to lure rats away from homes and buildings.

Growing Valerian

Valerian prefers full sun to partial shade and fertile, moist garden soil. Valerian self-sows and spreads by root runners once it is established.

Planting

In April, sow seeds shallowly outdoors, or transplant to a garden, once small plants are established. Seeds germinate poorly. It is easier to plant roots (in the spring or fall) in a pot or directly in the garden with the crown at the surface of the soil. Space new plants one foot apart. Valerian quickly becomes crowded, so dig and renew the plants every three years.

The roots of valerian attract earthworms, so they are helpful in the garden for soil aeration. Because of its height, valerian is best suited to the back of the herb garden.

Harvesting

When growing valerian to harvest as an herb, the top branches are generally cut off in the spring to retain strength in the root throughout the growing season and to keep it from dissipating when flowering. The root should be collected in spring, before the stem begins to shoot upwards, or in the autumn when the leaves decay.

The roots and rhizomes should be dug carefully (the numerous brittle rootlets are spread out) and cleaned. The odor of fresh roots is rather faint until they begin to dry.

Drying and Storage

Care should be taken to preserve the volatile oils. Dry quickly at 120° F until brittle. Pack tightly and keep in a dry environment to prevent deterioration. Valerian roots store well.

Wild Lettuce

Latin Name: *Lactuca virosa*

Also known as: Prickly Lettuce, Horse Thistle, Green Endive, Compass Plant, Poor Man's Opium, Opium Lettuce

Scientific Classification

Wild varieties of lettuce have some percentage of narcotic sap (induces sleep or stupor and relieves pain without the addictive qualities of opiates) and, among them, Lactuca virosa has the greatest concentration of narcotic juice. Other medicinal varieties of lettuce include L. scariola (also commonly known as prickly lettuce), L. altissima, L. Canadensis (also called wild lettuce and commonly found in America), and L. sativa (known as garden lettuce). Cultivation of garden lettuce has significantly reduced the narcotic sap content, but the herb is still used as an ingredient for lotions to heal skin disorders caused by sunburn and coarseness.

Family: Asteraceae – aster, daisy and sunflower family
Compositae – in earlier classifications

Genus Lactuca – lettuce

Species L. virosa – bitter lettuce

Influence on the Body	(PRINCIPAL ACTIONS are listed in CAPITAL LETTERS)
Blood and Circulatory System	heart palpitations
Body System	LOOSENS CATARRH (inflamed and congested mucous membranes) • HARDENED MUCUS
Digestive Tract	bitter (stimulates digestive juices and improves appetite) • dyspepsia (indigestion) • colic (severe abdominal pain) • irritated gastro-intestinal tract • diarrhea • intestinal worms
Eyes	Eyesight
Infections and Immune System	ERRATIC FEVER • diaphoretic (promotes perspiration) • Candida albicans (yeast infection) • whooping cough (also known as pertusis, a contagious disease characterized by severe coughing and 'whooping' sound upon inhalation)
Inflammation	arthritic joints

Lungs and Respiratory System	asthma • BRONCHITIS • CONGESTIVE COUGHS • LOOSENS PHLEGM • EXPECTORANT (loosens and removes phlegm from the respiratory tract) • TUBERCULOSIS
Nervous System	NERVINE (strengthens nervous system function) • anxiety • mild sedative • insomnia • restlessness • hypnotic (induces sleep) • narcotic (induces sleep or stupor and relieves pain without the addictive qualities of opiates) • relieves pain • anodyne (relieves pain and reduces nerve excitability) • spasms • antispasmodic (relieves cramping, spasms, and convulsions)
Skin, Tissues and Hair	chapped skin
Urinary Tract	diuretic (increases urine flow) • urinary tract infections

Key Properties:

NERVINE	*strengthens nerve function, quiets nerve excitability, eases pain, induces sleep*
Primarily affecting	*NERVES*

History	The ancients held lettuce in high esteem for its cooling and refreshing properties. Legend claims the Roman emperor Augustus built a statue of the physician who had prescribed lettuce for him, as he believed the plant had cured him of a serious illness. No doubt it was prickly lettuce.
	The Roman naturalist Gaius Plinius Secundus (23-79 AD), better known as Pliny the Elder, wrote extensively of Lactuca in his work *Naturalis Historia*:
	'This lettuce has the property of stanching blood, and of healing phagedænic [skin ulcer] sores and putrid spreading ulcers, as well as tumours before suppuration. Both the root as well as the leaves are good, too, for erysipelas [type of skin infection]; and a decoction of it is drunk for affections of the spleen.'
	The plant's genus name 'Lactuca' is derived from the classical Latin name for the milky juice, and 'virosa' means poisonous. It is called 'compass plant' because its leaves turn toward the sun during the day.

Wild Lettuce has been called 'poor man's opium' and was considered an opium substitute by 19th century physicians. They recommended wild lettuce preparations for nervous disorders, irritable coughs (even in children), and for its calming, sedative properties.

Wild Lettuce had a surge of popularity as a recreational drug in the 1970's but was abandoned for stronger psychotropic drugs.

Attributes	**Key Components: (including, but not limited to)**
Nutrients	Bitter • Lactucarium including: Lactucopicrin and Lactucin
	A thick, milky sap called lactucarium results from breaking or cutting the stem or leaf of wild lettuce. Young plants have relatively low amounts of lactucarium. Concentration in the plant peaks when it begins to flower.
	Wild Lettuce was studied extensively by the Council of the Pharmaceutical Society of Great Britain in 1911. They discovered two chemicals, lactucopicrin and lactucin, largely responsible for the herbal qualities of L. virosa.
Nervous System	Preparations made with dried lactucarium of the wild lettuce plant are often used to induce sleep and treat severe nervous disorders. It is known to calm restlessness, anxiety, and cramps.
	The leaves contain sedative and pain-relieving properties which, though milder, act like morphine. As a tranquilizer, wild lettuce preparations may be given to adults and children alike to ensure sound sleep at night.
	Sometimes, wild lettuce is called 'little opium,' due to its use as a sedative and hypnotic. Once dried, the sap is often referred to as 'lettuce opium', though it contains no opiates. Wild Lettuce is milder than opium and does not have the addictive qualities or digestive problems that are associated with opium. The effects of wild lettuce are felt quickly but do not last very long (30 minutes to a couple of hours).
Anodyne	Wild Lettuce is known to relieve pain. It has been used for arthritic joints and soothing inflamed, chapped skin.

Coughs	Wild Lettuce is frequently used in the form of a syrup to quiet irritable coughs. It has been used effectively for whooping cough and brings relief to those suffering from bronchitis.
Urinary Tract	Wild Lettuce is a diuretic that increases urine flow, soothes sore, inflamed mucous membranes, and helps to heal urinary tract infections.
Infections	Wild Lettuce extract has shown activity against Candida albicans. It is also a mild diaphoretic, promoting perspiration and cooling the body.
Digestion	As a bitter, wild lettuce induces gastric secretions, aids digestion, and eases colic and spasms of the digestive tract.
Herb Parts Used	Milky sap and leaves (the whole plant contains the milky latex sap)
Preparations and Remedies	The milky sap is not easily powdered and is only slightly soluble in boiling water (though it softens). Leaves may be purchased in bulk in the cut or powdered form.
Infusions	To prepare an infusion with wild lettuce, add 1-2 teaspoons of the herb's leaves to a cup of boiling water and steep for 10-15 minutes. Drink 1 cup 3 times a day.

A tincture or tea consisting of equal parts wild lettuce and valerian may be taken internally, or massaged on sore areas for minor pain relief. It is a natural sedative and soothes nerves. |
| *Poultices* | Wild Lettuce is used in poultice applications for its soothing and pain-relieving qualities. |
| **Safety** | No health hazards or adverse side effects are known.

To sensitive individuals, the sap of the plant may be irritating to the touch. |
| **Plant Profile** | *Natural Habitat:*
Indigenous to Western and Southern Europe and cultivated in Germany, Austria, France, Scotland, North America, and |

elsewhere. Wild Lettuce grows on banks and waste places in dry, sandy, rocky soils.

Description

Wild Lettuce is a large, stout plant with abundant milky sap. It is a biennial herb (has a two-year growth cycle), reaching a maximum height of six feet. The erect stem springs from a brown taproot. The stem is smooth, pale green, and sometimes spotted with purple. There are a few prickles on the lower part of the stem and the short horizontal branches above.

The plant has numerous, large, oblong leaves (from 6-18 inches long) growing at the base, and fewer, smaller, sharply-toothed leaves along the stem. Veins that contain the milky juice of the leaves are connected in a web-like formation. Pale-yellow flower heads are numerous and grow on elongated branches in August through October.

The rough, black fruit is oval, with a broad wing along the edge, and prolonged. Above it grows a white, propeller-like shoot with silvery tufts of hair.

The whole plant is rich in a milky juice that flows freely from any wound. When dry, the juice hardens and turns brown. The sap has a narcotic odor that resembles opium and a bitter flavor (although horses love the taste).

Harvesting Wild Lettuce

The herb is harvested in summer when the plant is in blossom.

Collectors cut the heads of the plants and scrape the juice into china vessels several times daily until it is exhausted. The sap is then warmed a little and tapped to release it from the container. The resulting lactucarium is cut into small parts and dehydrated for future use.

Commercially, the medicinal qualities from the sap can be extracted many ways, but the most common is by soaking the gathered plant material in alcohol. After several weeks, the plant material is filtered out, leaving an infused liquid extract.

Wild Yam

Latin Name: *Dioscorea villosa*

Also known as: Mexican Wild Yam, Colic Root, Rheumatism Root, Liver Root, China Root, Yuma, Devil's Bones

Scientific Classification

Yams are herbaceous vines whose stems twine consistently to the right or left, depending on the species. Of the approximate 800 known species, 4 are native to the United States and Canada.

Family: Dioscoreaceae – yam family

Genus Dioscorea – yam

Species D. villosa – wild yam

Influence on the Body	(PRINCIPAL ACTIONS are listed in CAPITAL LETTERS)
Blood and Circulatory System	blood purifier • lowers cholesterol
Body System	reduces inflammation • ANTICATARRHAL (eliminates mucous conditions) • restlessness • stimulant (increases internal heat, dispels chill, and strengthens metabolism and circulation).
Digestive Tract	bitter (stimulates digestive juices and improves appetite) • digestive disorders • stomach catarrh • ulcers • GAS • nausea • anti-emetic (relieves nausea and vomiting) • emetic (induces vomiting in large doses) • carminative (brings warmth and circulation, relieves intestinal gas discomfort, and promotes peristaltic movement) • laxative • BOWEL SPASMS • abdominal pains • BILIOUS COLIC (severe abdominal pain due to sluggish liver or gallstones) • diverticulitis (inflammation of out-pouches of the bowel wall) • IBS (irritable bowel syndrome) • intestinal irritation
Endocrine System	Addison's disease (impaired adrenal gland function) • exhaustion
Infections and Immune System	allergies • diaphoretic (promotes perspiration) • cholera (serious infectious disease with vomiting, diarrhea, cramps, fever, and dehydration)
Inflammation	Anti-inflammatory • ARTHRITIS • rheumatism • bursitis

Liver	gallbladder • gallbladder tonic (increases energy and strength) • hepatic (supports and stimulates the liver, gallbladder, and spleen, and increases the flow of bile) • LIVER PROBLEMS • hepatitis (liver inflammation) • hardening and blocking of liver • cholagogue (promotes bile flow) • jaundice
Lungs and Respiratory System	expectorant (loosens and removes phlegm from the respiratory tract) • bronchitis • spasmodic hiccup • SPASMODIC ASTHMA • whooping cough (also known as pertussis, a contagious disease with severe coughing and 'whooping' sound upon inhalation) • lung congestion
Muscles	cramps • MUSCLE PAIN
Nervous System	nervine (improves nerve function) • nerves • nervous disorders • neuralgia (sharp, stabbing pains) • pain • anodyne (relieves pain and reduces nerve excitability) • sciatica (nerve pain in lower back, sometimes radiating downward) • SPASMS • ANTISPASMODIC • relaxant • sedative (relieves tension of nerves and muscles)
Poisons	brown recluse spider bites • insect stings
Reproductive System	*Female:* female problems • MENSTRUAL CRAMPS • dysmenorrhea (painful or difficult menstruation) • birth control • ovarian and uterine pain • uterine cramps • uterine tonic (increases energy and strength of uterus) • helps prevent miscarriage • MORNING SICKNESS • pregnancy • after-birth pains
Skin, Tissues and Hair	boils • scabies (a contagious skin condition) • contact dermatitis • psoriasis
Urinary Tract	urinary problems • diuretic (increases urine flow)
Other Uses	contains raw source material for producing many of the steroid hormones, cortisone, and hydrocortisone used in modern medicine

Key Properties:

CHOLAGOGUE and digestive	stimulates the activity of the liver and natural flow of bile, improves digestive function
ANTI CATARRHAL	very valuable in catarrhal conditions of the pulmonary system, urinary and digestive tracts, and female organs

nervine	beneficial in cases of nervous excitability, enhances nerve health, relaxes nerve firing, soothes painful inflammation and spasms
hormone-like	enhances progesterone activity, has steroid precursor components which reduce inflammation and relax muscles
Primarily affecting	*MUSCLES • MUCOUS MEMBRANES • LIVER • REPRODUCTIVE ORGANS*
History	The genus name Dioscorea honors the Roman physician and naturalist Dioscorides (ca. 40-90 AD). Wild Yam's common name is derived from the West African word 'nyami', meaning 'to eat.' Many of the roots in the Dioscorea genus are edible, although *D. villosa* is quite bitter. There is no record of how wild yam came to be called 'Devil's Bones', but when the name is applied to the roots, it makes more sense. They are long and thin (have a skeletal appearance) and are twisted as they meander below the surface of the soil. The Chinese used wild yam to brighten the eyes and as an elixir, while the Aztec and Mayan natives used wild yam as a pain reliever. Aztec records show 'chipahuacxihuitl', or 'the graceful plant' (we know as wild yam), was used for skin ailments such as scabies and boils. In both Mexico and America, natives used wild yam for birth control and to prevent miscarriage. Native Americans used a root tea to relieve labor pains, and European settlers found in wild yam a remedy for colic (hence its common name 'colic root'). Wild Yam roots were employed for bilious (liver) colic and abdominal cramps by physicians in the Confederate Army during the Civil War. Eclectic physicians, a branch of American medicine popular in the early 1900's, made use of botanical remedies along with other substances and physical therapy in their practices. They found wild yams useful for treating gastro-intestinal problems (such as irritation of the digestive tract and chronic 'gastritis of drunkards'), asthma, and rheumatism. The herb was considered to be an antispasmodic and anodyne by Eclectic doctors.

Attributes	Key Components: (including, but not limited to)
Nutrients	• <u>Bitter</u> • <u>Saponins</u> including <u>Dioscin</u> and <u>Diosgenin</u> • <u>Alkaloids</u> including <u>Dioscorin</u> The outer bark of the wild yam root is high in saponins (steroid-like components), including dioscin and diosgenin, and alkaloids such as dioscorin. Each of these components have anti-inflammatory and muscle-relaxant properties that seem to work on the muscles of the abdomen and pelvis, nutritionally support the reproductive organs, and effectively treat arthritic and rheumatic conditions.
Nervine Antispasmodic	Wild Yam root yields an important alkaloid substance which relaxes the muscles of the stomach walls and the entire abdomen region. This alkaloid also acts as a sedative on the nerves governing these areas and gives relief from pain. Dried wild yam is relaxing and soothing to the nerves. It is valuable in cases of nervous excitability as a relaxant and anti-spasmodic that prevents cramping. It is used for abdominal, menstrual, and uterine cramps and for bowel spasms.
Digestion	Wild Yam provides excellent benefits to the function of the gallbladder and liver. It helps to promote the flow of bile and is used for biliary colic, pains of gallstones, and irritation and spasms of the abdomen and intestines. It also relieves chronic problems associated with flatulence (gas) and counteracts nausea.
Anticatarrhal	Wild Yam is one of the best herbal remedies to reduce mucous membrane congestion and inflammation. It is valuable in pulmonary, digestive, uterine, and urinary catarrhal conditions.
Blood Purifier and Circulation	Wild Yam stimulates the removal of waste and congestion in the body and relieves stiff, sore joints. Wild Yam has the ability to dilate (open) blood vessels and lower blood pressure and serum cholesterol levels. These properties indirectly improve liver health by increasing its efficiency and reducing liver stress. The therapeutic effect of saponins on patients with atherosclerosis and hypertension was confirmed in clinical practice. A study of elderly adults found an extract of wild yam showed antioxidant properties and raised HDL (High Density Lipoprotein, the good cholesterol) levels.

Research has also shown the diosgenin in wild yam extract has good to excellent anti-inflammatory activity and can soothe stiff arthritic joints and relieve rheumatic pain.

Adrenal Glands

Wild Yam has been used historically for those with exhausted adrenal glands. It is indicated for problems with the adrenal glands and low blood sugar.

Women

Wild Yam soothes ovarian and uterine pain and menstrual cramps. It is a glandular-balancing agent that counteracts nausea in women when given in small, frequent doses throughout pregnancy. Wild Yam has a potent tonic effect on the uterus and alleviates pregnancy pain, nausea, and cramping. It particularly relieves cramps in the region of the uterus during the last trimester of pregnancy.

The herb also reduces the threat of miscarriage and can relieve after-birth pains. Wild Yam root powder is often combined with powdered ginger, false unicorn, and red raspberry in herbal preparations to further help prevent miscarriage.

Mexican wild yam has been used as a contraceptive for many years by Mexican and Native American women. They claim if the roots are eaten every day for over two months, conception will not occur. Ovulation and the menstrual cycle will not be interrupted, but women's eggs are resistant to fertilization during the period the wild yam is ingested. When a woman wanted to become pregnant, she merely stopped eating the yam and, within one month, she would be fertile again. It is my observation this is effective only if you have the purest of diets and take no chemical medications.

Mexican wild yam was the source of the original contraceptive pill before pharmaceutical companies started making them synthetically. There are clinics in California who have used Mexican wild yam in balancing out the masculine hormones of females. The herb also helps with hot flashes and vaginal discharge.

It is believed by many the efficacy of wild yam for helping the body heal premenstrual syndrome (PMS), symptoms associated with menopause, and other hormonal imbalances is due more to the antispasmodic, tonic, and nutritive qualities; not because the herb is a 'progesterone precursor.

It appears the body may not directly change the hormone precursors found in wild yam into active hormones (as is done in the chemical lab). Rather, the body uses the nutritional support provided naturally in wild yams to support the reproductive organs and promote hormone balance.

Steroid-Like

It is believed the steroidal effects wild yam has on the body are not because it contains steroidal hormones, but because the nutrients found in wild yam have similar effects. The body recognizes them as food and does not mistake them for its own hormones, but it uses them in a similar manner. Steroidal saponins in wild yam can help alleviate muscle strain and stress.

Most wild yam hormone creams on the market contain synthetic progesterone. Synthetic progesterone in cream form does indeed have a strong hormonal influence, but it forces hormonal reactions and is not as healing to the body.

Creams made with natural wild yam alone have a gentler hormonal influence on the body that nurtures and assists the body in balancing and healing the hormone functions of the body. It is my belief it is much more effective to ingest wild yam than to take it trans-dermally (through the skin) in creams. However, this is truly a personal choice. Some people love wild yam cream and have great results with it.

Other Uses

The root of wild yam contains dioscin, from which the steroidal saponin 'diosgenin' is extracted. Diosgenin's discovery by Japanese researchers in 1936 later led to lab synthesis of the hormone progesterone and to the first birth-control pill. In the lab, the precursor diosgenin is converted chemically into progesterone.

Great quantities of wild yam were collected in the wild or cultivated in Mexico to supply diosgenin. It became the substance which labs used to make the following products: human sex hormones (birth control pills); drugs to treat menopause, dysmenorrhea, premenstrual syndrome, testicular deficiency, impotency, prostate hypertrophy, and psycho-sexual disorders; high blood pressure, arterial spasms, migraines, and other ailments.

Since 1970, diosgenin has been completely synthesized in the laboratory for commercial products.

	Widely prescribed cortisones and hydrocortisones were indirect products of Dioscorea plants used for Addison's disease, some allergies, bursitis, contact dermatitis, psoriasis, rheumatoid arthritis, sciatica, brown recluse spider bites, insect stings, and other disorders.
Herb Parts Used	Rhizomes (underground stems) and roots are used
Preparations and Remedies	Wild Yam is found in bulk for making teas. Do not try grinding wild yam root in the blender. It is very tough and may break the blades. It is easier to buy the herb already powdered or cut and sifted.
Powdered Formula	*Liver Formula:* (see MILK THISTLE preparations)
Infusions and Decoctions	Place wild yam root (cut) in a saucepan and cover with cold water. Bring to a boil, then turn heat down and simmer for about 20 minutes. Strain and drink the infusion 1-3 times a day for irritable bowel syndrome (IBS) or pain associated with labor, diverticulitis, or menstruation. The decoction will strengthen if allowed to sit for at least 8 hours, then returned to the stove to a simmer for another 20 minutes. Take 1 tablespoon of the warm decoction every 30 minutes for colic, abdominal and intestinal irritation, spasms, spasmodic asthma, vomiting, and hepatic congestion until symptoms are relieved. To counteract nausea, take frequent, small, 2-ounce doses (with honey added, if desired) until feeling better. Take one to three cups of cold wild yam decoction during the day for liver disorders, rheumatic pains, and spasms. *Pregnancy Decoction* 1 teaspoon Wild Yam root, cut 1/2 teaspoon Ginger, dried 1 teaspoon Red Raspberry leaves 1 teaspoon False Unicorn Combine herbs and steep in one pint of hot water for twenty minutes. When threatened by miscarriage, strain and take a mouthful every half hour to strengthen the uterus. *Liver / Jaundice Tonic:* (see DANDELION preparations)

Herb Combinations	Wild Yam combines well with other herbs. When using wild yam as a uterine agent, combine with ginger, red raspberry leaves, and false unicorn. For pulmonary and stomach areas, mix with cayenne and goldenseal root.

Due to the hardness of the root, macerating time (soaking to soften and release constituents) needs to be continued for up to five weeks (with daily agitation). |
| **Safety** | No health hazards or adverse side effects are known. The roots must be dried before use. Ingestion of fresh roots may cause irritation of mucous membranes, nausea, and/or vomiting. Overdose of the dried root may also cause vomiting. |
| **Plant Profile** | Natural Habitat:
A native of North and Central America, wild yam is now found in many regions of the world. It grows in damp woodlands, running over bushes and fences and twining about the growths in thickets and hedges. |
| *Description* | Wild Yam is a perennial vine (grows back from a persistent rootstock in the spring) with a smooth, reddish-brown stem that climbs up to 20 feet. It is one of the prettiest vines in all of horticulture with its stunning display of heart-shaped leaves like the scales of a dragon. The leaves average 2-4 inches in length. Their width is about three-quarters that of their length. They have conspicuous veins and are hairy on the underside.

Wild Yam root has separate male and female flowers. The female flowers sit on top of triangular-winged, green fruits. Each cell of the fruit capsule holds one or two flat seeds. Numerous, small, male flowers grow on separate, trailing vines. These tiny, pale, greenish-yellow flowers appear from June through July.

Wild Yam's large, tuberous root looks somewhat like a sweet potato root but are not related to the family of sweet yams found in supermarkets. The roots, rhizomes, and tubers are the source of the plant's medicinal qualities.

On average, the *D. villosa* species root weighs about four pounds. It is a long, pale brown, branched, woody, cylindrical tube that is often compressed, crooked, bent, and nodular. The flesh inside is moist, fibrous, and faintly rose colored. Once the root is dried and powdered, it has a whitish color. The starchy |

root lacks flavor at first, then has an acrid, pungent aftertaste. The root has very little odor.

Growing Wild Yam

Wild Yam is propagated by seed sown in the spring or by division of tubers in autumn or spring. The plant prefers a cool, moist, shaded area to grow. Seedlings are very small at first and need to be grown for a year or two and transplanted up to larger pots (as needed), before transplanting to the woodland or shaded garden. Trellis the vine or allow it to ramble. Space plants one foot apart.

Harvesting

If possible, gather and dry the root each year. Rhizomes are harvested in autumn. The plant is dug while dormant, washed and thinly sliced while still fresh, and then dried. Roots must be dried before they are used as an herb.

Yarrow

Latin Name: *Achillea millefolium*

Also known as: Yarroway, Thousand-leaf, Thousand Seed, Milfoil, Bloodwort, Soldier's Woundwort, Staunchweed, Nosebleed, Carpenter's Weed, Old Man's Pepper, Ladies' Mantle, Devil's Nettle, Englishman's Quinine

Scientific Classification

Yams are herbaceous vines whose stems twine consistently to the right or left, depending on the species. Of the approximate 800 known species, 4 are native to the United States and Canada.

Family: Asteraceae – aster, daisy and sunflower family
Compositae – in earlier classifications

Genus: Achillea – yarrow

Species: A. millefolium – common yarrow

Influence on the Body	(PRINCIPAL ACTIONS are listed in CAPITAL LETTERS)
Blood and Circulatory System	alterative (purifies the blood, cleanses, and induces efficient removal of waste products) • BLOOD CLEANSER • blood purifier • reduces blood pressure • blood coagulant • hemostatic (stops bleeding)
Blood Sugar	Diabetes
Body System	stimulant (increases internal heat, dispels chill, and strengthens metabolism and circulation) • tonic (increases energy and strength throughout the body) • mucous membranes • ANTI CATARRH (soothes inflamed mucous membranes and eliminates congestion) • ASTRINGENT (increases the tone and firmness of tissues, reduces mucous discharge from the nose, intestines, vagina, and draining sores) • insomnia
Cancer	Cancer
Digestive Tract	aromatic (contains volatile oils which aid digestion and relieve gas) • bitter (stimulates digestive juices and improves appetite) • digestant • stomachic • stomach problems • ulcers • gas • carminative (brings warmth and circulation, relieves intestinal gas discomfort, and promotes peristaltic movement) • diarrhea • infant diarrhea • colic (severe abdominal pain) • dysentery (bowel inflammation) • colon • BOWEL HERMORRHAGE • bleeding bowels • bleeding hemorrhoids

Ears	ear infections
First Aid	bruises • abrasions • cuts • wounds • vulnerary (promotes healing of wounds by protecting against infection and stimulating cellular growth) • burns • fractures
Infections and Immune System	COLDS • FLU • antibacterial • antiseptic • promotes sweating • DIAPHORETIC (promotes perspiration, increasing elimination through the skin) • FEVERS • ANTIPYRETIC (reduces fever) • night sweats • MEASLES • chicken pox • smallpox • malaria • typhoid • yeast infections • spleen
Inflammation	anti-inflammatory • bursitis • arthritis • rheumatism
Liver	liver problems • jaundice
Lungs and Respiratory System	respiratory catarrh • bronchitis • LUNGS • pleurisy • pneumonia • HEMORRHAGE
Mouth, Nose and Throat	sore throat • NOSE BLEEDS
Nervous System	nervous disorders • cramps • antispasmodic • epilepsy • congestive headaches • hysteria
Reproductive System	*Female:* female problems • sore breasts • uterus • vaginal discharge • leucorrhea (vaginal discharge due to infection) • douche • profuse or irregular menstrual bleeding • emmenagogue (promotes menstrual flow) • menstrual cramps • yeast infections
Skin, Tissues and Hair	skin problems • dandruff • hair loss preventative
Urinary Tract	urinary problems • urine retention • diuretic (increases urine flow) • kidney problems • Bright's disease (chronic kidney inflammation) • bladder disorders

Key Properties:

CLEANSING	purifies the blood, improves circulation, cleanses toxins and congestion, quiets inflammation, increases elimination, and gradually detoxifies and strengthens the spleen, liver, kidneys, and bowels
STIMULATING DIAPHORETIC	increases circulation and elimination, relaxes, opens, and cleanses pores, releases blocked passages, induces perspiration, lowers fevers

HEMOSTATIC strengthens blood vessels and helps arrest bleeding, hemorrhaging, and draining wounds, both externally and internally

Primarily affecting *CIRCULATION SYSTEMS*

History	Yarrow has accumulated many names through the years. Some refer to the physical characteristics of the plant and others refer to how it is used.
	In Homer's *The Iliad*, the centaur Chiron (who conveyed herbal secrets to his human pupils) taught Achilles to use yarrow to bind the wounds of his soldiers on the battle grounds of Troy. Yarrow's genus name 'Achillea' is said to have come from this tradition. Some say, however, it was named after the person Achillea, who discovered the plant.
	The name 'millefolium' is derived from the many segments of its foliage; 'mille' is the Latin word for thousand. This also accounts for its popular names, 'milfoil' and 'thousand weed.'
	The herb came to be connected with fortune telling and witchcraft. It was used in charms and spells. In some areas, it was supposedly dedicated to the evil one, from which arose the common name 'devil's nettle'. The Druids (an early Celtic priesthood in the area of the current British Isles) used the stems of the plant to foretell the weather, and the Chinese used them as 'stalks of divination' to predict the future.
	In Eastern European countries, the herb was known as 'yarroway.' It was said one could know their beloved was true if their nose began to bleed when quoting a charm while tickling their nose with the feathery leaves of yarroway. A similar tale said it was possible to ensure seven years of love after marriage, by tucking yarrow flowers into the wedding bouquet.
	During the Middle Ages, yarrow was made into an herbal mixture known as gruit and used in the flavoring of beer (prior to the use of hops). At one time, its pungent leaves were dried and used as inexpensive snuff, leading to the name 'old man's pepper.'
	English botanist, herbalist, and physician Nicholas Culpepper, (1616–1654), recommended yarrow for wounds and as being 'profitable in cramps.'
	While the English explored and colonized the world, they were

exposed to many cultures and diseases. At the time, quinine was the drug of choice in Europe for fevers. If quinine was not available, yarrow was used as a substitute, and it became known as the Englishman's Quinine.

The plant was used in traditional Native American herbal medicine. They used it as a tonic for run-down conditions and indigestion. The leaves made a poultice for skin rashes, rheumatic joints, chest colds, and applied to breasts following childbirth to desensitize them.

The Pawnee used the stalk for pain relief. The Chippewa inhaled the steam for headaches and chewed the roots as a tonic. The Cherokee drank yarrow tea to reduce fever and aid sleep. The Piute called yarrow 'wound medicine.' The Navajo considered yarrow to be a 'life medicine' and chewed the leaves to stop toothache pain. They also made infusions of the plant tops and poured it into the ears for earaches.

The Shakers knew of yarrow and included it in treatments for a variety of complaints from hemorrhages to flatulence.

Historically, yarrow's virtues have been used to relieve fevers, clean the blood, and heal wounds. These same attributes apply today.

Attributes	Key Components: (including, but not limited to)
Nutrients	Vitamins A • Choline (B complex) • C • E • K • Copper • Iron • Manganese • Linoleic acid • Tannins • Azulene (in the essential oil) • Achilleine (a bitter alkaloid) • Salicylic Acid (aspirin precursor) • Flavonoids • Bitter

Azulene has anti-inflammatory and antibacterial activities. Achilleine stimulates the appetite and relieves stomach and gallbladder disorders. It also has antispasmodic and astringent qualities (helps to slow heavy bleeding). Flavonoids may also have antispasmodic properties. |
| Tonic | Yarrow is one of the best multi-purpose herbal teas that may be used regularly in large amounts, and as a general restorative and tonic for run-down conditions. |
| Blood Purifier and System Cleanser | Yarrow promotes the removal of toxins from the blood and moves them through the digestive system. It improves digestive |

evacuation by supporting and regulating liver and pancreas functions and secretions. Blood circulation is thus improved, and the herb helps lower blood pressure.

Yarrow flowers contain an oil which easily infiltrates the bloodstream. It helps rid the body of uric acid impurities (a primary cause of gout) and morbid waste materials (by-products of disease and the healing process).

Yarrow's invigorating tonic action stimulates removal of mucous congestion and disease. Aromatic compounds found in yarrow help shrink inflamed tissues and promote sweating, which eliminates waste through the pores.

Mucous Membranes

Yarrow has a soothing and healing effect on mucous membranes of the urinary tract, respiratory tract, digestive tract, and female organs.

Use of the herb relieves kidney problems, infections, and mucous discharge from the bladder.

An infusion of the plant's leaves helps relieve congestion in the respiratory tract from colds, bronchitis, and lung disorders. A chest rub can be made with yarrow's essential oil to ease congestion. Yarrow also alleviates hemorrhage and bleeding of the lungs.

Colds and Infections

The herb has been used for centuries to 'sweat out' fever, flu, colds, and pneumonia. When taken at the first sign of symptoms, yarrow can often break up a cold within 24 hours.

Yarrow is considered very effective where there are symptoms of chills, constant nasal drip, catarrh, and sensations of alternate chills and fever. It helps to alleviate hay fever, and the herb is remarkably effective for relieving flu and fevers. It may be one of the best healing agents in dealing with plagues of flu-type diseases.

The tannins in the flowers are antiseptic and powerful virus inhibitors. Yarrow's essential oil has astringent, antibacterial, and some anti-inflammatory properties.

Yarrow is an excellent fever remedy for childhood diseases with skin eruptions such as measles, chicken pox, and smallpox.

YARROW— 343

Digestion	The herb acts as a bitter tonic and is highly recommended with other digestive herbs to help relax the bowels and improve digestion. Yarrow counteracts nausea, relieves gas, balances the function of the liver, and has an influence on secretion production throughout the digestive tract. It is healing to the glandular system and tones the mucous membranes of the stomach and bowels. It is excellent for shrinking hemorrhoids and for relieving diarrhea of infants and adults.
Women	Yarrow is excellent for menstrual problems, soothing, cleansing, and healing catarrhal conditions of the female organs. It is effective in controlling fungus and yeast infections in the female reproductive system.
Blood Vessels	Yarrow has blood-regulating effects that help strengthen vein walls. They reinforce tiny blood vessels and reduce blood clotting time. The herb's astringent action helps contract blood vessels, stop hemorrhage, and promote circulation.
	Use the tea both internally and externally to help stop bleeding and accelerate the healing process. Yarrow's beneficial effects on wounds are legendary. Combined with its anti-inflammatory properties, yarrow both helps repair varicose veins and alleviates their discomfort.
	Yarrow has seemingly conflicting actions, regulated by the needs of the body: it will quickly stop a nose bleed when inserted into the nostril. However, to ease a severe sinus headache, inserting a roll of yarrow into the nostril relieves pressure by causing the nose to bleed.
Other Uses	Yarrow intensifies the medicinal action of other herbs and is considered a catalyst in herb combinations.
	Swedish scientists have found yarrow extract repels mosquitoes.
Herb Parts Used	Leaves, flowering tops, and stems are used both fresh and dried. The aromatic properties are strongest in the flowers, astringency is greatest in the leaves.
Preparations and Remedies	*Fresh:* Chewing yarrow leaves will frequently ease the pain of a toothache.

Powdered Formula

Infusions

Infection Formula: (see GOLDENSEAL preparations)

Yarrow tea is bitter to the taste but very effective.

Yarrow Tea:
Pour 1 cup of boiling water over one to two teaspoons of dried or fresh yarrow. Cover and let steep for about 15 minutes.

– Drink one large cup of the unsweetened tea before every meal for gastritis, nausea, poor appetite, gallbladder pain, and as a digestive aid.

– For sweating out a fever, the tea must be taken warm (or take capsules with warm water or peppermint tea). This will initially increase body temperature, relax, and open skin pores, stimulate free perspiration, and ultimately reduce the fever.

– Drink cool tea for bronchitis and other respiratory afflictions. Taking cold yarrow tea at night can help to alleviate night sweats.

Yarrow, Chamomile and Fennel Tea:
Mix two parts yarrow flowers and one part each of chamomile blossoms and fennel seeds to relax stomach mucous membranes and prevent inflammation. Fennel improves the taste and reduces flatulence.

Yarrow and Mullein Tea:
Mix 1 part mullein leaves and 2 parts yarrow for infusion and cover well for 15 minutes in a proportionate amount of water (typically 1-3 teaspoons of combined herbs to 1 cup of water). Strain, sweeten, cool, bottle, and keep in a cool place. Take 1 cupful 2-3 times daily for hemorrhoids.

Yarrow and Calendula Tea:
Mix equal parts of yarrow and calendula flowers (or hawthorn) for weak veins, light nosebleeds, hemorrhoids, and menstrual conditions.

Yarrow and Red Raspberry Leaf Tea:
Equal parts yarrow and red raspberry make a good tea for varicose veins and weak vessels. Drink three cups daily.

Cold and Flu Tea:

Make a tea blend of equal parts yarrow, elder flowers, lemon balm, and mint. For fastest relief, drink two cups of the tea and rest in bed, as soon as cold or flu symptoms are felt.

Yarrow and Licorice Root Tea:
Prepare a tea with a mixture of three parts yarrow flowers and one part dried licorice root. Drink three cups a day during heavy menstrual bleeding. Drinking one cup of the tea daily relieves chronic sinus congestion in both adults and children.

Inhalation	Inhale the steam of fresh yarrow herbs in boiling water for hay fever and mild asthma.
Fomentations	Apply a towel soaked in yarrow tea (as hot as possible) and place a hot water bottle over the towel for chronic lower-back pain, external hemorrhoids, or other areas of discomfort.
	For stubborn wounds, apply a fomentation made with double-strength yarrow tea. It will help alleviate bleeding and accelerate blood capillary healing.
Poultices	The bruised or mashed leaves make an excellent first-aid poultice for treating traumatic injuries, especially deep cuts.
Shampoo Additive	Add yarrow tea to shampoo to help stop hair loss.
Enemas	Use one ounce of the tea in a retention enema for internal hemorrhoids. If there is swelling or bleeding, insert two ounces into the colon after each bowel movement. Use warm yarrow tea to soothe and ease inflammation.
	For diarrhea in children, insert one cupful or more (according to age) of the infusion.
Douche	Use the cool tea as a douche for vaginal irritation and discharge.
Bath	As a tea and bath additive, yarrow relieves vaginal inflammations, eases menstrual pain, and helps regulate menstrual flow.
Essential Oil	Yarrow essential oil is pale yellow to brilliant blue (azulenes turn blue upon distillation). Massage essential oil on area of concern in a carrier oil (almond oil, extra virgin olive oil, etc.). Use of yarrow essential oil is indicated for prostate or menstrual problems, neuralgia, acne, eczema, and inflamed tissues. It

minimizes varicose veins, reduces scars, and stimulates bladder nerves.

Ointment

Yarrow - Red Raspberry Ointment:
1/2 ounce Red Raspberry leaves, powder
1/2 ounce Yarrow flowers and stems, powder
3 ounces Extra Virgin Olive Oil
1 ounce Wheat Germ Oil
Approx. 1/2 ounce Beeswax

Fold herbs into warm olive oil and stir for 15 minutes over low heat. To make a stronger salve, heat for up to 3 days (use crock pot on warm setting for this longer maturation).

Remove from heat and strain herbs out. Put the infused oil back into the pot and add wheat germ oil and enough beeswax (around 1/2 ounce) to stiffen the ointment when at room temperature. Continue stirring over low heat until the beeswax is melted, take off heat and, while still stirring, let cool until it starts to thicken. Pour into clean container, let sit until set up, and store in a cool place.

Apply externally as needed, for accelerated blood vessel and tissue repair of closed wounds, bruises, and varicose veins. It helps reduce scars and relieves inflammation and discomfort.

Safety

No health hazards or adverse side effects are known.

This herb is a mild abortifacient and should not be taken during pregnancy, except in combination with other herbs and under the direction of a health care professional.

Essential oils are potent. Only a small amount is needed. They should never be put into the eyes nor directly contact mucous membranes. If contact burning occurs, soothe the area with a carrier oil such as almond or olive oil. Be careful to purchase only pure essential oils when using for therapeutic purposes.

Plant Profile

Natural Habitat:
Native to the coast of Oregon and California, yarrow is now found throughout North America, Europe, and Asia. It grows by roadsides and in wastelands, pastures, meadows, and dry fields.

Description

This perennial plant (grows back from a persistent rootstock each year) has a single, grayish-green stem (one to three feet high) that branches toward the top. The entire plant is covered with white, silky hairs. Lacy, fern-like leaves are narrow and oblong (three to four inches long and one inch broad). Each dark-green leaf has many finely cut segments.

Small, grayish-white (or rose-colored), daisy-like flowers are packed in dense clusters of terminal flower heads. Each cluster has an overall flat-topped appearance. Yarrow blooms throughout the summer and fall.

The plant has a hardy, horizontal rootstock and self-propagates by underground runners. Yarrow has a peculiar, pleasant aroma and a rough, bitter, astringent taste.

Growing Yarrow

Yarrow prefers full sun and fast draining soils. The plant will rot if the soil remains wet for long periods.

Planting

Yarrow will propagate by division of the creeping root stock, or by sowing seed and transplanting after the seedlings are big enough to thrive on their own. The herb is hardy and grows quite easily. Growing yarrow in stressful growing conditions will produce flowers with higher essential oil content. Plant in poor soil and water sparingly.

Sow seeds shallowly indoors in early spring or outdoors in late spring. To promote flowering, pick blossoms often. The life of the plant may be prolonged by dividing it every other year and planting 12-18 inches apart. Common yarrow is a weedy species and can become invasive.

Harvesting

Harvest leafy stems and flowers on dry mornings when plants are in the early stages of full bloom.

Drying

Pick flowers with plenty of stem and hang, upside down, in bunches in a dry, dark, airy location (when drying for floral arrangements, hang each flower separately).

Storage

When stems are dry, remove the flowers and leaves. Crumble the leaves and break stems into small pieces. Mix stems, leaves, and flowers together and store the mixture in airtight containers. Yarrow is not suitable for freezing.

Yellow Dock

Latin Name: *Rumex crispus*

Also known as: Curled Dock, Narrow Dock, Sour Dock, Rumex, Garden Patience

Scientific Classification

There are about 200 species in the Rumex genus, consisting principally of docks and sorrels. Yellow Dock is considered to be one of the most therapeutic variety of the dock species, although there are at least three other varieties of dock that may be used medicinally:
Rumex aquaticus (great water dock),
R. britannica (water dock), and *R. obtusifolius* (blunt-leaved dock).

Family:	Polygonaceae – buckwheat family
Genus:	Rumex – dock Docks were formerly placed in the genus Lapathum, a name derived from the Greek, lapazein, meaning 'to cleanse'
Species:	R. crispus – curly dock

Influence on the Body	(PRINCIPAL ACTIONS are listed in CAPITAL LETTERS)
Blood and Circulatory System	ANEMIA • IRON DEFICIENCY • CHLOROSIS (type of anemia chiefly affecting girls and young women) • ALTERATIVE (purifies the blood, cleanses, and induces efficient removal of waste products) • BLOOD CLEANSER • BLOOD PURIFIER • depurative (cleanses blood by promoting eliminative functions) • BLOOD DISORDERS • hemorrhage • bleeding • SCURVY (Vitamin C deficiency disease with symptoms of anemia, weakness, bleeding gums, etc.) • varicose veins • lymphatic system • spleen
Body System	energy • tonic • endurance • stamina • lack of vitality • fatigue • mucus • expels mucus • anticatarrhal (eliminates mucous inflammation and congestion) • ASTRINGENT (increases the tone and firmness of tissues, reduces mucous discharge from the nose, intestines, draining sores, etc.)
Cancer	CANCER • glandular tumors • leukemia
Digestive Tract	bitter • nutritive • digestive disorders • sour stomach • ulcers • bowel regulator and normalizer • dysentery (bowel inflammation) • constipation • laxative • cathartic (strong laxative, causing rapid evacuation) • diarrhea • expels worms • external

	hemorrhoids • bleeding hemorrhoids
Ears and Eyes	ear infections • earache • ULCERATED EYELIDS
Endocrine System	swollen glands • pancreas • pituitary gland • thyroid glands
First Aid	SORES • muscle strains • swellings • wounds • fractures • poison ivy • poison oak
Infections and Immune System	COUGH • flu • fever • hay fever • scarlet fever • chicken pox • athlete's foot • scrofula (tuberculosis inflammation of lymph nodes of the neck in children) • leprosy
Inflammation	inflammation • gout • arthritis • RHEUMATISM
Liver	LIVER CONGESTION • jaundice • hepatitis • cholagogue (promotes the flow of bile) • gallbladder
Lungs and Respiratory System	chronic bronchitis • lungs
Nervous System	pain • mental fatigue • paralysis
Reproductive System	syphilis • venereal disease *Female:* IRON SUPPLEMENT FOR PREGNANCY • leucorrhea (vaginal discharge due to infection) • vaginal infections
Skin, Tissues and Hair	acne • chafed skin • BOILS • HIVES • ITCHING • eczema • psoriasis • SKIN ERUPTIONS • SKIN DISEASES • CHICKEN POX ITCH
Mouth, Nose and Throat	mouth sores • laryngitis
Urinary Tract	Bladder

Key Properties:

TONIC	*builds, tones, and strengthens the entire system, resulting in general sense of well-being*
EXCELLENT IRON SOURCE	*provides components for red blood cells and builds the blood, the iron and other nutrients in yellow dock are easily digested and assimilated by the body*
ALTERATIVE - BLOOD PURIFIER	*cleanses toxins from the blood and strengthens eliminative organs to rid the body of wastes*
Primarily affecting	*BLOOD • SKIN • LIVER*

History	The genus name 'Rumex', is derived from Latin meaning 'a lance', referring to the shape of its leaves. The species name 'crispus' is the Latin word for 'crisped', referring to its leaves being crisped (wavy) at the edges. The plant's root is yellow and was used as a dye at one time. The name dock is applied to the plant family of similar, broad-leaved, wayside weeds that have roots with astringent qualities.

The ancients celebrated yellow dock as a cure for scurvy and diseases of the skin. The young leaves were eaten like spinach.

The herb was a favorite of Native Americans, old-time doctors, early settlers, and herbal practitioners. Native Americans applied crushed leaves as a poultice to boils and pounded the root into a compress for cuts and wounds.

Around the turn of the 20th century, American Eclectic physicians (practiced with a philosophy of 'alignment with nature') prescribed yellow dock preparations to purify the blood, rejuvenate the liver, relieve upset stomachs, help heal skin disorders, and as a laxative. |
| **Attributes**
Nutrients | **Key Components: (including, but not limited to)**

Vitamins A • C (good source) • Iron (excellent source) • Manganese • Potassium • other Trace Minerals

Anthraquinone glycosides • Tannins • Oxalates (in the leaves) • Bitter

Anthraquinones can arrest the growth of ringworms and other fungi, stimulate bile flow, and induce toxin elimination.

Oxalates are mild diuretics found in the fresh leaves of yellow dock and spinach. They help control bleeding and assist in healing skin ailments. |
| *Tonic* | Yellow dock tones the entire body and increases energy, strength, and endurance through its astringent purification of the circulatory and glandular systems. It also helps tighten and heal varicose veins. |
| *Blood Builder* | The roots of yellow dock have been found to contain as much as 40 percent iron compounds, making yellow dock one of the best sources of iron in nature. The roots take up the iron present in the |

soil and fix it into organic iron compounds that are easily absorbed in the body without causing constipation. They readily enrich the blood.

Iron is an essential component of red blood cells. Women lose iron during menstruation, and pregnancy exacts a toll on mothers to build a blood supply for the growing fetus. Midwives often suggest pregnant women use yellow dock to keep their bowels regular and improve their red blood cell count.

Yellow dock is recommended in all cases of anemia and iron deficiency. It also helps nourish and strengthen the spleen. Using yellow dock as an iron supplement will not cause constipation, as can sometimes happen when taking synthetic iron.

Cleansing

Yellow dock increases the ability of the liver and related organs to filter and purify the blood, glands, and lymph system. It is used to nourish, strengthen, and heal the liver, gallbladder, and glands. Yellow dock helps dissolve mucus and move it through the kidneys.

The skin is sensitive to toxins and waste in the blood. When the skin breaks out in rashes, eruptions, acne, itchy patches, boils, or disease, it indicates the liver is backed up or compromised and unable to adequately filter and cleanse the blood. Yellow dock helps cleanse the body inside and out. For skin problems and wounds, it should be taken internally and used externally with a wash, bath, or as a salve.

Cancer

When accumulated waste matter progresses to swelling or tumors, use yellow dock both internally and externally. It helps dissolve glandular and other tumors. It also builds the immune system and kills parasites, which contribute to cancer.

Digestive Tract

The root is a magnificent bowel balancer and helps to heal ulcers and bleeding hemorrhoids. Add yellow dock to formulas to help cleanse parasites and worms from the intestines and to perk up the appetite.

The herb can act as a digestive laxative because it stimulates the flow of bile. Yellow dock may loosen bowels when taken in greater amounts or relieve diarrhea if used in smaller quantities. Individuals can benefit from the herb if they have either constipation or loose stools.

Herb Parts Used	Roots dug during dormancy and dried. Fresh leaves for poulticing and as a tonic.
Preparations and Remedies Decoctions	*Fresh:* The young leaves are edible and may be used as a tonic and nutritive. Tough roots, like yellow dock, need to be processed longer than simple teas before they release their healing constituents. The most common method for doing this is heating the root infusion for a longer period of time (usually simmering, not boiling) and letting the roots remain soaking in the water for a period of time (eight hours or more). Additional simmering will concentrate the medicinal potency by evaporating the water of the infusion. The following decoction is adapted from *Polly Block's Birth Book*. I discovered it while apprenticing to be a midwife. After using all types of herbs to increase women's iron levels to normal, I found Polly's formula. It is by far the most effective for raising iron hematocrit levels. I also have found it effective in rejuvenating anyone that has a loss of vitality and strength or just wants to renew their liver quickly. Tastes bad but works GREAT! *Yellow Dock Decoction:* 2 ounces Yellow Dock root, cut 1 quart Distilled Water Honey, if desired Put yellow dock root in a glass quart jar and cover with boiling distilled water. Cap the jar and allow to sit overnight. In the morning, empty the contents into a clean pan and, using low heat, simmer uncovered. Reduce liquid to about one and a half cups. Strain and squeeze through a prepared broad cloth (pre-rinse new cloth in hot water to get rid of commercial stiffening agents). Two tablespoons of honey may be added (although I don't notice it helps the taste that much, because yellow dock has a strong flavor). Refrigerate. Take one tablespoon per day (two tablespoons if symptoms are severe). This formula builds blood and restores healthy iron levels. Doctors and midwives have double-checked the Iron count on patients, as week by week, they watch it normalize.

	Yellow dock is also used to cleanse the blood of impurities, support the liver. and improve acne and skin disorders. Women use it during menstruation and pregnancy to raise anemic iron levels to normal.
Gargle	Use the decoction as a gargle and drink the tea internally for cough, laryngeal irritation, and catarrh.
Externally	Apply a yellow dock ointment topically or use the tea as a wash or bath for skin ulcers, hard tumors, eruptive skin diseases, burns, and reducing skin inflammation caused by insect bites or allergies.
Wash	*Plantain and Yellow Dock Wash:* Make a strong tea of equal parts plantain and yellow dock. Bathe the affected area frequently as a wash.
Fomentation	Saturate a natural fiber cloth in a strong decoction, wring out excess liquid, and apply a fomentation for glandular tumors and inflammations.
Poultice	Apply fresh leaves that are bruised or mashed to oily skin, swellings, cuts, and scrapes. Use yellow dock topically as a poultice for cleansing, astringent action, and pain relief.
Ointments	The root simmered in oil makes an excellent ointment for scrofulous disorders (tuberculosis type infections), itching, and indolent glandular tumors. Olive oil is commonly used as the base oil. To make a rectal suppository, use coconut oil for the base, as it hardens when cold.
Safety	No health hazard or adverse side effects are known with proper dosages. For delicate stomachs, give the infusion in smaller amounts, gradually increasing dosages to tolerance. Yellow dock root is beneficial during pregnancy, as it aids iron assimilation and will help to prevent infant jaundice. Abstain from coffee and black or Chinese teas, as these are incompatible with iron tonics. The root of yellow dock does not contain oxalate compounds, and most herbal preparations use the root of the plant. However, it should be noted if extremely large amounts of the leaves are consumed in a short amount of time, oxalates, found in the leaves, may cause oxalate poisoning.

Plant Profile

Natural Habitat:
Yellow dock is native to Europe and Africa and is now common to the United States and many regions of the world. It grows in waste areas, cultivated soils, and along roadsides. The plant thrives wherever iron is present.

Description

Yellow dock has fleshy, leathery leaves that form a rosette at the base of the plant in its first year. It then develops a large taproot and sends up a tall stem (1-4 feet high). From this central point come long wavy leaves (6-14 inches long, decreasing in size towards the top) that are crisped along the edges. The leaves and stalk have a sour taste.

The plant's tall spike is covered with pale green, drooping flowers that are interspersed with leaves along the stalk. Flowers appear June through August and turn into masses of rust-brown, three-winged seed capsules in the fall. The plant produces triangular, brown-black nuts, enclosed by the wing-like capsules. Each plant produces 3,000-4,000 seeds.

Yellow dock has a perennial (plant grows back from a persistent rootstock in the spring), spindle-shaped root (8-12 inches long) that is somewhat twisted. The root is yellowish-brown on the outside and dusty and fibrous internally. Once dried and ground, the powdered root is brownish. Yellow dock has little or no odor and a rather bitter, astringent taste.

Growing Yellow Dock

Yellow dock needs full sun and thrives despite poor soil and neglect. It freely self-propagates and can take over a garden if growth is not controlled. It keeps other kinds of plants from crowding its space by releasing inhibitory substances into the soil or air.

Planting

Yellow dock can be propagated by seed or by division. Sow seeds in shallow beds in the spring, then thin plants to six inches apart.

Harvesting and Storage

Dig roots in spring or fall. Clean and slice the roots lengthwise before drying in the sun, or artificially with another, controlled low-heat source. Leaves are picked when young and used fresh or dried. Store in tightly sealed containers.

References

Alfalfa

- Phyllis A. Balch, Prescription for Herbal Healing (2002)
- Linda B. White, M.D., The Herbal Drugstore (2003)
- Phytoestrogen content and estrogenic effect of legume fodder. PMID 7892287
- James Duke, The Green Pharmacy Herbal Handbook (2000)
- Dr. Jeffrey Bland at the University of Puget Sound

Aloe

- http://www.ncbi.nlm.nih.gov/pubmed/12001972
- Gertrude B. Foster, Herbs for Every Garden (Dutton, 1966)
- Sumbul Shamim, S. Waseemuddin Ahmed, Iqbal Azhar (2004) Antifungal activity of Allium, Aloe, and Solanum species. Pharmaceutical Biology 42 (7) 491-498.
- S. Satish, K.A. Raveesha, G.R. Janardhana (1999) Antibacterial activity of plant extracts on phytopathogenic Xanthomonas campestris pathovars Letters in Applied Microbiology 28(2), 145-147 doi:10.1046/j.1365-2672.1999.00479.
- Maenthaisong R, Chaiyakunapruk N, Niruntraporn S et al. (2007). The efficacy of aloe vera for burn wound healing systematic review. Burns. 33:713-718.
- Steven Foster, Aloe Vera: The Succulent with Skin-Soothing, Cell-Protecting Properties. www.desertharvest.com (2009)
- Choi SW, Son BW, Son YS, Park YI, Lee SK, Chung MH. 2001. The wound-healing effect of a glycoprotein fraction isolated from aloe vera. Br J Dermatol. 2001 Oct; 145 (4): 535-45.
- Steven Bratman, M.D., Natural Health Bible, 2nd Edition. The Natural Pharmacist. www.TNP.com
- Vogler BK, Ernst E. (1999). "Aloe vera: a systematic review of its clinical effectiveness." Br J Gen Prac. 49:823-828.
- Langmead L. Feakins RM, Goldthorpe S, et al (April 2004). "Randomized, double-blind, placebo-controlled trial of oral aloe vera gel for active ulcerative colitis". Alimentary pharmacology & therapeutics 19 (7): 739-47, doi:10.1111/j.1365-2036.2004.01902.x. PMID 15043514.
- de Oliveira SM, Torres TC, Pereira SL et al. (2008). "Effect of a dentifrice containing Aloe vera on plaque and gingivitis control: A double-blind clinical study in humans.
- Yongchaiyudha S, Rungpitarangsi V, Bunyapraphatsara N, Chokechaijaroenporn O. (1996) Antidiabetic activity of Aloe Vera Juice. I. Clinical trial in new cases of diabetes mellitus, Phytomedicine 3:241-243.
- Bunyapraphatsara N, Yongchaiyudha S, Rungpitarangsi V, Chokechaijaroenporn O. (1996) Antidiabetic activity of Aloe very juice. II. Clinical trial in diabetes mellitus patients in combination with glibenclamide. Phytomedicine 3: 245-248.

- www.Florahealth.com (2009)
- Agarwal OP. Prevention of atheromatous heart disease. Angiology 36:485-492, 1985.
- Nassiff HA, Fajardo F, Velez F. (1993) Effecto del aloe sobre la hiperlipidemia en pacientes refractorios a la dieta. Rev Cuba Med Gen Integr 9:43-51

Barley
- Anderson JW, Hanna TJ, Peng X, Kryscio RJ. Whole grain foods and heart disease risk. J Am Coll Nutr 2000 Jun;19(3 Suppl):291S-9S 2000. PMID:17670.
- Behall KM, Scholfield DJ, Hallfrisch J. Diets containing barley significantly reduce lipids in mildly hypercholesterolemic men and women. Am J Clin Nutr. 2004 Nov;80(5):1185-93. 2004. PMID:15531664.
- Cleland JG, Loh H, Windram J, et al. Threats, opportunities, and statins in the modern management of heart failure. Eur Heart J. 2006 Mar;27(6):641-3. 2006. PMID:16490737.
- Delaney B, Nicolosi RJ, Wilson TA et al. Beta-glucan fractions from barley and oats are similarly antiatherogenic in hypercholesterolemic Syrian golden hamsters. J Nutr; 2003 Feb 133(2):468-75 2003.
- Djoussé L, Gaziano JM. Breakfast cereals and risk of heart failure in the physicians' health study I. Arch Intern Med. 2007 Oct 22;167(19):2080-5. 2007. PMID:17954802.
- Nilsson, A.; et al. (2006). Effects of GI and content of indigestible carbohydrates of cereal-based evening meals on glucose tolerance at a subsequent standardized breakfast. European Journal of Clinical Nutrition 60: 1092–1099. doi:10.1038/sj.ejcn.1602423.
- van Dam RM, Hu FB, Rosenberg L, Krishnan S, Palmer JR. Dietary calcium and magnesium, major food sources, and risk of type 2 diabetes in U.S. Black women. Diabetes Care. 2006 Oct;29(10):2238-43. 2006. PMID:17003299.
- Maria Cristina Casiraghi, Marcella Garsetti, Giulio Testolin, and Furio Brighenti Post-Prandial Responses to Cereal Products Enriched with Barley Beta-glucan, Journal of the American College of Nutrition August 2006; (Reported a reduction of glucose and insulin response to 52% in a study of 26 subjects.)
- Jinesh Kochar, Luc Djoussé and J. Michael Gaziano, Breakfast Cereals and Risk of Type 2 Diabetes; Obesity December 2007; (Showed 40% less likely to develop type 2 diabetes.)
- Tabak C, Wijga AH, de Meer G, Janssen NA, Brunekreef B, Smit HA. Diet and asthma in Dutch school children (ISAAC-2). Thorax. 2006 Dec;61(12):1048-53. Epub 2005 Oct 21. 2006. PMID:16244092.
- Liu RH. New finding may be key to ending confusion over link between fiber, colon cancer. American Institute for Cancer Research Press Release, November 3, 2004. 2004.
- Cade JE, Burley VJ, Greenwood DC. Dietary fibre and risk of breast cancer in the UK Women's Cohort Study. Int J Epidemiol. 2007 Jan 24; [Epub ahead of print] 2007. PMID:17251246.
- Suzuki R, Rylander-Rudqvist T, Ye W, et al. Dietary fiber intake and risk of postmenopausal breast cancer defined by estrogen and progesterone receptor status--a prospective cohort study among Swedish women. Int J Cancer. 2008 Jan 15;122(2):403-12. 2008. PMID:17764112.

- Food Intake and Energy Regulation Lab, Beneficial Health Effects of Consumption of Barley and Barley Components, USDA Agriculture Research Service.
- Behall KM, Scholfield DJ, Hallfrisch J. Comparison of hormone and glucose responses of overweight women to barley and oats. J Am Coll Nutr. 2005 Jun;24(3):182-8. 2005. PMID:15930484.
- Slavin, Joanne L. Ph.D., R.D., Study review, Nutrition March 2005; (Reported lower weight in individuals consuming the highest levels of fiber.)

Bilberry
- Bell DR, Gochenaur K. Direct vasoactive and vasoprotective properties of anthocyanin-rich extracts. J Appl Physiol. 2006 Apr;100(4):1164-70. Abstract.
- Roy S, Khanna S, Alessio HM, Vider J, Bagchi D, Bagchi M, Sen CK. Anti-angiogenic property of edible berries. Free Radic Res. 2002 Sep;36(9):1023-31.Abstract.
- Steven Bratman, M.D., wtih David Kroll, Ph.D., Natural Health Bible ((2000), see www.TNP.com

Black Cohosh
- Blumenthal M., et al, eds. S. Klein and R. S. Rister, translators. German Commission E Monographs: Therapeutic Monographs on Medicinal Plants for Human Use. Austin, Texas: American Botanical Council.1998.
- Düker, E.M.,et al. Effects of Extracts from Cimicifuga racemosa on Gonadotropin Release in Menopausal Women and Overiectomized Rats. Planta Medica, 1991, 57:420-424.
- Stolze, H. An Alternative to Treat Menopausal Complaints. Gyne. 1982, 3:14-16
- Stoll, W. Phytopharmacon Influences Atrophic Vaginal Epithelium. Double-blind Study-Cimicifuga vs. Estrogenic Substances. Therapeuticum. 1987, 1:23-31.
- Lloyd, J.U. and C.G. Lloyd. Drugs and Medicines of North America. 2 vols. Cincinnati: J.U. & C.G. Lloyd, 1884-85.
- HerbalGram. 2006; 69:31 American Botanical Council, see www.herbalgram.org

Burdock
- A B Niness (01 Jul 1999). "Inulin and Oligofructose: What Are They?". Journal of Nutrition 129 (7): 1402 (7): 1402. PMID 10395607. http://www.jn.nutrition.org/cgi/content/full/129/7/1402S. Retrieved on 2008-01-19.
- Abrams S, Griffin I, Hawthorne K, Liang L, Gunn S, Darlington G, Ellis K (2005). "A combination of prebiotic short- and long-chain inulin-type fructans enhances calcium absorption and bone mineralization in young adolescents". Am J Clin Nutr 82 (2): 471–6. PMID 16087995.
- Coudray C, Demigné C, Rayssiguier Y (2003). "Effects of dietary fibers on magnesium absorption in animals and humans". J Nutr 133 (1): 1–4. PMID 12514257.
- See Burdock Leaves an Innovative Burn Treatment. http://morechristlike.com/ burdock-leaves/

- See more about Renee Caisse's story and Essiac at: http://www.ivanfraser.com/articles/health/essiac_info.html

Chamomile
- Heneka N. Chamomilla recutita. Aust J Med Herbalism 1993;5:33-9.
- Safayhi H, et al. Chamazulene: an antioxidant-type inhibitor of leukotriene B4 formation. Planta Med 1994;60:410-13.
- Glowania HJ, et al. The effect of chamomile on wound healing--a controlled clinical-experimental double-blind trial. Z Hautkr 1987;62:1262-71.

Eyebright
- Bermejo BP, Diaz Lanza AM, Silvan Sen AM, et al. Effects of some iridoids from plant origin on arachidonic acid metabolism in cellular systems. Planta Med 2000;66(4):324-328.
- Ersoz T, Berkman MZ, Tasdemir D, et al. An iridoid glucoside from Euphrasia pectinata. J Nat Prod 2000;63(10):1449-1450.
- Salama O, Sticher O. Iridoid glucosides from Euphrasia rostkoviana. Part 4. Glycosides from Euphrasia species. Planta Med 1983;47:90-94.
- Recio MC, Giner RM, Manez S, et al. Structural considerations on the iridoids as anti-inflammatory agents. Planta Med 1994;60(3):232-234.

St. John's Wort
- Berner, Linde K, MM; Kriston, L, St. John's wort for major depression. Cochrane Database of Systematic Reviews 2008, Issue 4. Art. No.: CD000448. DOI: 10.1002/14651858.CD000448.pub3.

Bibliography & Resources

Airola, Paavo, N.D., Ph.D., *The Miracle of Garlic.* Sherwood, OR: Health Plus, Publishers (1978)

Balch, James F., M.D. and Phyllis A. Balch, C.N.C., *Prescription for Nutritional Healing.* Garden City Park, NY: Avery Publishing Group Inc. (1990)

Bauman, Edward, etal., *The Holistic Health Handbook.* Berkely, CA: And/Or Press (1978)

Bennett, Hal Zina, *Cold Comfort, Colds and Flu: Everybody's Guide to Self Treatment.* New York: Clarkson N. Potter, Inc./Publishers (1979)

Bergner, Paul, *The Healing Power of Echinacea, Goldenseal, and Other Immune System Herbs.* Prima Publishing (1997)

Block, Polly, *Obstetrics for the Home.* Homespun Publishers (1984) www.pollysbirthbook.com

Bloomfield, Harold HI, M.D., *Healing Anxiety with Herbs.* New York, NY: Harper Collins Publishers (1998)

Bricklin, Mark, *The Practical Encyclopedia of Natural Healing, New, Revised Edition.* Emmaus, PA: Rodale Press (1983)

Brill, "Wildman" Steve and Evelyn Dean, *Identifying and Harvesting Edible and Medicinal Plants in Wild (and Not So Wild) Places.* New York, NY: Harper Collins Books (1994)

Brown, Dr. O. Phelps, *The Complete Herbalist.* Jersey City, N.J.: Published by the Author (1858)

Buchman, Dian Dincin, *Herbal Medicine, The Natural Way to Get Well and Stay Well.* New York: Gramercy Publishing Co. (1979)

Buhner, Stephen Harrod, *Herbal Antibiotics, Natural Alternatives for Treating Drug-Resistant Bacteria.* Pownal, VT: Storey Books (1999)

Burroughs, Stanley and Alisa, *The Master Cleanser* (1993) revised edition

Castleman, Michael, *Nature's Cures.* Emmaus, PA, Rodale Press, Inc. (1996)

Cech, Richo, *Making Plant Medicine.* Williams, Oregon: Horizon Herbs Publication (2000)

Chaitow, Leon, D.O., N.D., *Candida Albicans, Could Yeast be Your Problem?* Rochester, VT: Healing Arts Press (1998)

Chishti, Hakim G.M., N.D., *The Traditional Healer, a Comprehensive Guide to the Principles and Practice of Unani Herbal Medicine.* Rochester, VT: Healing Arts Press (1998)

Christopher, Dr. John R., *School of Natural Health.* Provo, Utah: BiWorld Publishers, Inc. (1978) and 20th Revised and Expanded Anniversary Edition, Springville, Utah: Christopher Publications, Inc. (1996)

Clark, Hulda Regehr, Ph.D., N.D., *The Cure For All Cancers.* San Diego, CA: ProMotion Publishing (1993)

Clark, Hulda Regehr, Ph.D., N.D., *The Cure For All Diseases.* San Diego, CA: ProMotion Publishing (1995)

Clarkson, Rosetta E., *Herbs, Their Culture and Uses.* New York: The Macmillan Co. (1942)

Clarkson, Rosetta E., *The Golden Age of Herbs and Herbalists [formerly titled Green Enchantment].* New York: Dover Publications, Inc. (1972)

Clotfelter, *The Herb Tea Book.* Loveland, CO: Interweave Press

Colker, Carlon M., M.D., *Sex Pills A to Z, What Works & What Doesn't.* Hauppauge, NY: Advanced Research Press, Inc. (1999)

Comfrey and Chlorophyll. Santa Ana, California (1969)

Complete German Commission E Monographs, Therapeutic Guide to Herbal Medicines. Boston, Massachusetts (1998)

Culpeper, Nicholas, M.D. and Thomas Kelly, *The Complete Herbal, updated and revised; Compiled using additional writings from Culpeper legacy.* London: Thomas Kelly. (1846)

Dawson, Adele G., *Herbs Partners in Life, a Guide to Cooking, Gardening and Healing with Wild and Cultivated Plants.* Rochester, VT: Healing Arts Press (1991)

DeLuz, Roni, RN, ND, PhD, James Hester and Hilary Beard, *21 Pounds in 21 Days, The Martha's Vineyard Diet Detox.* New York, NY: Harper Collins Publishers Inc., (2007)

deWaal, Dr. M., *Medicinal Herbs in the Bible.* York Beach, ME: Samuel Weiser, Inc. (1984)

Dextreit, Raymond, *Our Earth Our Cure.*

DK Natural Care Library, *Saw Palmetto, Hormone Health Enhancer.* New York, NY: Dorling Kindersley, Inc. (2000)

Downey, Rhonda Pallas, *The Healing Power of Flowers.* Woodland Publishing (2007)

Elkins, Rita, M.H., *Medicinal Herbs of the Rain Forest, Uncovering the Rain Forest's Natural Medicines.* Pleasant Grove, UT: Woodland Publishing (1997)

England, Allison with Lola Borg, *Aromatherapy for Mother & Baby, Natural Healing with Essential Oils During Pregnancy and Early Motherhood.* Rochester, VT: Healing Arts Press (1994)

Felter, Harvey Wickes, M.D., and John Uri Lloyd, Phr. M., Ph.D., *King's American Dispensatory.* (1898)

Foster, Steven and Christopher Hobbs, *Peterson Field Guides: Western Medicinal Plants and Herbs.* Boston and New York: Houghton Mifflin Co. (2000)

Foster, Steven and James A. Duke, *Peterson Field Guides: Eastern/Central Medicinal Plants and Herbs.* Boston and New York: Houghton Mifflin Co. (2002)

Foster, Steven and Rebecca L. Johnson, *Desk Reference to Nature's Medicine.* Washington, D.C.: National Geographic (2006)

Foster, Steven, *101 Medicinal Herbs, An Illustrated Guide.* Loveland, Colorado: Interweave Press, Inc. (1998) – also see: www.herbphoto.com

Gladstar, Rosemary and Pamela Hirsch, *Planting the Future, Saving Our Medicinal Herbs.* Rochester, VT: Healing Arts Press (2000)

Glum, Dr. Gary L., "Essiac: Nature's Cure for Cancer, an Interview with Dr. Gary L. Glum" by Elisabeth Robinson. Herbal Healer Academy, Inc. Newsletter (1994)

Glum, Dr. Gary L., *Calling of an Angel, the Story of Rene Caisse and Essiac.* (1988)

Goodenoughs, Dr. Josephus, *Dr. Goodenough's Home Cures & Herbal Remedies, Comprising the Favorite Remedies of Over One Hundred of the World's Best Physicians and Nurses.* New York: Avenel Books (1982)

Gordon, Lesley, *A Country Herbal.* New York, NY: Webb & Bower (Publishers) Limited (1980)

Grieve, M., *A Modern Herbal, Vol I & II.* New York and London: Hafner Publishing Co. (1967)

Griffin, LaDean, *Is Any Sick Among You? (James 5:14).* Salt Lake City, UT: Hawkes Publishing Inc. (1993)

Griffin, LaDean, *Is Any Sick Among You? (James 5:14).* St. George, UT: Tree of Light Publishing (1974)

Hamilton, Rowan, MNIMH and Arnold Fox, M.D., *Discover the Power of Aged Garlic Extract.*

Harrar, Sari and Sara Altshul O'Donnell, *The Woman's Book of Healing Herbs, Healing Teas, Tonics, Supplements, and Formulas.* Emmaus, PA: Rodale Press, Inc. (1999)

Harris, Ben Charles, *Better Health with Culinary Herbs.* Barre, MA: Barre Publishers (1971)

Heatherley, Ana Nez, *Healing Plants, A Medicinal Guide to Native North American Plants and Herbs.* New York, NY: The Lyons Press (1998)

Herbal Healing, *A Practical Introduction to Medicinal Herbs.* Great Britain: Ashgrove Press Limited (1994)

Herbalgram web site, see: www.herbalgram.org

Hermann, Matthias, *Herbs and Medicinal Flowers.* Geneve, West German (1973)

Hobbs, Christopher, *Milk Thistle: The Liver Herb, Second Edition.* Capitola, CA: Botanica Press (1984)

Horizon Herbs, LLC, Williams, OR. (Certified organic seeds and plant starts) www.horizonherbs.com (2009)

Huson, Paul, *Herbalism, A Practical Guide.* Briarcliff Manor, NY: Stein and Day/Publishers/Scarborough House (1974)

Hutchens, Alma R., *A Handbook of Native American Herbs.* Boston, Massachusetts: Shambhala Publications, Inc. (1992)

Hutchens, Alma R., *Indian Herbalogy of North America.* Boston, MA: Shambhala Publications, Inc. (1973)

Hutchens, Alma R., *Indian Herbalogy of North America.* Ontario, Canada (1982)

Kadans, Dr. Joseph M., *Doctor Kadans' Herbal Weight-Loss Diet.* West Hyack, NY: Parker Publishing Company, Inc. (1982)

Kadans, Joseph M., N.D., Ph.D., *Modern Encyclopedia of Herbs with the Herb-O-Matic Locator Index.* New York, NY: Simon & Schuster, Inc. (1993)

Keith, Velma J. and Monteen Gordon, *The How To Herb Book.* Pleasant Grove, Utah: Mayfield Publications (1996)

Lau, Dr. Benjamin, M.D., Ph,D., *Garlic and You: The Modern Medicine.* Canada: Apple Publishing Company Ltd. (1997)

Lavabre, Marcel F., *Aromatherapy Workbook.* Rochester, VT: Healing Arts Press (1990)

Lee, John R., M.D. with Virginia Hopkins, *What Your Doctor May Not Tell You about Menopause, The Breakthrough Book of Natural Progesterone.* New York, NY: Warner Books, Inc. (1996)

Ley, Beth M., Ph.D., *Flax! Fabulous Flax!! Nature's Best Source of Omega-3 Fatty Acids and Lignan Fiber!* Detroit Lakes, MN: BL Publications (2003)

Leyel, C.F., *Compassionate Herbs.* London: Faber & Faber Limited (1946)

Little, Elbert L., former Chief Dendrologist, U.S. Forest Service, *The Audubon Society Field Guide to North American Trees, Eastern Region.* New York: Alfred A. Knopf, Inc. (1980)

Livingston-Wheeler, Virginia, M.D. and Edmond G. Addeo, *The Conquest of Cancer, Vaccines and Diet.* New York: Franklin Watts (1984)

Lockard, Allen and Alice Q. Swanson, *A Digger's Guide to Medicinal Plants.* Eolia, Missouri (2004)

Mars, Brigitte, Herbalist AHG, *Natural First Aid.* Pownal, VT: Storey Books (1999)

McKenna, Dr. John, *Natural Alternatives to Antibiotics.* Garden City Park, NY: Avery Publishing Group (1998)

McVicar, Jekka, *Herbs for the Home, A Definitive Sourcebook to Growing and Using Herbs.* New York, NY: Viking Studio Books, a division of Penguin Books USA Inc. (1994)

Meyer, Joseph E., *The Herbalist.* U.S. (1934) & (1970)

Mindell, Dr. Earl, *Garlic, The Miracle Nutrient.*

Mojay, Gabriel, *Aromatherapy for Healing the Spirit.* New York, NY: Henry Holt and Company, Inc. (1996)

Moore, Michael, *Medicinal Plants of the Mountain West.* Santa Fe, New Mexico: Museum of New Mexico Press (1979)

Morton, Julia F., D.Sc., *Folk Remedies of the Low Country.* Miami, FL: E. A. Seemann Publishing, Inc. (1974)

National Geographic Society, *Nature's Healing Arts from Folk Medicine to Modern Drugs.* (1977)

Nature's Miracle Healing Medicine, *Garlic Can Cure or Prevent Many Serious Illnesses.* Woodbridge, NJ: Globe Communications Corp. (1984)

O'Brien, Marian Maeve, *The Bible Herb Book.* St. Louis, MO: The Bethany Press (1960)

Ody, Penelope, *The Holistic Herbal Directory, a Directory of Herbal Remedies for Everyday Health Problems.* Edison, New Jersey: Chartwell Books Inc. (2001)

Olsen, Cynthia, *Essiac, a Native Herbal Cancer Remedy.* Twin Lakes, Wisconsin: Lotus Press (1998)

PDR (Physician's Desk Reference) for Herbal Medicines. Montvale, New Jersey: Medical Economics Company, Inc. (1998)

PDR for Herbal Medicines, Third Edition. Mantvale, NJ: Thomson PDR (2004)

Pedersen, Mark, *Nutritional Herbology, Volume II, Herbal Combinations.* Spanish Fork, UT: Pedersen Publishing (1990)

Percival, James, *The Essiac Handbook, a Shaman's Blessing.* Orlando, FL: Rideout Publishing Company (1994)

Pitchford, Paul, *Healing with Whole Foods, Oriental Traditions and Modern Nutrition.* Berkeley, CA: North Atlantic Books (1993)

Richardson, Joseph G., M.D., *Medicology or Home Encyclopedia of Health.* New York, Philadelphia, London: University Medical Society (1907)

Ritchason, Jack, N.D., *The Little Herb Encyclopedia.* Pleasant Grove, Utah: Woodland Health Books (1995)

Rodale's All-New Encyclopedia of Organic Gardening, The Indispensable Resource for Every Gardner. Pennsylvania: Rodale Press, Emmaus (1992)

Rose, Jeanne, *375 Essential Oils and Hydrosols.* Berkeley, California: Frog, Ltd. (1999)

Rose, Jeanne, *Herbs and Things, Jeanne Rose's Herbal.* New York: Grosset & Dunlap Workman Publishing Company (1972)

Rosenthal, Norman, M.D., *St. John's Wort, The Herbal Way to Feeling Good.* New York, NY: Harper Collins Publishers (1998)

Rothenberg, Robert E, M.D., F.A.C.S., *The New American Medical Dictionary and Health Manual, 6th edition.* New York, NY: Penguin Books (1992)

Royal, Penny C., *Herbally Yours.* Hurricane, Utah: Sound Nutrition (1982)

Santillo, Humbart, N.D., *Natural Healing with Herbs.* Prescott, AZ: Hohm Press (1993)

Schnaubelt, Kurt, PhD., *Advanced Aromatherapy, the Science of Essential Oil Therapy.* Rochester, VT: Healing Arts Press (1998)

Scholl, B. Frank, Ph.G., M.D., *Library of Health, Complete Guide to Prevention and Cure of Disease.* Philadelphia, PA: Historical Publishing Co. (1923)

Schulick, Paul, *Ginger, Common Spice & Wonder Drug, Revised Edition.* Herbal Free Press Ltd. (1994)

Schulick, Paul, *The Immune System Health Guide Book.* (1986)

Schulze, Dr. Richard, *Lecture on Top Ten Herbs for Medical Emergencies.* Charlottesville, Virginia: University of Natural Healing (1998)

Scott, Julian and Susan, *Natural Medicine for Women.* New York, NY: Avon Books (1991)

Shealy, C. Norman, M.D., Ph.D., *The Illustrated Encyclopedia of Healing Remedies.* London, England: Harper Collins Publishers Ltd (1998)

Simpson, Caryl, *The International Garlic Festival Cookbook.* Arizona Garlic Festival, Verde Valley, Arizona

St. Claire, Debra, *Pocket Herbal Reference Guide.* Freedom, CA: The Crossing Press (1992)

St. Claire, Debra, *The Herbal Medicine Cabinet, Preparing Natural Remedies at Home.* (1997-2006)

Starck, Marcia, *The Complete Handbook of Natural Healing.* St. Paul, MN (1991)

Stary, Frantisek, *The Natural Guide to Medicinal Herbs and Plants.* New York: Barnes & Noble Books (1991)

The Doctors Book of Home Remedies for Women. Emmaus, Pennsylvania: Rodale Press, Inc. (1997)

Thomas, Lalitha, *10 Essential Herbs.* Prescott, AZ: Hohm Press (1992)

Tisserand, Robert B., *The Art of Aromatherapy, the Healing and Beautifying Properties of the Essential Oils of Flowers and Herbs.* New York: Inner Traditions International Ltd. (1977)

Trudeau, Kevin, *Natural Cures "They" Don't Want You to Know About.* Elk Grove Village, IL: Alliance Publishing Group, Inc. (2004)

Tyler, Varro E., PhD, *The Honest Herbal, a Sensible Guide to the Use of Herbs and Related Remedies, Third Edition.* New York: Haworth Press, Inc., (1993)

United States Dispensatory, 20th Edition. published by the American Pharmacy (1917)

USDA U.S. Dept. of Agriculture, Natural Resources Conservation Services, see http://plants.usda.gov/index.html for reported locations of wild and naturalized populations in North America and for scientific classifications of plants.

USDA *U.S. Dept. of Agriculture*, see www.usda.gov for nutrient composition of foods

Vigfirdas, Ray S. and Edna M. Rey-Vigfirdas, *Wild Plants of the Sierra Nevada.* Reno & Las Vegas, NV: University of Nevada Press (2006)

Weeden, Norman F., Ph.D., *A Sierra Nevada Flora.* Berkeley, CA: Wilderness Press (1996)

Weiner, Dr. Michael A., *The People's Herbal, a Family Guide to Herbal Home Remedies.* Toronto, Canada: General Publishing Co. Limited (1984)

White, Linda B., M.D. and Sunny Mavor, A.H.G., *Kids, Herbs, and Health: A Parents' Guide to Natural Remedies.* Loveland, CO: Interweave Press (1998)

White, Martha, *Traditional Home Remedies.* Yankee Publishing, Inc. (1997)

Wigmore, Ann, *The Sprouting Book.* San Fidel, New Mexico: Avery, a member of Penguin Putnam, Inc. (1986)

Wilen, Joan and Lydia, *Chicken Soup and Other Folk Remedies, Revised Edition.* New York: Ballantine Publishing Group (2000)

Wilen, Joan and Lydia, *Garlic, Nature's Super Healer.*

Wilen, Joan and Lydia, *Healing Remedies.* New York: Ballantine Books (2008)

Wilen, Joan and Lydia, *More Chicken Soup and Other Folk Remedies, Revised Edition.* New York: Ballantine Publishing Group (2000)

Williams, Jude C., Master Herbalist, *Jude's Herbal Home Remedies, Natural Health, Beauty & Home-Care Secrets.* St. Paul, MN: Llewellyn Publications (1996)

Wren, R.C., F.L.S., *Potter's New Cyclopaedia of Botanical Drugs and Preparations.* New York, Toronto and London: Potter & Clarke, LTD. (1956)

Yance, Donald R., Jr., C.N., M.H., A.H.G., with Arlene Valentine, *Herbal Medicine, Healing & Cancer, A Comprehensive Program for Prevention and Treatment.* New York: McGraw Hill (1999)

Young, D. Gary, N.D., *Essential Oils, Integrative Medical Guide.* USA: Essential Science Publishing (2003)

Zimmerman, Marcia, C.N., *The ADD Nutrition Solution, a Drug-Free Thirty-Day Plan.* New York: Henry Holt and Company (1999)

Glossary

Scientific Classification

Carolus Linnaeus is recognized as the first to develop a workable system of categorizing nature into similar groups. In his great work, *the Systema Naturae* (1st ed. 1735), nature was divided into three kingdoms: mineral, vegetable, and animal, then subdivided into five ranks: class, order, genus, species, and variety.

Today, there are seven major ranks that are generally recognized: kingdom, phylum, class, order, family, genus, species, with intermediate rankings used as needed.

Latin Name Also called the 'Scientific Name,' is the system of binomial nomenclature (two-name identification) classifying individual species. The genus is capitalized and species is lowercase, both are written formally in italics. For example: *Echinacea angustifolia.* Higher rankings are always written in plain text.

Abbreviation The two-part scientific name is usually written in full, with the exception of shortening the genus name to an initial (and period) when written several times, or if different species from the same genus are being listed or discussed in the same paper or report. The genus is written in full when first used, then abbreviated.

For example, when discussing the three medicinal species of the genus Echinacea, they may be appropriately listed as: **Echinacea angustifolia, E. purpurea and E. pallida**

Acyclic Not cyclic.

Adaptogen Increases resistance to stress.

Addison's Disease Serious disease caused by insufficient or non-function of the adrenal glands.

Alterative Purifies the blood, cleanses, and induces efficient removal of waste products. With time, substance will help detoxify the spleen, liver, kidneys, and bowels. Overall, this results in improved digestion, assimilation, glandular secretions, organ function, skin health, and general well-being.

Amenorrhea Menstrual failure.

Analgesic Relieves pain.

Angina Chest pain thought to be due to inadequate supply of oxygen to the heart muscle. Get help immediately, as this may be life threatening.

Anodyne Relieves pain and reduces nerve excitability.

Antacid Neutralizes acidity, especially in stomach and duodenum.

Anthelmintic Kills parasites and worms.

Anticatarrhal Eliminates mucous conditions.

Antidote Substance used to counteract a poison.

Antiemetic Calms stomach, helps prevent vomiting.

Antigalactagoge Limits the production and secretion of mother's milk.

Antioxidant Protects against oxygen-free radical damage at the cellular level (a major cause of disease, premature deterioration, and aging).

Anti-periodic Prevents regular recurrences of a disease or symptoms.

Antipyretic Reduces fever.

Antiseptic Fights pathogenic bacteria and prevents infection.

Antispasmodic Relieves muscular spasms, convulsions and cramps.

Antitussive Inhibits the cough reflex.

Aperient Mild laxative without purging.

Aperitive Improves appetite.

Aphrodisiac Stimulates sexual desire.

Aromatic Has a spicy taste, contains volatile oils which aid digestion and relieve gas.

Arrhythmia Irregular heart beat.

Arteriosclerosis Hardening of the arteries.

Astringent Increases tone and firmness of tissues, reduces swelling and mucous discharge.

Atherosclerosis Hardening of the inner lining of arteries.

Athlete's Foot Fungal infection, most often occurring between the toes.

Ayurvedic Medicine Ancient Hindu science of health and medicine native to the Indian Subcontinent and practiced in other parts of the world as a form of alternative medicine.

Bactericide Kills bacteria.

Bell's Palsy Facial nerve paralysis of one side of the face. Many recover, although some do not achieve a complete recovery.

Bilious Colic Severe abdominal pain due to sluggish liver or gallstones.

Bitter Stimulates digestive juices and improves appetite. The 'bitter' principle was named 'cnicin' by Nativelle in 1839. He proposed bitter foods increased appetite and improved digestion by first stimulating the 'bitter' taste buds on the tongue, activating secretion of saliva and digestive juices, thus supporting efficient digestion, protecting digestive tract tissues, and enhancing bile flow and pancreatic functions.

Bladder Incontinence Involuntary urinary voiding.

Bolus Vaginal or rectal suppository.

Bright's Disease Chronic kidney inflammation.

Calmative Gently calms nerves.

Carbuncle Type of large boil on the skin and underlying tissues, with several possible points of pussy discharge.

Carminative Brings warmth and circulation, relieves intestinal gas discomfort, and promotes peristaltic movement.

Catalyst Improves circulation and accelerates the effectiveness of other herbs.

Catarrh Inflamed and congested mucous membranes, which can result in mucous drainage and discharge.

Cathartic Strong laxative causing rapid evacuation.

Cell Proliferant Enhances the formation of new tissue and speeds the healing process.

Cellulitis Inflammation of connective tissues just beneath the skin surface.

Chlorosis Type of anemia seen most often in girls and young women.

Cholagogue Promotes the flow of bile.

Cholera Serious infectious disease. Symptoms may include vomiting, diarrhea, cramps, fever, and dehydration.

Cholestasis Suppression of bile flow.

Chorea A nervous disease characterized by involuntary movements.

Cirrhosis Inflammatory disease of the liver accompanied with the replacement of liver cells by fibrous tissue, sometimes called 'hardening of the liver'. Blood circulation through the liver may eventually be obstructed by cirrhosis.

Colic Severe abdominal pain.

Consumption Older term meaning tuberculosis of the lungs.

Counterirritant Causes irritation in one area to relieve pain in another part of the body.

Croup Inflammation of the larynx, accompanied by cough, difficult breathing, and fever.

Cushing's Disease Hyperfunction of adrenal gland cortex, characterized by marked increase in blood pressure, obesity, etc.

Cystic Fibrosis Childhood disease with glandular secretion failure (pancreas), progressive disability and often early death, causing marked susceptibility to lung infections and difficulty breathing.

Cystitis Bladder inflammation.

Decoction An infusion of medicinal properties from roots or bark into a liquid. It takes more time to pull nutrients out of roots and bark than it does leaves. A weak decoction can be made by simmering the herb root for 15-45 minutes in water. A much more effective decoction requires a three-step process:

1) Simmer roots or bark for 15-45 minutes in water (distilled water is preferred).

2) Allow infusion to sit covered for at least eight hours or overnight.

3) Simmer again to concentrate nutrients. Discard solids and store decoction in refrigerator.

Delirium Tremens Condition brought on by alcohol poisoning. Symptoms include noticeable trembling, hallucinations, feelings of persecution and ultimately, exhaustion.

Demulcent Softens and soothes inflammation of mucous membranes.

Deobstruent Removes obstructions.

Depurative Cleanses blood by promoting eliminative functions.

Diaphoretic Promotes perspiration, increases elimination through the skin.

Diphtheria Contagious disease characterized by difficult breathing, sore throat, and system toxicity.

Diuretic Increases urine flow.

Diverticulitis Bowel wall 'outpouch' inflammation. An inflamed outpouch of the bowel wall is called a diverticula.

DNA Deoxy-ribonucleic acid. Contains genetic instructions for development and function of living organisms.

Doctrine of Signatures Belief that medicinal properties are revealed symbolically by an herb's outward appearance.

Dropsy Older term describing water retention causing swelling to tissues, thought to be due to heart insufficiency in some cases.

Dysentery Bowel inflammation.

Dysmenorrhea Painful or difficult menstruation.

Dyspepsia Indigestion.

Dyspnea Shortness of breath.

Dysuria Impaired ability to pass urine with painful voiding.

Eclectic Medicine Branch of American medicine popular at the turn of the 20th century. These physicians (called 'Eclectics') believed in a philosophy of 'alignment with nature'. Eclectics made use of botanical plants and other substances, practiced a type of physical therapy and, in general, employed methods and concepts they found to be beneficial to their patients. They opposed the techniques of bleeding, chemical purging, and the use of mercury compounds common among the 'conventional' doctors of their time.

Emmenagogue Promotes menstrual flow.

Emollient Softens and soothes skin externally and mucous membranes when taken internally.

Emphysema Disease characterized by enlarged air spaces in the lungs, making breathing difficult.

Emetic Causes vomiting.

Endometriosis Condition of having cells which ordinarily line the uterus in unusual places (such as in the bladder or intestinal wall). May produce irregular or painful menstruation and sterility.

Enteritis Inflammation of the intestinal tract.

Epilepsy Brain disorder accompanied by periodic convulsions and loss of consciousness.

Erysipelas Streptococcal infection of the skin and underlying tissues, characterized by red appearance and accompanied by high fever and marked toxic reaction.

Expectorant Loosens and removes phlegm from the respiratory tract.

Extract Also known as a tincture, it is concentrated active constituents that are obtained from herbs using a liquid solvent (glycerin, raw apple cider vinegar, or alcohol are commonly used).

FDA or USFADA U.S. Federal Drug Administration. An agency of the United States responsible for protecting and promoting public health through regulation and supervision of food safety, tobacco products, dietary supplements, prescription and over-the-counter pharmaceutical drugs, vaccines, biopharmaceuticals, blood transfusions, medical devices, electro-magnetic radiation emitting devices (ERED), veterinary products, and cosmetics.

The beginnings of the FDA go back to 1883 when Harvey W. Wiley, chief chemist of the Department of Agriculture's (USDA) Division of Chemistry, was assigned to conduct research on the adulteration and misbranding of food and drugs on the American market. The Division published its findings from 1887-1902 and, in June 1906, President Theodore Roosevelt signed into law the Food and Drug Act. The act prohibited, under penalty of seizure of goods, the adulteration or misbranding of food and drugs. The responsibility for examining food and drugs was given to Wiley's USDA Bureau of Chemistry.

A 1912 amendment to the Food and Drug Act added language that further prohibited false and fraudulent claims of curative or therapeutic effect to the Act's definition of misbranded. In 1927, the Bureau of Chemistry's regulatory powers were reorganized under a new USDA body, the Food, Drug, and Insecticide organization. This was shortened to the Food and Drug Administration (FDA) three years later in 1930.

Febrifuge Reduces fever.

Felons Type of abscess on the fingertip surface. If left untreated, it may infect the underlying bone.

Fibrositis Overgrowth of fibrous tissues due to injury or inflammation. Often interferes with normal range of motion and may be very painful.

Flatulence Excessive gas in bowels.

Fomentation Towel soaked in tea infusion or decoction and placed on affected area.

Galactagogue Enhances lactation of nursing mothers.

Gardening Terms

Annuals Plants which die each year and must be planted again from seeds.

Biennials Plants that die within a two-year cycle, at which time new plants must grow from seed.

Perennials Plants that die down in the winter but grow back from a persistent rootstock each year.

Herbaceous Plants without woody stems (in other words, they are not trees or shrubs).

Scarification To roughen the seedcoat (with sandpaper, or by chipping with a knife or razor) in order to improve moisture absorption. Take care not to damage the inner embryo.

Stratification Chilling of seeds before planting to mimic winter. See Echinacea for step-by-step instructions on how to stratify seeds for planting.

Gastritis Inflammation of the lining of the stomach.

German Commission E Monographs These monographs (plant profiles based on research, experience, and medical studies) serve as the basis for recommendations that influence the regulation of herbal medicines in Germany. They were first instituted in 1978, when the Commission (consisting of professionals in pharmacy, medicine, industry, and science, as well as lay persons) was organized. One of the first monographs produced was of hawthorn.

Gingivitis Inflammation of the gums.

Goiter An enlargement of the thyroid gland, often related to iodine deficiency.

Greens As referenced in our text, herbs containing chlorophyll, especially found in concentrated form in alfalfa grass and barley grass.

HDL (High Density Lipoprotein) Lipoproteins are lipids (fats) and proteins joined to transport lipids in the blood. HDLs transport cholesterol from the tissues of the body to the liver to be combined with the bile and removed from the body through digestion. Some experts believe HDL removes excess cholesterol from arterial plaque, slowing its buildup. HDL cholesterol is considered the 'good' cholesterol.

Hemorrhoid Varicose veins of the rectum or anus. Some protrude from the anal opening (external hemorrhoids), while others are within the anal canal (internal hemorrhoids).

Hemostatic Arrests bleeding.

Hepatic Supports and stimulates the liver, gallbladder, and spleen, and increases the flow of bile.

Hepatitis Inflammation of the liver caused by a virus.

Humours It was once thought the balance of the fluids in the body were of primary importance to an individual's well-being. Diagnosis of ill health was given based on various types of human temperament (humours) that indicated an imbalance in the body. Principally, the four fluids considered were blood, choler (yellow bile), phlegm, and melancholy (black bile). Thus a preponderance of blood would make a person 'sanguine', while excess of phlegm would make him or her 'phlegmatic'; too much choler (or yellow bile) would give rise to a 'choleric' disposition, while an excess of black bile would produce a 'melancholic' one.

Hypermenorrhea Excessive menstruation.

Hypertensive Increases blood pressure.

Hypertrophy Enlargement of the heart muscle caused by increased workload.

Hypnotic Induces sleep.

Hysteria Extreme emotional state.

Immuno-stimulant Stimulates the body's defense system.

Infusions Process of infusing active constituents into a liquid. For our purposes, this includes teas, decoctions, and infused oils.

Impetigo Highly contagious skin disease.

LDL (Low Density Lipoprotein) A type of lipoprotein that transports cholesterol and triglycerides from the liver to peripheral tissues. When too much LDL cholesterol circulates in the blood, it can slowly build up on the inner walls of the arteries that feed the heart and brain. Together with other substances, it can form plaque (a thick, hard deposit) that can narrow arteries and make them less flexible. This condition is known as atherosclerosis. If a clot forms and blocks a narrowed artery, heart attack or stroke may result. Since high levels of LDL cholesterol can signal medical problems like cardiovascular disease, it is often called the 'bad' cholesterol.

Leucorrhea Vaginal discharge due to infection.

Lithotriptic Dissolves urinary stones.

Lumbago Lower back pain.

Lupus Erythematosus Skin disease evident mainly on hands and face, typically presenting a facial 'butterfly' rash.

Lymphangitis Inflammation of lymph vessels.

Macerate To soak in a liquid to soften and release constituents. Solar maceration includes exposure to direct sunlight for a few hours for the first three days.

Mastitis Breast inflammation.

Mastodynia Breast pain noted chiefly just before onset of menstrual periods.

Miasm Older term meaning unhealthy vapors or unwholesome atmosphere.

Menorrhagia Excessive bleeding during menstruation.

Mucilage Soft, slippery substance that soothes mucous membrane inflammation.

Mucus without an 'o' A noun: a thick fluid produced by the lining of some tissues of the body.

Mucous with an 'o' An adjective that modifies a noun or pronoun, as in: mucous membrane, mucous discharge, mucous conditions, etc.

Multiple Sclerosis Disease of the myelin sheath of the nerves with symptoms that include various degrees of numbness, weakness, loss of muscle coordination, and problems with vision, speech, and bladder control.

Myalgia Muscular pain.

Myasthenia Gravis Disease characterized by the wasting of muscles, particularly those associated with swallowing.

Myopia Short or near sightedness.

Oxytocic Stimulates contractions and accelerates childbirth.

Narcolepsy Chronic sleep disorder.

Narcotic Induces sleep or stupor and relieves pain without the addictive qualities of opiates.

Necrosis Death of cells or tissues.

Nephritis Inflammation of the kidneys.

Nervine Improves nerve function.

Neuralgia Sharp, stabbing pains due to deposits or congestion putting pressure on nerves.

Neurasthenia Lack of energy.

Neuritis Inflamed and weakened nerves.

Neuropathy Any disease of nerve tissue.

Nutritive Supplies substantial amount of nutrients and aids in building and toning the body.

Opthalmia Eye inflammation.

Parasiticide Kills parasites and worms.

Parkinson's Disease Nervous condition involving a rhythmic tremor, rigidity of muscle action, and slowing of all body motion. Also called shaking palsy.

Parturient Stimulates uterine contractions, which induces and assists labor.

Pectoral Healing to problems in the bronchio-pulmonary area.

Periostitis Inflammation or infection of the tissue covering bones (the periosteum).

Peristalsis Intestinal contractions that propel bowel contents onward.

Peritonitis Inflammation or infection of the peritoneum (abdominal lining).

Phlebitis Inflammation of veins.

Pleurisy Painful inflammation of chest cavity lining.

Positively Inotropic Increased strength of muscular contractions.

Prebiotics Helps restore the balance of bacteria in the digestive tract. Prebiotics are generally foods that make their way through the digestive system and help good bacteria grow and flourish. Prebiotics help keep beneficial bacteria healthy.

Probiotics are beneficial bacteria that can be found in various foods. Beneficial bacteria aids digestion and helps keep the intestinal tract healthy. Common strains of beneficial bacteria include Lactobacillus and Bifidobacterium.

Prolactin Pituitary hormone that stimulates development and growth of mammary glands during pregnancy and is essential for the initiation and maintenance of milk production of nursing mothers.

Prostatitis Prostate inflammation.

Purgative Causes rapid, watery evacuation of intestinal contents (diarrhea).

Pyelitis Infection of the pelvic outlet of the kidneys.

Pyorrhea Inflammation of the gums with possible pus formation.

Raynaud's Disease Illness known for pain and spasms in the fingers and toes when cold.

Refrigerant Produces coolness, reduces fever.

Relaxant Relaxes nerves and muscles, relieves tension.

Rhinitis Inflammation of the membrane lining the nose.

Rhizomes Underground stems.

Rickets Vitamin D deficiency disease evidenced in marked cases by bone deformities.

Ringworm Contagious fungal disease typically appearing in the shape of a ring.

Rosacea Enlargement and redness of the entire nose. Also called whiskey nose, although it is not limited to heavy drinkers.

Rubefacient Increases blood flow to the skin. May cause local reddening.

Scabies Contagious skin condition caused by an insect, causing great itching.

Sciatica Nerve pain in lower back, sometimes radiating down leg.

Scrofula Tuberculosis inflammation of lymph nodes of the neck in children.

Scrofuloderma Tuberculosis infection of the skin.

Scurvy Vitamin C deficiency disease with common symptoms of weakness, bleeding, and anemia.

Seborrhea Skin disease due to oversecretion of sebaceous glands. May lead to baldness when on the scalp.

Sedative Exerts calming, soothing, or tranquilizing effect. May be general, local, nervous, or vascular.

Septicemia Serious bacterial infection of the blood.

Sialagogue Promotes an increase flow of saliva.

Stimulant Increases internal heat, dispels internal chill, and strengthens metabolism and circulation.

Stomachic Strengthens stomach function.

Strangury Difficult, painful urination, with passage of only a small amount at a time.

St. Vitus' Dance A nervous disease characterized by involuntary movements.

Styptic Contracts blood vessels and stops hemorrhage by astringent, tightening action.

Tea Infusion of medicinal qualities of herbs into water. Leaves and other plant parts are usually used to make a tea. Thicker roots and bark require a longer infusion time (see decoctions).

A general recipe for herb tea is to pour a cup of boiling water over one to three teaspoons of herb, cover with lid, and let steep (stand) for twenty minutes. Strain out plant parts and enjoy. Refrigerate unused portion.

Thrush Fungal infection of the mouth.

Tincture Also called an extract, tinctures are concentrated, active constituents that are obtained from herbs using a liquid solvent. Glycerin, raw apple cider vinegar, or alcohol are most commonly used.

Tonic Increases energy, strengthens muscular and nervous systems, improves digestion and assimilation, and imparts a general sense of well-being.

Typhoid Disease usually caused by infected water or food, accompanied by high fevers, ulcers, diarrhea, headache, and hemorrhages.

Urethritis Inflammation of urethra.

Urolithiasis Process of forming stones in the urinary tract.

Vaginitis Vaginal inflammation.

Vasoconstrictor Substance that narrows blood-vessels, restricting the flow of blood.

Vasodilator Agent that causes blood vessels to relax and widen (dilate), often decreasing blood pressure and reducing the workload for the heart.

Vermifuge Expels or repels intestinal worms.

Volatile Substance easily converted into a vapor.

Vulnerary Promotes healing of wounds by stimulating cellular growth and warding off infection.

Whooping Cough Also known as pertussis, a contagious disease characterized by severe coughing and 'whooping' sound upon inhalation.

Index

Herbs in ALL CAPITAL LETTERS indicate a primary herb function

A

abscesses, herbs for
  burdock, 61
  CHAMOMILE, 91
  dandelion, 122
  echinacea, 131, 135
  garlic, 160
  licorice, 221
  lobelia, 232
  SLIPPERY ELM, 288, 294
abrasions. *See* first aid, herbs for
acidity, herbs for. *See* pH balance, herbs for
acne, herbs for
  alfalfa, 2
  ALOE, 13, 16
  barley, 27
  burdock, 62, 65
  catnip, 73
  chaparral, 100
  chaste tree, 108
  COMFREY, 113
  DANDELION, 123
  ECHINACEA, 131
  garlic, 160, 173
  goldenseal, 189, 194
  juniper, 208
  kelp, 215
  RED CLOVER, 268, 270
  valerian, 317
  yellow dock, 350
addiction, herbs for
  barley, 26
  black cohosh, 43
  capsicum, 84
  catnip, 72
  CHAMOMILE, 91, 95
  chaparral, 102
  goldenseal, 188
  lobelia, 231
  valerian, 321
Addison's Disease, herbs for
  LICORICE, 221
  wild yam, 330, 336
adrenal glands, herbs for the
  hawthorn, 201
  slippery elm, 288, 290
  wild yam, 334
adrenal weakness, herbs for
  hawthorn, 201
  juniper, 207
  KELP, 215
  LICORICE, 221, 222
age spots
  BARLEY, 27
  DANDELION, 123
AIDS, herbs for
  ALOE, 13
  BARLEY, 26
  red clover, 267
  St. John's wort, 297
air pollution, herbs for
  chamomile, 91
alcoholism, herbs for
  alfalfa, 2
  capsicum, 84
  CHAMOMILE, 91
  lobelia, 231
  milk thistle, 242
  saw palmetto, 280
  valerian, 316, 321
alfalfa
  history of, 3
  influence and properties of, 1–2
  nutrients in, 4, 8
  preparation and remedies, 8–10
  safety and profile, 10–11
  uses for, 4–7
alkalizers
  ginger, 181
allergic reaction, herbs for
  brigham tea, 59
  LOBELIA, 232
  milk thistle, 246

allergies, herbs for
  alfalfa, 1–11
  ALOE, 13
  barley, 26
  brigham tea, 55
  burdock, 61
  chaparral, 99
  COMFREY, 112
  dandelion, 125
  EYEBRIGHT, 141
  garlic, 160
  goldenseal, 189
  juniper, 207
  mullein, 249
  slippery elm, 288
  wild yam, 330
  yarrow, 343
  yellow dock, 350
aloe
  history of, 14–15
  influence and properties of, 12–14
  nutrients in, 15
  preparation and remedies, 20–23
  safety and profile of, 23–25
  uses for, 15–23
aloin, 18–19. See also aloe
alopecia, herbs for
  saw palmetto, 284
alteratives
  burdock, 62, 65
  chaparral, 99, 100
  comfrey, 113
  dandelion, 123
  eyebright, 142
  GARLIC, 159
  goldenseal, 190
  kelp, 214, 215
  peppermint, 257
  RED CLOVER, 268
  red raspberry, 274
  uva ursi, 308
  yarrow, 339
  YELLOW DOCK, 349
anal fissures, herbs for
  ALOE, 13
analgesics
  capsicum, 80
  lobelia, 231
  peppermint, 258
anemia, herbs for
  alfalfa, 1
  aloe, 12
  BARLEY, 26
  catnip, 72
  COMFREY, 112
  DANDELION, 122, 125, 126
  garlic, 159
  kelp, 214
  red clover, 269
  St. John's wort, 297
  uva ursi, 208
  yellow dock, 350, 352
  YELLOW DOCK, 349
angina, herbs for
  black cohosh, 43
  BLESSED THISTLE, 50
  HAWTHORNE, 200, 203
  lobelia, 231
anodynes
  chamomile, 92
  chaparral, 100
  ginger, 177
  juniper, 208
  MULLEIN, 249
  peppermint, 258
  wild lettuce, 326, 327
  wild yam, 331
antacid
  flaxseed, 148
  ginger, 176
  red raspberry, 274
anthocyanosides
  bilberry, 39, 40
anti-aging, herbs for
  aloe, 14
  barley, 26
  BARLEY, 27
  chaparral, 103
  dandelion, 122
  garlic, 159, 161, 164
  licorice, 221
anti-catarrhal. See catarrh, herbs for
anti-coagulants. See blood thinners
anti-inflammatory herbs. See inflammation, herbs for
anti-periodics
  goldenseal, 189
anti-spasmodic. See spasms, herbs for
antibacterial herbs
  aloe, 13

comfrey, 116
mullein, 249, 252
peppermint, 257
St. John's wort, 297
valerian, 316
yarrow, 340, 343
antibiotic herbs
chamomile, 92
dandelion, 126
ECHINACEA, 130, 133
GARLIC, 160, 164–65
GOLDENSEAL, 189
kelp, 215, 217
red clover, 267
uva ursi, 308
antidotes. *See* poison antidotes
antifungal herbs
aloe, 13
chamomile, 92
chaparral, 99, 103
echinacea, 134
GARLIC, 164
GOLDENSEAL, 189
juniper, 207
JUNIPER, 207, 211
antimicrobial herbs
aloe, 13
chaparral, 100
echinacea, 131
GARLIC, 161, 164–65
peppermint, 257
red clover, 267
St. John's wort, 303
antioxidants
bilberry, 37, 40
CHAPARRAL, 99, 103
GARLIC, 159, 161
licorice, 226
milk thistle, 246
slippery elm, 291
antipyretics. *See* fever, herbs for
antiseptic herbs
aloe, 13
bilberry, 37
capsicum, 80
chamomile, 95
chaparral, 99, 103
ECHINACEA, 130, 134
eyebright, 142
GARLIC, 160, 162, 164

ginger, 182
GOLDENSEAL, 189, 194
kelp, 215
mullein, 249, 252
peppermint, 257
saw palmetto, 280
uva ursi, 312
yarrow, 340
antitussive herbs
MULLEIN, 250, 252
antivenomous herbs
black cohosh, 44, 48
lobelia, 232
antiviral herbs
aloe, 13, 16, 20
GARLIC, 160, 164
licorice, 222, 224, 225
peppermint, 257
red clover, 267
St. John's wort, 297
anxiety, herbs for
barley, 27
chaste tree, 108
goldenseal, 194
St. John's wort, 298, 302
valerian, 319–20
wild lettuce, 326, 327
aphrodisiac, female
black cohosh, 44
licorice, 222
saw palmetto, 280
appendicitis, herbs for the
slippery elm, 287
appetite stimulants
ALFALFA, 1
blessed thistle, 50
burdock, 61
CAPSICUM, 78, 79
catnip, 72
CHAMOMILE, 91, 92
DANDELION, 122, 123, 126
eyebright, 142
garlic, 159, 161, 165
GINGER, 176
goldenseal, 188, 190, 195
juniper, 207, 211
milk thistle, 242, 246
PEPPERMINT, 257
St. John's wort, 297
uva ursi, 308

INDEX— 378

wild lettuce, 325
yellow dock, 352
appetite suppressants
BARLEY, 27
lobelia, 236
red clover, 267
arteriosclerosis, herbs for
capsicum, 78
GARLIC, 159
HAWTHORN, 200, 201, 203
juniper, 207
kelp, 214
licorice, 221
arthritis, herbs for
ALFALFA, 2
aloe, 13, 18
BARLEY, 26
black cohosh, 43
blessed thistle, 50
BURDOCK, 62, 64
capsicum, 79, 83
CHAPARRAL, 99, 102
COMFREY, 113, 116
DANDELION, 123, 125
GARLIC, 160, 165, 170
ginger, 177, 182
hawthorn, 201
juniper, 208
kelp, 215
licorice, 226
LOBELIA, 232
slippery elm, 288, 290
St. John's wort, 297, 300
uva ursi, 308
valerian, 317
wild lettuce, 325
WILD YAM, 330, 334
yarrow, 340
yellow dock, 350
asthma, herbs for
ALFALFA, 2
aloe, 13
barley, 27, 30
BLACK COHOSH, 43
BRIGHAM TEA, 55, 58
chaparral, 99
DANDELION, 123
flaxseed, 148
GARLIC, 160, 165
goldenseal, 189, 193

licorice, 222
LOBELIA, 232, 235
mullein, 250
saw palmetto, 280
SLIPPERY ELM, 288
wild lettuce, 326
wild yam, 331
astringents
alfalfa, 5
bilberry, 37
BILBERRY, 37–38, 40
black cohosh, 43
brigham tea, 56
comfrey, 112, 113, 116
eyebright, 141, 142, 144
goldenseal, 188
hawthorn, 200
juniper, 208
lobelia, 231
mullein, 250
peppermint, 257
red raspberry, 274, 275
slippery elm, 287, 289
St. John's wort, 298
uva ursi, 308
YARROW, 339, 343, 344
yellow dock, 349
atherosclerosis, herbs for
alfalfa, 6
bilberry, 37
GARLIC, 166–67
athlete's foot, herbs for
aloe, 13
chaparral, 100, 103, 104
COMFREY, 112
garlic, 160, 173
red clover, 267, 272
yellow dock, 350
autonomic function, herbs for
black cohosh, 48

B
back ache, herbs for
chaparral, 100
bacterial infections, herbs for
alfalfa, 2
dandelion, 122
bactericides
burdock, 61
chamomile, 95

bad breath, herbs for
  alfalfa, 5
  echinacea, 131
baldness. *See* hair growth, herbs for
barley
  history of, 27–28
  influence and properties of, 26–28
  nutrients in, 29
  preparation and remedies, 33–35
  safety and profile, 35–36
  uses for, 29–34
bathing, herbs for
  chamomile, 96–97
  ginger, 184–85
  uva ursi, 313
  valerian, 322
  yarrow, 346
bedwetting, herbs for
  chamomile, 92, 94
  JUNIPER, 208
  ST. JOHN'S WORT, 298
  uva ursi, 309, 311
bee stings. *See* insect bites and stings, herbs for
Bell's Palsy
  ALFALFA, 2
benign prostatic hyperplasia (BPH), herbs for
  saw palmetto, 283
bilberry
  history of, 38–39
  influence and properties of, 37–38
  nutrients in, 39
  preparation and remedies, 41
  safety and profile, 41–42
  uses for, 39–41
bile flow promotion, herbs for. *See* cholagogues
binding agents
  slippery elm, 291, 294
birth control, herbs for
  blessed thistle, 51
  wild yam, 331, 334, 335
bites. *See* insect bites and stings, herbs for snake bites, herbs for
bitter. *See* appetite stimulants
black cohosh
  history of, 44–45
  influence and properties of, 43–45
  nutrients in, 45

  preparation and remedies, 48–49
  safety and profile, 49
  uses for, 45–48
bladder problems, herbs for
  aloe, 14
  BURDOCK, 62
  chamomile, 92
  chaparral, 100
  COMFREY, 113
  dandelion, 123
  echinacea, 131
  flaxseed, 149, 153
  garlic, 161
  GOLDENSEAL, 189, 193
  JUNIPER, 208
  licorice, 222
  RED CLOVER, 268
  red raspberry, 275
  saw palmetto, 280, 284
  slippery elm, 288
  St. John's wort, 303
  UVA URSI, 309
  valerian, 317
  yarrow, 340
bladder stones, herbs for
  bilberry, 37
  dandelion, 123
bladderwrack, 214, 217, 218
bleeding, herbs to stop
  alfalfa, 1
  ALOE, 12
  CAPSICUM, 82, 85, 88
  GOLDENSEAL, 188, 194
  JUNIPER, 207
  yarrow, 339, 344
  yellow dock, 349
blessed thistle
  history of, 51
  influence and properties, 50–51
  preparation and remedies, 53
  safety and profile of, 53–54
  uses for, 52–53
bloating
  chaste tree, 108
blood builder
  alfalfa, 1, 2, 6
  dandelion, 126
  ECHINACEA, 130
  yellow dock, 351–52
blood circulation. *See* circulation

INDEX— 380

blood cleanser/purifier
  ALFALFA, 1, 5
  ALOE, 12–13, 14
  BARLEY, 26, 31
  BLACK COHOSH, 43
  BLESSED THISTLE, 50, 52
  BURDOCK, 61, 64
  chamomile, 91
  chaparral, 99, 102, 103
  COMFREY, 112
  DANDELION, 122, 123, 125, 126
  ECHINACEA, 130
  EYEBRIGHT, 141, 142
  GARLIC, 159, 161, 165–67
  juniper, 207, 210
  LICORICE, 221
  RED CLOVER, 267, 268, 270
  St. John's wort, 297, 302–3
  uva ursi, 312
  wild yam, 330, 333
  YARROW, 339, 340, 342–43
  YELLOW DOCK, 349
blood clots, herbs for
  hawthorn, 200
blood disorders, herbs for
  chamomile, 91
  YELLOW DOCK, 349
blood neutralizer. *See* pH balance, herbs for
blood poisoning, herbs for
  burdock, 61
  chaparral, 99
  ECHINACEA, 130, 134
  GARLIC, 159
  lobelia, 231
blood pressure, herbs for
  alfalfa, 1
  aloe, 12
  black cohosh, 43
  CAPSICUM, 78, 82
  catnip, 74
  chaparral, 99
  DANDELION, 122, 126
  flaxseed, 152–53
  FLAXSEED, 148
  garlic, 161, 166, 171
  HAWTHORN, 200
  kelp, 214
  licorice, 221, 224
  milk thistle, 242
  red clover, 270
  VALERIAN, 316
  yarrow, 339
blood sugar. *See* diabetes
blood thinners
  aloe, 12
  bilberry, 37
  garlic, 166
  GINGER, 181
  red clover, 270
blood toxicity. *See* toxin cleanse, herbs for
blood vessels. *See* vascular system, herbs for
body odor. *See* deodorant
boils, herbs for
  alfalfa, 2
  BARLEY, 27
  BURDOCK, 62
  chaparral, 100
  COMFREY, 113
  dandelion, 123
  ECHINACEA, 131, 134, 135
  FLAXSEED, 149
  ginger, 177
  goldenseal, 189
  juniper, 208
  lobelia, 232
  milk thistle, 242
  mullein, 250
  peppermint, 258
  RED CLOVER, 268, 270
  slippery elm, 288, 291
  St. John's wort, 298
  wild yam, 331
  YELLOW DOCK, 350
bolus. *See* suppositories
bone loss, herbs for
  red clover, 272
bowel hemorrhage, herbs for
  YARROW, 339
bowels, herbs for the
  alfalfa, 1, 5
  aloe, 13
  black cohosh, 43
  chaparral, 99
  dandelion, 123, 125
  ginger, 176
  goldenseal, 188
  juniper, 207

kelp, 216
licorice, 221
mullein, 249, 253
RED RASPBERRY, 274, 277
wild yam, 330
yarrow, 344, 352
yellow dock, 349
brain function, herbs to promote
blessed thistle, 50, 52
flaxseed, 153
garlic, 168
juniper, 208, 211
milk thistle, 246
breast cancer prevention, herbs for
kelp, 217–18
breast cancer, herbs for
dandelion, 122, 126
flaxseed, 148, 154
milk thistle, 246
breast milk. *See* lactation, herbs for
breasts, herbs for the
aloe, 13
comfrey, 116
mullein, 250
red clover, 268, 272
SAW PALMETTO, 280
St. John's wort, 298
yarrow, 340
breath freshening, herbs for
capsicum, 79
goldenseal, 189
brigham tea
history of, 56–57
influence and properties of, 55–56
preparation and remedies, 59
safety and profile of, 59–60
uses for, 57–59
Bright's disease, herbs for
saw palmetto, 280
UVA URSI, 309
yarrow, 340
broken bones. *See* fractures, herbs for
bronchitis, herbs for
barley, 27
black cohosh, 43
burdock, 62
CAPSICUM, 79
catnip, 72
CHAMOMILE, 92
chaparral, 102

COMFREY, 113
dandelion, 123
echinacea, 131
flaxseed, 148
GARLIC, 160
GINGER, 177
GOLDENSEAL, 189, 192
licorice, 222
LOBELIA, 232, 236
MULLEIN, 250
PEPPERMINT, 258
RED CLOVER, 267, 270
saw palmetto, 280
SLIPPERY ELM, 288
ST. JOHN'S WORT, 298, 303
uva ursi, 308
wild lettuce, 328
WILD LETTUCE, 326
yarrow, 340, 343
yellow dock, 350
bruises. *See* first aid, herbs for
burdock
history of, 63
influence and properties of, 61–63
nutrients in, 63–64
preparations and remedies, 67–70
safety and profile, 70–71
uses for, 64–67
burning, herbs for. *See* smudges
burns, herbs for
ALOE, 13, 16, 21–22
BURDOCK, 61, 65
COMFREY, 112
flaxseed, 149
goldenseal, 189
red clover, 267, 272
SLIPPERY ELM, 288, 291
St. John's wort, 297, 301
yarrow, 340
bursitis, herbs for
ALFALFA, 2
aloe, 13
BURDOCK, 62
chaparral, 99
COMFREY, 113, 116
juniper, 208
kelp, 215
lobelia, 232
mullein, 250
wild yam, 330, 336

INDEX— 382

yarrow, 340

C
Caisse, Renee, 65–66
callouses, herbs for
  aloe, 13
  chamomile, 92
  dandelion, 126
cancer, herbs for. *See also* specific cancer types.
  barley, 26, 32
  BLESSED THISTLE, 50, 53
  BURDOCK, 61, 65
  CHAPARRAL, 99, 103
  comfrey, 112
  echinacea, 130
  GARLIC, 159, 168–69
  slippery elm, 287
  ST. JOHN'S WORT, 297
  yarrow, 339, 352
  YELLOW DOCK, 349
candida, herbs for
  chaparral, 99, 103
  echinacea, 134
  GARLIC
  wild lettuce, 325
canker sores, herbs for
  ALOE, 13, 19
  BURDOCK, 62
  GOLDENSEAL, 189
  licorice, 225
  LOBELIA, 232
capsicum
  history of, 80–81
  influence and properties, 78–80
  nutrients in, 81
  preparations and remedies, 84–88
  safety and profile of, 88–90
  uses for, 81–84
carbuncles, herbs for
  burdock, 62
  echinacea, 131, 134, 135
  flaxseed, 153
  garlic, 160
carcinogen inhibitors
  alfalfa, 5
cardiac weakness. *See* heart, herbs for the
  uva ursi, 208
carminatives. *See* gas relief, herbs for

cat stimulants, 75
catalysts
  capsicum, 79, 83
  ginger, 178, 181, 182
  licorice, 222
  wild yam, 337
  yarrow, 344
cataracts, herbs for
  chaparral, 99
  EYEBRIGHT, 141
catarrh, herbs for
  echinacea, 131
  eyebright, 141
  goldenseal, 191–92, 193
  juniper, 207
  licorice, 221
  LOBELIA, 231
  MULLEIN, 249
  saw palmetto, 280
  SLIPPERY ELM, 288
  ST. JOHN'S WORT, 297, 303
  UVA URSI, 309
  wild lettuce, 325
  WILD YAM, 330, 333
  yarrow, 340
  YARROW, 339
  yellow dock, 349
catnip
  history of, 73
  influence and properties of, 72–73
  nutrients in, 73–74
  preparations and remedies, 75–76
  safety and profile, 77
  uses for, 74–75
cattle feed, herbs used for
  kelp, 215
  red clover, 268
cayenne. *See* capsicum
cell regeneration. *see* tissue repair, herbs for
cellulitis, herbs for
  St. John's wort, 297
chamomile
  history of, 93
  influence and properties, 91–93
  nutrients in, 93
  preparations and remedies, 96–97
  safety and profile, 97–98
  uses for, 93–96
chaparral

INDEX— 383

history of, 100–101
influence and properties of, 99–100
nutrients in, 101
preparations and remedies, 104–6
safety and profile of, 106–7
uses for, 102–3
chapped skin. *See* skin chafing, herbs for
chaste tree
history of, 108–9
influence and properties, 108
preparations and remedies, 110
safety and profile of, 110–11
uses for, 109–10
chemotherapy, herbs for
milk thistle, 242
chest congestion, herbs for
brigham tea, 58
CAPSICUM, 79
catnip, 72
COMFREY, 113
eyebright, 141
GARLIC, 160
goldenseal, 190, 193
licorice, 225
lobelia, 231
saw palmetto, 280
ST. JOHN'S WORT, 298, 303
uva ursi, 308
WILD LETTUCE, 326
wild yam, 331
yarrow, 343
chicken pox, herbs for
ALOE, 14
BURDOCK, 62
catnip, 72
chaparral, 99
ginger, 177
goldenseal, 189
LOBELIA, 232
yarrow, 340, 343
yellow dock, 350
childbirth, herbs for
black cohosh, 44
chamomile, 95
lobelia, 236
RED RASPBERRY, 275, 276
St. John's wort, 298, 303
uva ursi, 309
childhood diseases, herbs for
catnip, 72, 73, 74

chamomile, 92, 94
garlic, 160
GINGER, 177
LOBELIA, 232
mullein, 249
peppermint, 257
red clover, 267
cholagogues
alfalfa, 5
aloe, 13
blessed thistle, 51
burdock, 62
DANDELION, 123, 125
garlic, 160
ginger, 176
goldenseal, 189, 190
milk thistle, 242, 243, 244
peppermint, 258
wild yam, 331, 333
yellow dock, 350, 351
cholera, herbs for
black cohosh, 43
GARLIC, 160
GINGER, 177
GOLDENSEAL, 189
milk thistle, 242
peppermint, 257
red raspberry, 274
wild yam, 330
cholesterol, herbs for
alfalfa, 6
barley, 26, 29, 32
capsicum, 82
dandelion, 126
FLAXSEED, 148, 153
garlic, 161, 166–67
ginger, 181
licorice, 226
red clover, 270
wild yam, 330, 333
chorea, herbs for
lobelia, 232, 235
circulation, herbs for
ALOE, 12
black cohosh, 47
blessed thistle, 50, 52
brigham tea, 58
CAPSICUM, 81, 82
catnip, 72, 74
CHAMOMILE, 91

chaparral, 99, 102
echinacea, 130
GARLIC, 159, 160, 166–67
GINGER, 176, 180–81
GOLDENSEAL, 188
HAWTHORN, 200, 201, 203–5
licorice, 226
LICORICE, 221
lobelia, 231, 236
milk thistle, 243, 246
peppermint, 258
red clover, 268
yarrow, 343, 344
cirrhosis, herbs for
DANDELION, 123, 125
licorice, 222, 225
MILK THISTLE, 242, 245
cleanse, toxin. *See* toxin cleanse, herbs for
cleansing (digestive), herbs for. *See* digestive aids
clover honey nectar, 268
coagulants. *See* bleeding, herbs to stop
cold sores, herbs for
COMFREY, 113
colds, herbs for
alfalfa, 2
burdock, 61
capsicum, 84
catnip, 72, 74
chamomile, 92, 94
chaparral, 99, 102
comfrey, 112
ECHINACEA, 130, 134
EYEBRIGHT, 141
GARLIC, 160, 171
GINGER, 177
GOLDENSEAL, 189, 192
JUNIPER, 207
LICORICE, 222, 225
LOBELIA, 232
mullein, 249
PEPPERMINT, 257
red clover, 267
RED RASPBERRY, 274
saw palmetto, 280
valerian, 316
YARROW, 340, 343
cholestasis, herbs for
milk thistle, 242

colic, herbs for
catnip, 72, 74
CHAMOMILE, 91, 94
garlic, 159
GINGER, 176
juniper, 207
lobelia, 231
mullein, 249
PEPPERMINT, 257, 260
red raspberry, 274, 277
St. John's wort, 297, 303
valerian, 316
wild lettuce, 325
wild yam, 330, 333
yarrow, 339
colitis, herbs for
ALOE, 13, 18
chamomile, 91
comfrey, 112
GARLIC, 159
GINGER, 176
GOLDENSEAL, 188
KELP, 215
PEPPERMINT, 257, 261
SLIPPERY ELM, 287, 290
colon cancer prevention
alfalfa, 1
flaxseed, 148, 154
garlic, 168
colon, herbs for the
alfalfa, 1
ALOE, 13
CAPSICUM, 79
comfrey, 112
ginger, 176
GOLDENSEAL, 188
SLIPPERY ELM, 287, 290
yarrow, 339
comfrey
history of, 113–15
influence and properties of, 112–13
nutrients in, 115
preparations and remedies, 117–19
safety and profile, 119–21
uses for, 115–17
Commission E (Germany), 41, 46, 93, 151, 179, 244, 251, 318
complexion, herbs for the
KELP, 215
compresses

chamomile, 96
peppermint, 263
concentration, herbs for
blessed thistle, 51
congestion. *See* chest congestion, herbs for nasal congestion, herbs for
congestive heart failure, herbs for, 202. *See* edema, herbs for
juniper, 210
conjunctivitis, herbs for
EYEBRIGHT, 141, 144
goldenseal, 188, 193
slippery elm, 290
constipation, herbs for
alfalfa, 1
ALOE, 13–18
barley, 26
BLESSED THISTLE, 50
BURDOCK, 61
catnip, 72
chamomile, 91
dandelion, 122, 125
FLAXSEED, 148, 151
ginger, 176
goldenseal, 188
licorice, 221
lobelia, 231
mullein, 249
peppermint, 257
red clover, 267
red raspberry, 274
SLIPPERY ELM, 287
valerian, 316
yellow dock, 349, 352
consumption. *See* tuberculosis, herbs for
contact healers
ALOE, 13
convulsions, herbs for
black cohosh, 44
CAPSICUM, 79
CATNIP, 73
juniper, 208
LOBELIA, 232, 235
milk thistle, 242
peppermint, 258
VALERIAN, 317
corns, herbs for
aloe, 13
CHAMOMILE, 92
dandelion, 123, 126

cortisone, herbs for
licorice, 221, 222, 224
cough syrups
capsicum, 88
garlic, 172
ginger, 184
hawthorn, 205–6
licorice, 228
slippery elm, 294–95
coughs, herbs for
black cohosh, 43
burdock, 61
catnip, 72
chamomile, 92
COMFREY, 112
eyebright, 142
flaxseed, 148, 153
GARLIC, 160, 171
GINGER, 177
GOLDENSEAL, 189
juniper, 211
LICORICE, 222, 224, 225
LOBELIA, 232
MULLEIN, 250, 252
PEPPERMINT, 257
red clover, 267, 270
red raspberry, 274
SLIPPERY ELM, 288
St. John's wort, 298
valerian, 316
wild lettuce, 328
YELLOW DOCK, 350
cramps, menstrual. *See* menstruation, herbs for
croup, herbs for
catnip, 72
LOBELIA, 232, 236
MULLEIN, 250
slippery elm, 288
Cushing's disease
alfalfa, 2
licorice, 221
cuts, herbs for. *See* first aid, herbs for
cystic fibrosis, herbs for
juniper, 208
cystitis. *See* bladder problems, herbs for
cysts, herbs for
dandelion, 125

D

dandelion
  history of, 124
  influence and properties, 122–23
  nutrients in, 124–25
  preparations and remedies, 127–28
  safety and profile, 128–29
  uses for, 125–26
dandruff, herbs for
  burdock, 62
  chamomile, 92, 95
  chaparral, 100
  comfrey, 113
  yarrow, 340
decoctions
  barley, 34–35
  chaparral, 104–6
  hawthorn, 205
  mullein, 254
  wild yam, 336
  yellow dock, 353–54
decongestants
  brigham tea, 58
  capsicum, 79
delirium, herbs for
  black cohosh, 43
  lobelia, 232
  milk thistle, 242
demulcents
  ALOE, 12
  barley, 26
  burdock, 61, 62
  comfrey, 112, 113
  flaxseed, 149
  KELP, 215
  LICORICE, 221, 222, 224
  milk thistle, 242
  SLIPPERY ELM, 287
deobstruents
  dandelion, 123
  red clover, 267
deodorants
  alfalfa, 1, 5
  ALOE, 13
  barley, 26
  slippery elm, 287
depression, herbs for
  BLESSED THISTLE, 51, 59
  brigham tea, 55, 59
  chaste tree, 108

  licorice, 226
  milk thistle, 242
  peppermint, 258
  ST. JOHN'S WORT, 298, 301–2
depuratives
  alfalfa, 1
  ALOE, 13
  BURDOCK, 61
  DANDELION, 122
  ECHINACEA, 130
  goldenseal, 188
  red clover, 267
dermatitis, herbs for
  dandelion, 123
  licorice, 222, 226
  red clover, 270
  wild yam, 331, 336
detoxifiers
  blessed thistle, 52
  dandelion, 123
  kelp, 219
diabetes, herbs for
  ALFALFA, 1, 6
  aloe, 13, 19
  barley, 26, 29–30
  BILBERRY, 37
  black cohosh, 43
  CAPSICUM, 78
  dandelion, 122, 125, 126
  EYEBRIGHT, 141
  flaxseed, 148
  garlic, 159, 167–68
  GOLDENSEAL, 188, 194
  JUNIPER, 207, 211–12
  kelp, 214
  LICORICE, 221
  milk thistle, 242, 246
  red raspberry, 274
  saw palmetto, 280
  slippery elm, 287
  UVA URSI, 308, 312
  valerian, 316
  yarrow, 339
diaper rash, herbs for
  comfrey, 113
  SLIPPERY ELM, 288
diaphoretics. *See* perspiration, herbs for causing
diarrhea, herbs for
  BILBERRY, 37

BLACK COHOSH, 43
capsicum, 84
catnip, 72
chamomile, 91
comfrey, 112
garlic, 159
GINGER, 176, 180
GOLDENSEAL, 188
MULLEIN, 249, 253
PEPPERMINT, 257, 261
RED RASPBERRY, 274, 277
SLIPPERY ELM, 287
St. John's wort, 297, 303
uva ursi, 308
wild lettuce, 325
yarrow, 339, 344
yellow dock, 349, 352

diarrhea(infant), herbs for
yarrow, 339, 344

digestion, herbs for
ALFALFA, 2, 4
ALOE, 13, 14, 18–19
barley, 26, 29, 32
black cohosh, 43
BLESSED THISTLE, 50, 52–53
capsicum, 78, 83
CATNIP, 72, 73, 74
CHAMOMILE, 91, 94
COMFREY, 112, 116
dandelion, 122, 123
echinacea, 130
eyebright, 141, 142
flaxseed, 148, 151
garlic, 161, 164
GINGER, 176, 177, 180
goldenseal, 190, 195
juniper, 207, 208, 211
kelp, 215, 216
lobelia, 231
milk thistle, 242
PEPPERMINT, 257, 258, 260–61
red clover, 267, 271
red raspberry, 274, 275
SAW PALMETTO, 280
slippery elm, 287, 289–91
uva ursi, 308
valerian, 316, 321
wild lettuce, 325, 328
yarrow, 339, 344
yellow dock, 349

diosgenin, 335–36
diphtheria, herbs for
capsicum, 79
ECHINACEA, 130
goldenseal, 189
lobelia, 232
slippery elm, 288

disinfectants
uva ursi, 308

diuretics
alfalfa, 2
BILBERRY, 37
black cohosh, 44
blessed thistle, 51
brigham tea, 56, 59
burdock, 62, 64
catnip, 74
chamomile, 92
chaparral, 100
dandelion, 123, 125
garlic, 160, 161, 165
ginger, 177, 181
goldenseal, 189
hawthorn, 201
juniper, 210
kelp, 215
licorice, 222
lobelia, 232
mullein, 250, 253
red clover, 268, 270
saw palmetto, 281
St. John's wort, 298, 303
UVA URSI, 309, 311
valerian, 317
wild lettuce, 326, 328
wild yam, 331
yarrow, 340

diverticulitis, herbs for
aloe, 13
chamomile, 91
FLAXSEED, 148
peppermint, 257
slippery elm, 287
wild yam, 330

dizziness, herbs for
chamomile, 92
garlic, 160
GINGER, 177
peppermint, 258

douche, vaginal. *See* vaginal douche

red clover, 272
slippery elm, 291
dropsy. *See* edema, herbs for
drug withdrawal, herbs for
catnip, 72
CHAMOMILE, 91
LICORICE, 221
lobelia, 231
valerian, 316
dysentery, herbs for
aloe, 13
BILBERRY, 37
comfrey, 112, 116
FLAXSEED, 148
juniper, 207
lobelia, 231
MULLEIN, 249
PEPPERMINT, 257
red raspberry, 274, 277
slippery elm, 287
St. John's wort, 297, 303
uva ursi, 308
yarrow, 339
yellow dock, 349
dysmenorrhea. *See* menstruation, herbs for
dyspepsia. *See* digestion, herbs for
dysuria, herbs for
alfalfa, 2
mullein, 250
uva ursi, 309

E
ear infection, herbs for
aloe, 13
ECHINACEA, 130
garlic, 160
LICORICE, 221
LOBELIA, 232
MULLEIN, 249, 253
yarrow, 340
yellow dock, 350
earaches, herbs for
chamomile, 92
echinacea, 130
EYEBRIGHT, 141
garlic, 172
goldenseal, 188
LOBELIA, 231
MULLEIN, 249, 253

peppermint, 257
yellow dock, 350
echinacea
history of, 131–33
influence and properties of, 130–31
nutrients in, 133
preparations and remedies, 136–37
safety and profile, 137–40
uses for, 133–36
eczema, herbs for
ALOE, 14
barley, 27, 33
BURDOCK, 62, 64
CHAMOMILE, 94
chaparral, 100
comfrey, 113
DANDELION, 123, 125
ECHINACEA, 131, 134
garlic, 160
goldenseal, 189
juniper, 208
KELP, 215
licorice, 226
lobelia, 232
red clover, 270, 272
slippery elm, 288
yellow dock, 350
edema, herbs for
bilberry, 37
BLACK COHOSH, 43
blessed thistle, 50
chamomile, 91
dandelion, 122, 125
echinacea, 131
garlic, 159
HAWTHORN, 200
JUNIPER, 207, 208, 210
licorice, 221
mullein, 249
uva ursi, 208
electrical shock
lobelia, 235
emesis therapy, 237, 239–40
emetics. *See* vomiting, herbs to induce
emmenagogues. *See* menstruation, herbs for
emollients
ALOE, 14
barley, 27
flaxseed, 149

kelp, 215
licorice, 222
SLIPPERY ELM, 288
emphysema, herbs for
brigham tea, 55
COMFREY, 113
ECHINACEA, 131
garlic, 160
licorice, 222
LOBELIA, 232
MULLEIN, 250
endangered herbs
goldenseal, 190–91
endocrine glands, herbs for the
KELP, 215, 217
endometrial cancer, herbs for
flaxseed, 148
endometriosis, herbs for
kelp, 215
endurance, herbs for
alfalfa, 1
DANDELION, 122, 126
garlic, 159
ginger, 176
hawthorn, 200
licorice, 221
yellow dock, 349
enemas
aloe, 13
capsicum, 88
catnip, 75–76
chamomile, 96
flaxseed, 148, 151
garlic, 163, 173–74
peppermint, 261, 263
red clover, 272
red raspberry, 278
slippery elm, 291, 293
yarrow, 346
enemas, administration of, 76
energy, herbs for. *See* tonics
environmental pollution, herbs to relieve
kelp, 219
ephedra, 56–59
epilepsy, herbs for
BLACK COHOSH, 44, 48
brigham tea, 55
catnip, 73
garlic, 160

juniper, 208, 211
LOBELIA, 232, 235
milk thistle, 242
valerian, 317, 320
yarrow, 340
essential oil
chamomile, 95–96, 97
garlic, 170
ginger, 183, 185
juniper, 213
peppermint, 263
valerian, 322
yarrow, 346–47
Essiac formula, 65–66, 69–70
estrogen deficiency, herbs for
BLACK COHOSH, 44, 45–47
licorice, 222
Euphrasia. *See* eyebright
expectorants
BLACK COHOSH, 43, 44, 48
BRIGHAM TEA, 55
chamomile, 92
CHAPARRAL, 99, 102
comfrey, 113, 117
GARLIC, 160, 161, 165
kelp, 215
licorice, 222
LOBELIA, 232, 236
MULLEIN, 250
red clover, 267, 270
saw palmetto, 280
slippery elm, 288
St. John's wort, 298, 303
wild lettuce, 326
wild yam, 331
yellow dock, 349
eye compresses
barley, 34–35
chamomile, 96
eyebright, 145–46
eye infections, herbs for
EYEBRIGHT, 141
GOLDENSEAL, 188
eye washes
chamomile, 96
eyebright, 145
GOLDENSEAL, 188, 192, 196–97
lobelia, 237
red clover, 267, 270
red raspberry, 274, 277

eyebright
  history of, 142–43
  influence and properties of, 141–42
  nutrients in, 143
  preparations and remedies, 144–46
  safety and profile, 146–47
  uses for, 143–44
eyesight, herbs for
  aloe, 13, 17
  BILBERRY, 37, 38, 39–40
  capsicum, 79
  chaparral, 99
  comfrey, 112
  EYEBRIGHT, 141, 142–43
  garlic, 160
  juniper, 207
  mullein, 249
  slippery elm, 288
  wild lettuce, 325

F
fainting, herbs for
  PEPPERMINT, 257
fatigue, herbs for
  alfalfa, 2
  catnip, 72
  comfrey, 112
  dandelion, 122
  GINGER, 176
  licorice, 221
  St. John's wort, 297
  valerian, 316
  yellow dock, 349
Federal Drug Administration (FDA)
  barley, 29
  brigham tea, 56–57
  chaparral warning, 104
  comfrey ban, 119–20
  lobeline ban, 236
fertility, herbs for
  flaxseed, 154
  kelp, 218
  licorice, 226
  red clover, 271
fertilizer, herbs used for
  kelp, 215
fever blisters, herbs for
  aloe, 13
fever, herbs for
  alfalfa, 2, 5

BARLEY, 26
BLACK COHOSH, 43
BLESSED THISTLE, 50
BURDOCK, 62, 64
catnip, 72, 74
CHAMOMILE, 92, 94
comfrey, 112
dandelion, 122
ECHINACEA, 130
flaxseed, 148
GARLIC, 160
GINGER, 177
goldenseal, 189, 193
licorice, 222
LOBELIA, 232
PEPPERMINT, 257
RED RASPBERRY, 274
slippery elm, 288
uva ursi, 308
wild lettuce, 325
YARROW, 340, 343
yellow dock, 350
fibrositis, herbs for
  chaparral, 100
fingernails, herbs for the
  KELP, 215, 217
first aid, herbs for
  ALOE, 13, 16–17
  black cohosh, 43
  capsicum, 79, 85
  chamomile, 92, 94
  chaparral, 99
  COMFREY, 112
  juniper, 207
  lobelia, 232
  mullein, 249
  red raspberry, 274
  yarrow, 340
flatulence. See gas relief, herbs for
flaxseed
  history of, 149
  influence and properties of, 148–49
  nutrients in, 151
  preparations and remedies of, 155–57
  safety and profile, 157–58
  uses for, 151–55
flu, herbs for
  ALOE, 13
  capsicum, 84
  catnip, 72, 74

chamomile, 92
chaparral, 99, 102
dandelion, 122
GARLIC, 160
licorice, 225
PEPPERMINT, 257
red clover, 267
RED RASPBERRY, 274, 277
YARROW, 340, 343
yellow dock, 350

fomentations
chamomile, 96
comfrey, 117
eyebright, 145
ginger, 185
goldenseal, 196
lobelia, 239
mullein, 254–55
red clover, 272
yarrow, 346
yellow dock, 354

food poisoning, herbs for
licorice, 221
LOBELIA, 231

fractures, herbs for
alfalfa, 1
COMFREY, 112, 115
dandelion, 122
kelp, 215
red raspberry, 274
slippery elm, 288
yarrow, 340
yellow dock, 350

frost bite, herbs for
aloe, 13
capsicum, 79

fungal infections, herbs for
alfalfa, 2
juniper, 207

G
galactagogue. *See* lactation, herbs for
gallbladder, herbs for the
aloe, 13
BLESSED THISTLE, 51
burdock, 62
comfrey, 113
DANDELION, 123
garlic, 160
goldenseal, 189

kelp, 215
milk thistle, 242, 243, 245
peppermint, 258
red clover, 267, 270
saw palmetto, 280
St. John's wort, 297
wild yam, 331, 333
yellow dock, 350, 352

gallstones, herbs for
black cohosh, 43
burdock, 62
chamomile, 92
dandelion, 123, 125
uva ursi, 308

gangrene, herbs for
chamomile, 92, 94
COMFREY, 112
ECHINACEA, 130, 135
slippery elm, 288

gargles
alfalfa, 9
comfrey, 113
juniper, 208
peppermint, 258, 264
red clover, 272
red raspberry, 277
yellow dock, 354

garlic
history of, 161–63
influence and profile of, 159–61
nutrients in, 164
preparations and remedies, 169–74
safety and profile of, 174–75
uses for, 164–69

gas relief, herbs for
BLESSED THISTLE, 50
burdock, 61
capsicum, 79, 83
catnip, 72
CHAMOMILE, 91, 92, 93
dandelion, 122
echinacea, 130
garlic, 161, 165
ginger, 177
GINGER, 176
juniper, 207, 208, 211
kelp, 215
milk thistle, 242
PEPPERMINT, 257, 258, 261
RED RASPBERRY, 274, 275

slippery elm, 287, 291
valerian, 316
WILD YAM, 330, 333
yarrow, 339, 344
gastritis, herbs for
  aloe, 13
  barley, 26
  flaxseed, 148, 151
  goldenseal, 195
  RED RASPBERRY, 274
ginger
  history of, 178–79
  influence and properties, 176–78
  nutrients in, 179–80
  preparations and remedies, 182–85
  safety and profile of, 186–87
  uses for, 180–82
gingivitis, herbs for
  aloe, 13, 19
  echinacea, 131
gland regulation, herbs for
  echinacea, 130
  garlic, 159, 160
  goldenseal, 188
  kelp, 215, 216
  licorice, 221
  MULLEIN, 249, 250, 252
  SAW PALMETTO, 280, 281
  yarrow, 344, 352
  yellow dock, 350
glaucoma, herbs for
  chaparral, 99
  EYEBRIGHT, 141
glycyrrhizin. *See* licorice
goiter, herbs for
  KELP, 215
goldenseal
  history of, 190–91
  influence and properties of, 188–90
  nutrients in, 191
  preparations and remedies, 195–98
  safety and profile of, 198–99
  uses for, 191–95
gonorrhea, herbs for
  burdock, 62
  echinacea, 131, 135
  GOLDENSEAL, 189
  juniper, 208, 212
  licorice, 222
  red raspberry, 275

  uva ursi, 308
gout, herbs for, St. John's wort 297
  ALFALFA, 2
  BURDOCK, 62, 64
  COMFREY, 113, 116
  dandelion, 123, 125, 126
  flaxseed, 148
  ginger, 177
  juniper, 208
  peppermint, 258
  red clover, 267
  slippery elm, 288, 291
  yarrow, 343
  yellow dock, 350
gripe, herbs for
  ginger, 177
  peppermint, 257, 260
ground cover crop, herbs used for
  red clover, 268, 272
gum disease, herbs for
  comfrey, 113
  echinacea, 131, 134
  GOLDENSEAL, 189, 192
  juniper, 208

H
hair growth, herbs for
  aloe, 14
  burdock, 66–67
  chaparral, 100
  juniper, 208
  kelp, 215, 217
hair health, herbs for
  chamomile, 95, 97
hair loss prevention, herbs
  yarrow, 340, 346
halitosis. *See* bad breath, herbs for
hangover, herbs for
  CAPSICUM, 78
  valerian, 316
hawthorn
  history of, 201–2
  influence and properties of, 200–201
  nutrients in, 202
  preparations and remedies, 205–6
  safety and profile, 206
  uses for, 203–305
hay fever, herbs for. *See* allergies, herbs for
headache, herbs for

alfalfa, 2
aloe, 13
black cohosh, 44
BLESSED THISTLE, 51, 52
capsicum, 79
chamomile, 92
comfrey, 113
echinacea, 135
eyebright, 142, 144
GINGER, 177
kelp, 215
LOBELIA, 232
PEPPERMINT, 258
valerian, 317
healing, herbs to promote
capsicum, 82
yarrow, 344
heart attack, herbs for
CAPSICUM, 78, 82, 85
garlic, 167
heart disease, herbs for
alfalfa, 1
aloe, 13, 19
barley, 26, 29
capsicum, 82
HAWTHORN, 200, 203–5
kelp, 214
heart palpitations
CAPSICUM, 78
lobelia, 231
VALERIAN, 316, 321
wild lettuce, 325
heart problems, herbs for
milk thistle, 242
heart, herbs for the
alfalfa, 1
aloe, 12, 19
black cohosh, 47
blessed thistle, 50
brigham tea, 58
CAPSICUM, 78
garlic, 166–67
GARLIC, 159
goldenseal, 188, 193
HAWTHORN, 200, 201, 203–5
juniper, 207
licorice, 221, 226
lobelia, 231, 236
PEPPERMINT, 257
RED RASPBERRY, 274

St. John's wort, 297
valerian, 321
heartburn, herbs for
ALOE, 13, 18–19
chamomile, 91
dandelion, 122
garlic, 159
GINGER, 176
milk thistle, 242
PEPPERMINT, 257
valerian, 316
heat stroke. *See* sunstroke, herbs for
hemorrhage, herbs for
alfalfa, 1
CAPSICUM, 78, 82
chamomile, 91
comfrey, 112
dandelion, 122
echinacea, 130
ginger, 176
GOLDENSEAL, 188, 193, 194
milk thistle, 242
MULLEIN, 249
slippery elm, 287
St. John's wort, 297
YARROW, 340, 344
yellow dock, 349
hemorrhoids, herbs for
alfalfa, 1
ALOE, 13
BILBERRY, 37
BURDOCK, 61
catnip, 72
chamomile, 91
chaparral, 99
comfrey, 112
flaxseed, 148, 151
garlic, 166, 170
GOLDENSEAL, 188
licorice, 221, 225
mullein, 249, 253
red raspberry, 274
uva ursi, 308
yarrow, 339, 344
yellow dock, 349
hemostatics
red raspberry, 275
hepatitis, herbs for
alfalfa, 2
barley, 27

DANDELION, 123
goldenseal, 189
licorice, 225
LOBELIA, 232
MILK THISTLE, 242, 245
St. John's wort, 297, 303
wild yam, 331
yellow dock, 350
herb combinations. *See* catalysts
hernias, herbs for
slippery elm, 287, 291
herpes, herbs for
ALOE, 13, 17
barley, 26
BURDOCK, 62
chaparral, 99
COMFREY, 112
licorice, 222
mullein, 249, 252
peppermint, 257
slippery elm, 288
St. John's wort, 297, 303
uva ursi, 308
herpes(genital), herbs for
goldenseal, 189
hiccups, herbs for
catnip, 72
peppermint, 258
wild yam, 331
high blood pressure remedies
aloe, 12
HIV, herbs for
chaparral, 99, 103
St. John's wort, 297, 303
hoarseness, herbs for. *See* sore throat, herbs for
hormone balance, herbs for
alfalfa, 2
BLACK COHOSH, 44, 45–47
blessed thistle, 51, 52
chaparral, 100
flaxseed, 154
red clover, 268, 271
red raspberry, 276
SAW PALMETTO, 280, 281–84
wild yam, 334–35
Hormone Replacement Therapy (HRT) study, 46–47
hot flashes, herbs for
BLACK COHOSH, 44

kelp, 215
hot sauce recipe, 84
hyaluronic acid, 135
hypnotics. *See* sleep, herbs for
hyperactivity, herbs for
LOBELIA, 231
hyperglycemia, herbs for
BURDOCK, 61
garlic, 167
LICORICE, 221
hypertension, herbs for
alfalfa, 1
GARLIC, 166
HAWTHORN, 200
kelp, 218
valerian, 321
VALERIAN, 316
hypochondria
valerian, 317, 319
hypoglycemia, herbs for
ALFALFA, 1, 6
BURDOCK, 61
catnip, 72
DANDELION, 122
garlic, 159
hawthorn, 200
JUNIPER, 207, 211
LICORICE, 221, 224
lobelia, 231
milk thistle, 242
valerian, 316
hypotension, herbs for
CAPSICUM, 78
hypothermia. *See* warmth, herbs for
hysteria, herbs for
BLACK COHOSH, 44
BLESSED THISTLE, 51
catnip, 73
CHAMOMILE, 92
lobelia, 232, 235
peppermint, 258
St. John's wort, 298
valerian, 317, 319, 320
yarrow, 340

I
illness, herbs for
BARLEY, 26
immune system, herbs for the
aloe, 19–20

barley, 26, 32
ECHINACEA, 130, 131, 133–35
GARLIC, 160, 161, 165
goldenseal, 189
kelp, 217–18
licorice, 225
red clover, 270
immuno-suppressants
mullein, 250, 252
impetigo, herbs for
BURDOCK, 62
impotence, herbs for
barley, 27
chaste tree, 108
licorice, 222
SAW PALMETTO, 280
wild yam, 335
incontinence, herbs for
juniper, 208
uva ursi, 309
indigestion. See digestion, herbs for
industrial uses of herbs
bilberry, 37, 41
chamomile, 95–96
flaxseed, 149, 154
kelp, 215
licorice, 226
peppermint, 258, 262
infection, herbs for
alfalfa, 5–6
barley, 26
bilberry, 37
burdock, 61
CAPSICUM, 79
COMFREY, 112
ECHINACEA, 130
GARLIC, 160, 164, 172
GOLDENSEAL, 189
JUNIPER, 207, 211
KELP, 215
milk thistle, 246
infectious diseases, herbs for
aloe, 13, 16
capsicum, 79
GARLIC, 160, 164
lobelia, 237
infertility, herbs for
catnip, 73
chaste tree, 108
saw palmetto, 280

inflammation, herbs for
alfalfa, 2
aloe, 13
BARLEY, 26
bilberry, 37
black cohosh, 43, 44, 48
blessed thistle, 53
burdock, 62, 64
capsicum, 79
catnip, 72
chamomile, 92, 93, 95
chaparral, 99, 102
COMFREY, 113
echinacea, 131, 133, 135
eyebright, 141
FLAXSEED, 148, 149
garlic, 165
ginger, 182
GOLDENSEAL, 189, 193
juniper, 208
licorice, 222, 224, 226
milk thistle, 246
red clover, 267
red raspberry, 277
saw palmetto, 280
slippery elm, 288, 290, 294
St. John's wort, 297, 300
uva ursi, 312
wild yam, 330, 333
yarrow, 340
yellow dock, 350
influenza, herbs gore
ginger, 177
mullein, 252
inhalants
peppermint, 263
yarrow, 346
insanity, herbs for. See mental illness, herbs for
insect bites and stings, herbs for
ALOE, 13
BLACK COHOSH, 43, 48
brigham tea, 59
burdock, 65
capsicum, 79
COMFREY, 112, 116
ECHINACEA, 130, 135
garlic, 160
juniper, 207
lobelia, 232

red clover, 268
St. John's wort, 298
wild yam, 331, 336
insect repellent
catnip, 74
garlic, 161, 169, 174
insomnia, herbs for
alfalfa, 2
black cohosh, 44
catnip, 73
CHAMOMILE, 92
chaparral, 100
dandelion, 123
garlic, 159
hawthorn, 200
LOBELIA, 231
MULLEIN, 249
peppermint, 257
red clover, 267
St. John's wort, 297
valerian, 316
wild lettuce, 326
yarrow, 339
insulin production, herbs for
GOLDENSEAL, 188, 194
juniper, 211
interferons, 134, 225, 246
internal bleeding, herbs for
capsicum, 88
St. John's wort, 297
intestinal irritation, herbs for
garlic, 159
wild yam, 330
intestinal parasites, herbs for
blessed thistle, 50
chamomile, 91, 94
chaparral, 99, 103
echinacea, 130
garlic, 159
goldenseal, 190
juniper, 207, 208
kelp, 215
mullein, 249
saw palmetto, 280
slippery elm, 291
valerian, 316
yellow dock, 352
inulin, 63–64, 125
iodine production, herbs for
kelp, 217

iron deficiency. *See* anemia, herbs for
Irritable Bowel Syndrome (IBS), herbs for
flaxseed, 150
peppermint, 261
wild yam, 330
itching, herbs for
aloe, 14
BURDOCK, 68
chamomile, 94
COMFREY, 113
goldenseal, 189
juniper, 208
licorice, 226
peppermint, 258
YELLOW DOCK, 350

J
jaundice, herbs for
alfalfa, 2
aloe, 13
blessed thistle, 51
capsicum, 79
chamomile, 92
DANDELION, 123, 125
eyebright, 141, 144
lobelia, 232
MILK THISTLE, 242
slippery elm, 288
St. John's wort, 297
wild yam, 331
yarrow, 340
yellow dock, 350
joint inflammation, herbs for. *See* arthritis, herbs for
alfalfa, 2
MULLEIN, 249, 250, 253
slippery elm, 288
juniper
history of, 209
influence and properties of, 207–8
nutrients in, 210
preparations and remedies, 212–13
safety and profile, 213
uses for, 210–12

K
kelp
history of, 216
influence and properties of, 214–16

nutrients in, 216
preparations and remedies, 219
safety and profile, 219–20
uses for, 216–19
kidney problems, herbs for
alfalfa, 2
aloe, 14
barley, 27
bilberry, 37
black cost, 44
blessed thistle, 51
BURDOCK, 62
capsicum, 79
chamomile, 92
chaparral, 100
comfrey, 113
DANDELION, 125
flaxseed, 153
garlic, 161
ginger, 177
GOLDENSEAL, 189
JUNIPER, 208, 210
kelp, 215, 216
licorice, 222
MILK THISTLE, 242, 246
red clover, 268
red raspberry, 277
slippery elm, 288
UVA URSI, 309, 311
yarrow, 340
kidney stones, herbs for
chaparral, 100
comfrey, 113
dandelion, 123
FLAXSEED, 149
juniper, 208
uva ursi, 309, 311

L
lactation, herbs for
promotion of
alfalfa, 2, 6–7
blessed thistle, 51, 52
chaste tree, 108, 109
dandelion, 123, 126
milk thistle, 242
red clover, 267
RED RASPBERRY, 275, 277
suppression of
aloe, 13

bilberry, 37, 41
saw palmetto, 280
laryngitis, herbs for
CAPSICUM, 79
echinacea, 131
licorice, 222, 225
lobelia, 232
red clover, 270
yellow dock, 350
laxatives
ALOE, 18–19
BURDOCK, 61
comfrey, 112, 116
dandelion, 122, 125, 126
flaxseed, 148, 149, 151, 156
garlic, 165
goldenseal, 188
licorice, 224, 227–28
red clover, 267
red raspberry, 274
uva ursi, 308
valerian, 316
wild yam, 330
yellow dock, 349
lead poisoning, herbs for
kelp, 215
learning problems, herbs for
GINGER, 177, 181
leg cramps, herbs for
kelp, 215
leprosy, herbs for
barley, 26
BURDOCK, 62
garlic, 160
juniper, 208
red clover, 267
yellow dock, 350
leukemia, herbs for
barley, 32
CHAPARRAL, 99
RED CLOVER, 267
yellow dock, 349
leukorrhea. See vaginal discharge, herbs for
libido, herbs for the
saw palmetto, 280
slippery elm, 288
licorice
history of, 223
influence and properties of, 221–22

INDEX— 398

nutrients in, 224
preparations and remedies, 226–28
safety and profile, 228–30
uses for, 224–26
lignans, 154
liniment rub, 86
capsicum, 86–87
lobelia, 238
linseed oil, 151, 155
lithotriptics
burdock, 62
dandelion, 123
juniper, 208
uva ursi, 309, 311
valerian, 317
liver spots. *See* age spots
liver, herbs for the
alfalfa, 2, 5
aloe, 13
black cohosh, 43
blessed thistle, 51
burdock, 62, 64
capsicum, 79
catnip, 72
chamomile, 92
chaparral, 102
DANDELION, 123, 125, 126
eyebright, 141, 144
GARLIC, 160, 168
GOLDENSEAL, 189, 193
hawthorn, 201
kelp, 216
licorice, 225
lobelia, 232
MILK THISTLE, 242, 243, 244–45, 246
peppermint, 258
RED CLOVER, 267, 271
uva ursi, 308
valerian, 317
wild yam, 331, 333
yarrow, 340, 343, 344
yellow dock, 350, 352
lobelia
history of, 233–34
influence and properties of, 231–33
nutrients in, 234
preparations and remedies, 238–40
safety and profile, 240–41
uses for, 235–38
lock jaw. *See* tetanus, herbs for

lucerne. *See* alfalfa
lumbago, herbs for
barley, 27
black cohosh, 43
garlic, 160
slippery elm, 288
valerian, 317
lung hemorrhage, herbs for
ginger, 177
slippery elm, 291
yarrow, 343
lungs, herbs for the
BLESSED THISTLE, 51
burdock, 62
chaparral, 100
COMFREY, 113, 114–15, 117
GARLIC, 160, 165
ginger, 181
goldenseal, 192, 193
LICORICE, 222
LOBELIA, 232, 236
MULLEIN, 250, 252
red clover, 267
SLIPPERY ELM, 288
YARROW, 340, 343
yellow dock, 350
lupus, herbs for
burdock, 61
echinacea, 132
goldenseal, 189
lymphatic congestion, herbs for
burdock, 61, 64
chaparral, 102
ECHINACEA, 130, 131, 133, 135
garlic, 165
goldenseal, 189
juniper, 207, 210
MULLEIN, 249, 252
red clover, 267

M
Ma Huang, 56–57
malaria, herbs for
BLACK COHOSH, 43
brigham tea, 55
capsicum, 79
goldenseal, 189
yarrow, 340
malnourishment, herbs for
saw palmetto, 281

INDEX— 399

slippery elm, 287, 290
mastitis. *See* breasts, herbs for the
measles, herbs for
   black cohosh, 43
   BURDOCK, 62
   catnip, 72
   chamomile, 92
   GOLDENSEAL, 189
   lobelia, 232
   peppermint, 257
   red raspberry, 274
   valerian, 316
   YARROW, 340, 343
memory, herbs to improve
   alfalfa, 2
   BLESSED THISTLE, 51
   CAPSICUM, 79
   dandelion, 123
   eyebright, 142
   flaxseed, 148
   juniper, 208, 211
   licorice, 221
   milk thistle, 246
men, herbs for. *See* impotence, herbs for; prostate problems, herbs for; testicles(swollen), herbs for
meningitis. *See* spinal meningitis, herbs for
menopause, herbs for
   alfalfa, 7
   BLACK COHOSH, 44, 46–47
   blessed thistle, 51, 52
   chaparral, 100
   CHASTE TREE, 108
   flaxseed, 148
   hawthorn, 201
   KELP, 215
   licorice, 222
   St. John's wort, 298, 303
   valerian, 317, 321
   wild yam, 335
menstruation suppression, herbs for
   milk thistle, 242
   peppermint, 258
menstruation, herbs for
   ALFALFA, 2, 6–7
   aloe, 13, 20
   BLACK COHOSH, 44, 46
   blessed thistle, 51, 52
   capsicum, 79

   catnip, 73
   chamomile, 92, 95
   CHASTE TREE, 108, 109–10
   comfrey, 113
   flaxseed, 148
   garlic, 160, 164
   ginger, 177, 182
   GOLDENSEAL, 189
   hawthorn, 201
   juniper, 208, 212
   kelp, 218
   licorice, 226
   lobelia, 232
   red clover, 268, 271
   RED RASPBERRY, 275, 276
   slippery elm, 288
   ST. JOHN'S WORT, 298, 303
   uva ursi, 309
   valerian, 317, 321
   wild yam, 331, 334, 335
   yarrow, 340, 344
mental illness, herbs for
   catnip, 73
   valerian, 317
metabolism, herbs to increase
   brigham tea, 55, 59
   capsicum, 80, 83
   dandelion, 122
   echinacea, 130
   kelp, 217
   milk thistle, 243, 244
   red clover, 270
metal poisoning, herbs for
   BARLEY, 26
   garlic, 160
midwives, herbs used by
   RED RASPBERRY, 276
   yellow dock, 352
migraine headaches, herbs for
   blessed thistle, 51
   chamomile, 92
   chaste tree, 108
   garlic, 160
   ginger, 181
   LOBELIA, 232
   peppermint, 258
   valerian, 317
milk thistle
   history of, 243–44
   influence and properties of, 242–43

nutrients in, 244
preparations and remedies, 247
safety and profile, 248
uses for, 244–46
miscarriage prevention, herbs for
catnip, 73
RED RASPBERRY, 275
wild yam, 331, 334
miscarriage, herbs for
LOBELIA, 232
mood elevators
catnip, 74
morning sickness, herbs for
alfalfa, 2
catnip, 73
GINGER, 177, 180, 182
goldenseal, 189
KELP, 215
peppermint, 258, 260
RED RASPBERRY, 275
WILD YAM, 331
mosquito bites, herbs for. *See* insect bites and stings, herbs for
mosquito repellants
yarrow, 344
motion sickness prevention, herbs for
GINGER, 176
PEPPERMINT, 257, 260
mouth cancer
flaxseed, 148
mouthwashes
COMFREY, 113
echinacea, 134
peppermint, 258
red raspberry, 277
mucous drainage, herbs for
ECHINACEA, 131
saw palmetto, 280
mucous membranes, herbs for. *See also* demulcent
BARLEY, 26
black cohosh, 48
COMFREY, 112, 116
echinacea, 131, 133, 135
eyebright, 141, 144
FLAXSEED, 148, 149
garlic, 160, 161, 165
GOLDENSEAL, 188, 190, 191–92
juniper, 207
licorice, 221, 222, 224, 225

lobelia, 231
milk thistle, 246
MULLEIN, 249, 252
RED RASPBERRY, 274, 277
saw palmetto, 285
slippery elm, 287, 290
uva ursi, 308
yarrow, 339, 343
yellow dock, 352
mullein
history of, 250–51
influence and properties of, 249–50
nutrients in, 252
preparations and remedies, 253–55
safety and profile of, 256
uses for, 252–53
multiple sclerosis, herbs for
St. John's wort, 298, 300
mumps, herbs for
catnip, 72
ginger, 177
LOBELIA, 232
mullein, 249
muscle cramps, herbs for
catnip, 72
chaparral, 100
comfrey, 113
dandelion, 123
garlic, 160
lobelia, 232
mullein, 249
red clover, 268
valerian, 316
wild lettuce, 327
wild yam, 331
yarrow, 340
muscle pain, herbs for
wild yam, 331
muscle relaxants
black cohosh, 43, 48
goldenseal, 189, 193
valerian, 321
muscle strain, herbs for
St. John's wort, 298
yellow dock, 350
muscle tone, herbs for
alfalfa, 2
muscular dystrophy, herbs for
barley, 27
myalgia, herbs for

St. John's wort, 298, 301
myasthenia gravis, herbs for
  brigham tea, 55

N
narcolepsy, herbs for
  brigham tea, 59
narcotics
  wild lettuce, 326
nasal congestion, herbs for
  mullein, 250
  valerian, 317
nasal douche
  alfalfa, 2
  goldenseal, 197
nausea, herbs for
  ALFALFA, 1
  chamomile, 91
  GINGER, 180
  goldenseal, 190
  PEPPERMINT, 257
  RED RASPBERRY, 274
  wild yam, 330, 333
  yarrow, 344
necrosis, herbs for
  garlic, 160
nephritis, herbs for
  lobelia, 232
  UVA URSI, 309
nerve damage, herbs for
  chamomile, 93–94
  St. John's wort, 298
  valerian, 316, 319
nervines
  black cohosh, 44, 47
  blessed thistle, 51
  brigham tea, 55, 58
  catnip, 73, 74
  chamomile, 92
  garlic, 160, 168
  ginger, 177
  juniper, 208
  LOBELIA, 232, 235
  milk thistle, 243
  PEPPERMINT, 258, 261
  saw palmetto, 280
  ST. JOHN'S WORT, 298, 300–301
  valerian, 317
  WILD LETTUCE, 326
  wild yam, 330, 333

nervous disorders, herbs for
  aloe, 13
  black cohosh, 44
  burdock, 62
  chamomile, 92, 93
  goldenseal, 189
  milk thistle, 242
  MULLEIN, 250
  RED CLOVER, 268
  red raspberries, 275
  St. John's wort, 298
  VALERIAN, 317
  wild yam, 331
  yarrow, 340
nervous system, herbs for the
  aloe, 13
  black cohosh, 44, 47–48
  brigham tea, 58
  burdock, 62
  capsicum, 81
  catnip, 72
  kelp, 218
  red clover, 268
neuralgia, herbs for
  BLACK COHOSH, 44
  saw palmetto, 280
  St. John's wort, 298
  valerian, 317
  wild yam, 331
neuritis, herbs for
  kelp, 215
nicotine addiction, herbs for
  barley, 26
  black cohosh, 43
  catnip, 72, 74
  CHAMOMILE, 91
  licorice, 221
  lobelia, 231, 236
  peppermint, 257
  slippery elm, 287
  valerian, 316
nicotine poisoning, herbs for
  garlic, 160
night blindness, herbs for
  BILBERRY, 37
nightmares, herbs for
  PEPPERMINT, 257
nose bleeds, herbs for
  alfalfa, 1
  CAPSICUM, 78

GOLDENSEAL, 189
mullein, 250
yarrow, 344
YARROW, 340
nursing aids. *See* lactation aids
nutritive
 ALFALFA, 1
 BARLEY, 26, 28–29
 bilberry, 37
 comfrey, 112, 113
 dandelion, 122, 125
 flaxseed
  149
 KELP, 215, 216, 217
 red clover, 267, 268, 269
 saw palmetto, 280
 SLIPPERY ELM, 287, 289, 290
 yellow dock, 349

O
obesity, herbs for
 alfalfa, 2
 barley, 27, 30
 BLACK COHOSH, 43
 BRIGHAM TEA, 55, 58
 burdock, 62
 CAPSICUM, 79
 chamomile, 92
 chaparral, 100
 comfrey, 113
 DANDELION, 123
 flaxseed, 153
 GARLIC, 160, 165
 goldenseal, 189, 193
 KELP, 215, 216
 licorice, 222
 LOBELIA, 232, 235
 mullein, 250
 saw palmetto, 280
 SLIPPERY ELM, 288
 uva ursi, 309
 wild lettuce, 326
 wild yam, 331
oil, essential. *See* essential oil
oils, infused
 garlic, 170, 172
 ginger, 185
 goldenseal, 197
 hypericum (St. John's wort), 304
 mullein, 255

oily skin, herbs for
 dandelion, 123
ointments
 burdock, 68
 capsicum, 87
 licorice, 228
 red clover, 273
 yarrow, 347
 yellow dock, 354
Omega-3 fatty acids, 152–53
ophthalmia, herbs for
 lobelia, 232, 237
 red raspberry, 274
 slippery elm, 288, 291
optic nerve weakness, herbs for
 JUNIPER, 207, 211
osteoarthritis, herbs for. *See* arthritis, herbs for
ovulation. *See* fertility, herbs for

P
pain relief, herbs for
 alfalfa, 2
 black cohosh, 44, 47–48
 capsicum, 79, 80
 catnip, 73, 74
 chamomile, 92, 94
 chaparral, 100, 102
 COMFREY, 113
 juniper, 208, 210
 LOBELIA, 231
 MULLEIN, 249, 250, 253
 slippery elm, 288
 VALERIAN, 317
 wild lettuce, 326, 327
 wild yam, 331
 yellow dock, 350
pain relief, topical
 ALOE, 13, 16–17
palsy, herbs for
 juniper, 208
 lobelia, 232
 St. John's wort, 298
 valerian, 317
pancreas, herbs for the
 capsicum, 79
 comfrey, 112
 dandelion, 122
 GOLDENSEAL, 188
 JUNIPER, 207

kelp, 215
licorice, 221
uva ursi, 208
yellow dock, 350
pancreatitis, herbs for
barley, 26
paralysis, herbs for
black cohosh, 44
capsicum, 79
garlic, 160
valerian, 317
yellow dock, 350
parasites. *See* intestinal parasites, herbs for
Parkinson's disease, herbs for
capsicum, 79
parturients. *See* childbirth, herbs for
Pasteur, Louis, 162
pelvic circulations, herbs for
ginger, !77
peppermint
history of, 259–60
influence and properties, 257–58
nutrients in, 260
preparations and remedies, 262–64
safety and profile, 264–66
uses for, 260–62
peristalsis, herbs for
garlic, 166
lobelia, 236
peritonitis, herbs for
echinacea, 130
flaxseed, 153
lobelia, 231
perspiration, herbs for causing
black cohosh, 44
blessed thistle, 50, 51, 53
burdock, 64
CAPSICUM, 78, 79, 81, 83
catnip, 74
chamomile, 94
chaparral, 102
echinacea, 131
garlic, 159, 160, 165
GINGER, 177, 181
lobelia, 232, 237
peppermint, 258, 261
red raspberry, 274
valerian, 316
wild lettuce, 325

wild yam, 330
YARROW, 340
pertussis. *See* whooping cough, herbs for
pH balance, herbs for
alfalfa, 1
aloe, 14, 16, 19
barley, 32
dandelion, 126
ginger, 181
hawthorn, 205
pharyngitis, herbs for
garlic, 160
phlebitis
capsicum, 78
phlegm, herbs for. *See* expectorants
pimples. *See* acne, herbs for
pin worms. *See* worms, herbs to expel
pink eye. *See* conjunctivitis
pituitary gland, herbs for the
ALFALFA, 2, 6, 11
burdock, 65
KELP, 215
yellow dock, 350
plague, herbs for
GARLIC, 160, 162
juniper, 208, 209
plaque, atherosclerotic. *See* atherosclerosis, herbs for
pleurisy, herbs for
capsicum, 79
comfrey, 113
flaxseed, 148, 153
LOBELIA, 232
MULLEIN, 250
slippery elm, 288
yarrow, 340
pneumonia, herbs for
burdock, 62
comfrey, 113
flaxseed, 153
garlic, 160, 171
ginger, 177
goldenseal, 192
licorice, 222
LOBELIA, 232
mullein, 250
slippery elm, 288
yarrow, 340, 343
poison antidotes
BLACK COHOSH, 44

burdock, 62, 64
ECHINACEA, 130
red clover, 269
poison ivy/oak remedies
ALOE, 13
BURDOCK, 62
goldenseal, 189
lobelia, 232
slippery elm, 288
yellow dock, 350
polyps, herbs for
BARLEY, 26
post-partum, herbs for
uva ursi, 312
valerian, 317
wild yam, 331, 334
poultices
ALOE, 13, 21
barley, 34
black cohosh, 48
burdock, 67–68
capsicum, 86
chamomile, 94, 96
comfrey, 116, 117–18
echinacea, 137
flaxseed, 153, 156–57
garlic, 173–74
juniper, 211
lobelia, 237, 239
mullein, 255
peppermint, 263
red clover, 273
slippery elm, 289, 292, 293–94
wild lettuce, 328
yarrow, 344
yellow dock, 354
prebiotics
burdock, 63
echinacea, 131, 134
pregnancy, herbs for
bilberry, 41
BLESSED THISTLE, 51, 52
burdock, 65
chamomile, 97
echinacea, 137
KELP, 215, 216, 217
RED RASPBERRY, 275, 276
wild yam, 331
yellow dock, 350
YELLOW DOCK, 350

premenstrual syndrome (PMS), herbs for
aloe, 13
chaste tree, 108, 109–10
DANDELION, 123
flaxseed, 154
valerian, 321
wild yam, 331, 334, 335
yarrow, 340
prolapsed uterus. *See* uterus, herbs for a prolapsed
prostate problems, herbs for
chaparral, 100
ECHINACEA, 131, 135
GARLIC, 160
GOLDENSEAL, 189
juniper, 208
kelp, 215, 218
uva ursi, 308, 312
prostate, herbs for the
red clover, 268, 271
SAW PALMETTO, 280, 283–84
psoriasis, herbs for
ALOE, 14, 19
barley, 27
BURDOCK, 62
chaparral, 100
comfrey, 113
dandelion, 123
echinacea, 134
garlic, 160
goldenseal, 189
kelp, 215
licorice, 246
RED CLOVER, 268, 270, 272
wild yam, 331, 336
yellow dock, 350
pulmonary disease, herbs for
MULLEIN, 250, 252
purgatives. *See* laxatives
pyorrhea, herbs for
alfalfa, 2
capsicum, 79
comfrey, 113
echinacea, 131
goldenseal, 195

R
rabies, herbs for
garlic, 160

radiation burns. See burns, herbs for
radiation poisoning, herbs for
  KELP, 215, 219
  milk thistle, 242
rashes. See skin conditions, herbs for
Raynaud's disease, herbs for
  bilberry, 37
rectal irritation, herbs for
  red clover, 267
red clover
  history of, 268–69
  influence and properties of, 267–68
  nutrients in, 269
  preparations and remedies, 272–73
  safety and profile of, 273
  uses for, 269–72
red pepper. See capsicum
red raspberry
  history of, 275
  influence and properties of, 274–75
  nutrients in, 276
  preparations and remedies, 277–78
  safety and profile of, 279
  uses for, 276–77
refrigerants
  catnip, 72
  red raspberry, 2i74
relaxants. See sedatives
renal ulcerations. See ulcerated kidneys
reproductive organs (female), herbs for
  alfalfa, 2, 6–7
  black cohosh, 44
  catnip, 73
  dandelion, 123
  RED RASPBERRY, 275, 276
  saw palmetto, 280, 283
  slippery elm, 288, 293
  wild yam, 331, 334
  yarrow, 340, 344
reproductive organs (male), herbs for
  saw palmetto283, 283
respiratory congestion, herbs for. See chest congestion, herbs for
respiratory infection, herbs for
  blessed thistle, 51
  echinacea, 133
  flaxseed, 148
  goldenseal, 189, 192
respiratory system. See lungs, herbs for the

rheumatism, herbs for
  ALFALFA, 1
  aloe, 13
  BLACK COHOSH, 43
  BURDOCK, 61, 62, 64
  CAPSICUM, 78, 79, 85
  CHAPARRAL, 99
  comfrey, 113
  dandelion, 123, 125
  flaxseed, 148
  garlic, 160, 165, 170
  hawthorn, 201
  juniper, 208
  kelp, 218
  lobelia, 232
  mullein, 250
  peppermint, 258
  red clover, 267
  red raspberry, 274
  St. John's wort, 297
  uva ursi, 308
  wild yam, 330, 334, 336
  yarrow, 340
  YELLOW DOCK, 350
rickets, herbs for
  red clover, 267, 271
ringworm, herbs for
  ALOE, 13, 16, 18
  garlic, 160
  goldenseal, 189, 195
  lobelia, 232
  yellow dock, 351
RNA stimulation, herbs for
  milk thistle, 245
rodent repellents
  peppermint, 264
rosacea, herbs for
  burdock, 62
rubefacients
  capsicum, 79, 82
  GINGER, 177
  peppermint, 258

S
saliva production, herbs to increase.
  See sialagogues
salves
  comfrey, 118–19
  goldenseal, 197–98
  hypericum (St. John's wort), 304

INDEX— 406

lobelia, 239
saw palmetto
  history of, 281–82
  influence and properties of, 280–81
  nutrients in, 282
  preparations and remedies, 285
  safety and profile of, 285–86
  uses for, 282–85
scabies
  wild yam, 331
scalds. See burns, herbs for
scar tissue, herbs for
  ALOE, 13
scarlet fever, herbs for
  black cohosh, 43
  goldenseal, 189
  lobelia, 232
  red clover, 267
  valerian, 316
  yellow dock, 350
sciatica, herbs for
  black cohosh, 44
  burdock, 62
  juniper, 208
  St. John's wort, 298
  wild yam, 330, 336
scrofuloderma, herbs for
  red clover, 268
  yellow dock, 350
scurvy, herbs for
  alfalfa, 1
  bilberry, 37
  burdock, 61
  dandelion, 122
  juniper, 207
  YELLOW DOCK, 349
sea sickness. See motion sickness prevention, herbs for
seasonal affective disorder (SAD), herbs for
  St. John's wort, 301
seborrhea, herbs for
  ALOE, 14, 17
  goldenseal, 189, 194
sedatives
  black cohosh, 44, 47
  catnip, 73, 74
  chamomile, 92
  hawthorn, 200, 205
  lobelia, 231, 235

peppermint, 258
  red clover, 267, 271
  saw palmetto, 280, 285
  St. John's wort, 298
  VALERIAN, 316, 319
  wild lettuce, 326, 327
  wild yam, 331, 333
senility. See memory, herbs to improve
septicemia. See blood poisoning, herbs for
sexual stimulants
  SAW PALMETTO, 280
shingles, herbs for
  aloe, 14
  capsicum, 79
  peppermint, 258
  St. John's wort, 298
  uva ursi, 309
shock, herbs for
  capsicum, 79, 82, 85
  catnip, 72
  ginger, 177
  lobelia, 232
  PEPPERMINT, 257
  valerian, 316
sialagogues
  echinacea, 130
  ginger, 176
  licorice, 222
silymarin, 244–45, 246
sinuses, herbs for the
  alfalfa, 2
  capsicum, 79
  comfrey, 113
  eyebright, 142
  garlic, 160
  ginger, 177
  GOLDENSEAL, 189, 196
  MULLEIN, 250, 252
skin cancer, herbs for
  flaxseed, 148
  GOLDENSEAL, 189, 194
skin chafing, herbs for
  garlic, 160
  wild lettuce, 326
  yellow dock, 350
skin conditions, herbs for
  alfalfa, 2
  ALOE, 13, 15–17
  barley, 32–33

black cohosh, 44
BURDOCK, 62, 64, 65
capsicum, 79
catnip, 73
chaparral, 100
COMFREY, 113
dandelion, 123, 125, 126
ECHINACEA, 131
flaxseed, 149
garlic, 173
GOLDENSEAL, 189, 194
milk thistle, 242, 246
mullein, 250
RED CLOVER, 286
slippery elm, 288, 291
St. John's wort, 298
valerian, 317
yarrow, 340
sleep, herbs for
black cohosh, 44
CHAMOMILE, 92
hawthorn, 200
lobelia, 236
valerian, 319–20
wild lettuce, 326, 327
slippery elm
history of, 289–90
influence and properties of, 287–89
nutrients in, 290
preparations and remedies, 292–95
safety and profile of, 295–96
uses for, 290–92
slippery elm gruel, 293
smallpox, herbs for
black cohosh, 43
garlic, 160
goldenseal, 189
yarrow, 340, 343
smoking. *See* nicotine addiction, herbs for
smudges
juniper, 209
mullein, 253
snake bites, herbs for
BLACK COHOSH, 44, 48
brigham tea, 59
chaparral, 99
echinacea, 131, 135
juniper, 207
milk thistle, 242

soaks
chaparral, 104
peppermint, 264
sore throat, herbs for
black cohosh, 43
burdock, 62
chamomile, 92
echinacea, 131
eyebright, 142
garlic, 160, 171
GINGER, 177
GOLDENSEAL, 189, 192
hawthorn, 201, 205
juniper, 208
LICORICE, 222
mullein, 250
peppermint, 258
saw palmetto, 280
slippery elm, 288, 291
yarrow, 340
sores. *See* first aid, herbs for; wounds, herbs for
spasms, herbs for
alfalfa, 2
BLACK COHOSH, 44, 48
capsicum, 79, 80
catnip, 73, 74
chamomile, 92, 94
garlic, 159, 161
ginger, 176, 180
goldenseal, 189, 193
hawthorn, 200
JUNIPER, 208
LOBELIA, 232, 233, 235
mullein, 249, 250, 252
peppermint, 258, 261
red clover, 268, 271
RED CLOVER, 268
RED RASPBERRY, 275
saw palmetto, 280
St. John's wort, 298
valerian, 316, 317, 321
wild lettuce, 326
wild yam, 331
yarrow, 340
spinal meningitis, herbs for
BLACK COHOSH, 44, 48
GARLIC, 160
goldenseal, 189
lobelia, 232

INDEX— 408

spleen, herbs for the
  blessed thistle, 50
  chamomile, 92
  dandelion, 122
  garlic, 165
  goldenseal, 189
  milk thistle, 242, 243
  UVA URSI, 308
  yarrow, 340
  yellow dock, 349, 352
sprains, herbs for
  capsicum, 79
  chamomile, 92, 94
  COMFREY, 112
  lobelia, 232
  mullein, 249
sprouting seeds
  alfalfa, 9–10
  milk thistle, 247
St. John's wort
  history of, 298–300
  influence and principals of, 297–98
  nutrients in, 300
  preparations and remedies, 303–5
  safety and profile of, 305–7
  uses for, 300–303
St. Vitus Dance, herbs for
  BLACK COHOSH, 44
  lobelia, 232
  red clover, 268
  valerian, 317, 320
stamina, herbs for. *See* endurance, herbs for
  yellow dock, 349
steroid-like properties, herbs with
  wild yam, 333, 335
stimulants
  aloe, 12
  blessed thistle, 50
  brigham tea, 55, 58
  capsicum, 80, 81–82
  catnip, 72
  chamomile, 91
  echinacea, 130
  kelp, 215
  licorice, 221
  lobelia, 231, 235
  milk thistle, 242, 243
  peppermint, 257, 261
  red clover, 267

  red raspberry, 274
  saw palmetto, 280
  wild yam, 330
  yarrow, 339, 343
stings. *See* insect bites and stings, herbs for
stomach ache, herbs for
  catnip, 72
  chamomile, 91
  GINGER, 176
  red raspberry, 277
  St. John's wort, 297, 303
stomach disorders, herbs for
  burdock, 61
  chaparral, 99
  SLIPPERY ELM, 287, 290–91
  yarrow, 339
stomach, herbs for the
  alfalfa, 1
  comfrey, 112
  dandelion, 123
  hawthorn, 200
  juniper, 207
  PEPPERMINT, 257, 260
  red raspberry, 274
  yarrow, 344
stool softener
  flaxseed, 148
  licorice, 224–25
stress, herbs for
  barley, 27
  catnip, 72
  goldenseal, 194
  hawthorn, 200, 205
  licorice, 221, 224
  valerian, 316, 319, 321
stroke, herbs for
  alfalfa, 2
  capsicum, 79
styes, herbs for
  burdock, 61
  eyebright, 141
sugar substitutes
  licorice, 222, 225
sunburn. *See* burn remedies
sunstroke, herbs for
  lobelia, 235
suppositories
  slippery elm, 293
  yellow dock, 354

surgery preparation, herbs for
  CAPSICUM, 78
swelling, herbs for
  BURDOCK, 62
  comfrey, 112, 115
  dandelion, 125
  goldenseal, 188, 194
  yellow dock, 350
syphilis, herbs for
  barley, 27
  black cohosh, 44
  BURDOCK, 62
  echinacea, 131, 135
  goldenseal, 189
  red clover, 268
  slippery elm, 288
  uva ursi, 308
  yellow dock, 350
system strength, herbs for
  uva ursi, 312

T
T-cell production, herbs for
  echinacea, 133
tapeworm. *See* worms, herbs to expel
teas
  alfalfa, 9
  bilberry, 41
  black cohosh, 49
  blessed thistle, 53
  brigham tea, 57, 59
  burdock, 68–69
  capsicum, 85
  catnip, 75–76
  chamomile, 96
  chaparral, 104–6
  comfrey, 117
  dandelion, 127–28
  eyebright, 144–45
  flaxseed, 156
  garlic, 172
  ginger, 183–84
  goldenseal, 196
  hawthorn, 205
  juniper, 212–13
  licorice, 227
  lobelia, 238
  milk thistle, 247
  mullein, 253–54
  peppermint, 262

  red clover, 272
  red raspberry, 277–78
  slippery elm, 289, 292
  St. John's wort, 303–4
  uva ursi, 312–13
  valerian, 321–22
  wild lettuce, 328
  wild yam, 336
  yarrow, 345–46
teething, herbs for
  catnip, 74
  chamomile, 92
  LOBELIA, 231, 237
tension, herbs for
  catnip, 72
  goldenseal, 193
testicles(swollen), herbs for
  mullein, 250
tetanus, herbs for
  capsicum, 79
  chaparral, 99
  LOBELIA, 232, 235
Thomson, Samuel, 233–34
throat cancer, herbs for
  mullein, 249
thyroid, herbs for the
  black cohosh, 43
  goldenseal, 188
  KELP, 215, 217
  yellow dock, 350
tinctures
  echinacea, 136–37
  goldenseal, 195–96
  lobelia, 238–39
tinnitus, herbs for
  aloe, 13
  black cohosh, 48
tissue repair, herbs for
  alfalfa, 2, 6
  ALOE, 13, 14
  COMFREY, 112, 113, 115
  echinacea, 134
  lobelia, 232
tongue paralysis, herbs for
  ginger, 177
tonics
  alfalfa, 1
  aloe, 13
  barley, 26
  blessed thistle, 50

burdock, 61
CAPSICUM, 78, 87
chamomile, 91
chaparral, 99
comfrey, 112
dandelion, 122, 125
eyebright, 141
GARLIC, 159, 161, 168
GINGER, 176
goldenseal, 190
hawthorn, 200
kelp, 215
KELP, 215, 217
LICORICE, 221, 222
milk thistle, 243
yarrow, 342
yellow dock, 349, 350
tonsillitis, herbs for
  alfalfa, 2, 5
  aloe, 13
  BURDOCK, 62
  CAPSICUM, 79
  comfrey, 113
  ECHINACEA, 131
  goldenseal, 189
  lobelia, 232
  mullein, 250
  slippery elm, 288
tooth decay. herbs for
  ALFALFA, 1, 6
  dandelion, 125
tooth infection, herbs for
  GOLDENSEAL, 189
toothache, herbs for
  capsicum, 84
  catnip, 73, 75
  chamomile, 92
  GARLIC, 160
  GINGER, 177
  LOBELIA, 231
  mullein, 250
  peppermint, 258
topical pain relief. *See* pain relief, topical
toxin cleanse, herbs for
  alfalfa, 1, 5
  BARLEY, 26, 31, 32
  BLESSED THISTLE, 50, 53
  burdock, 61, 65
  capsicum, 84
  chamomile, 95

CHAPARRAL, 99, 100, 102, 103
comfrey, 112
dandelion, 122, 123, 125, 126
echinacea, 130, 131, 135
eyebright, 144
flaxseed, 148, 154
GARLIC, 159, 165, 168
ginger, 181
JUNIPER, 211
kelp, 215, 216
milk thistle, 242, 244–46
mullein, 252
RED CLOVER, 267, 270
yarrow, 340, 342
yellow dock, 350, 351
tuberculosis, herbs for
  aloe, 13
  barley, 27
  BLACK COHOSH, 43
  burdock, 62
  chaparral, 99
  comfrey, 113
  GARLIC, 160, 165
  juniper, 208, 211
  MULLEIN, 250, 252
  red clover, 267
  slippery elm, 288
  WILD LETTUCE, 326
tumors, herbs for
  alfalfa, 1
  burdock, 61
  CAPSICUM, 78
  chamomile, 91
  CHAPARRAL, 99
  comfrey, 112
  echinacea, 130, 134
  GARLIC, 159, 168
  goldenseal, 194
  KELP, 215
  lobelia, 231
  mullein, 249, 252
  RED CLOVER, 267, 268, 271
  slippery elm, 287
  ST. JOHN'S WORT, 297, 303
  yellow dock, 352
typhoid, herbs for
  bilberry, 37
  black cohosh, 43
  chamomile, 92
  echinacea, 130, 134

garlic, 160
GINGER, 189
GOLDENSEAL, 189
valerian, 316
yarrow, 340

U

ulcerated bowels, herbs for
COMFREY, 112
ulcerated eyelids
YELLOW DOCK, 350
ulcerated kidneys
UVA URSI, 309
ulcerated skin, herbs for
bilberry, 37
goldenseal, 189
red clover, 268
slippery elm, 288, 291
ulcers, herbs for
alfalfa, 4–5
aloe, 13
barley, 26
burdock, 61
capsicum, 79, 83
chamomile, 91
comfrey, 112, 116
eyebright, 141
garlic, 160
licorice, 221, 224
mullein, 249
peppermint, 257, 261
red raspberry, 274
SLIPPERY ELM, 287
ST. JOHN'S WORT, 297
valerian, 316
wild yam, 330
yarrow, 339
yellow dock, 349, 352
urethritis
UVA URSI, 309
uric acid, herbs for, 218
alfalfa, 2
red clover, 270
uva ursi, 309
yarrow, 343
urinary tract infection, herbs for
DANDELION, 123
juniper, 208, 210
red raspberry, 277
saw palmetto, 281

slippery elm, 288
uva ursi, 309
wild lettuce, 326, 328
urinary tract, herbs for the
bilberry, 37
blessed thistle, 51, 52
CHAPARRAL, 100, 102
flaxseed, 153
goldenseal, 194
red clover, 268
red raspberry, 275
saw palmetto, 284
ST. JOHN'S WORT, 298, 303
UVA URSI, 311
wild yam, 331
yarrow, 340, 343
uterine ulceration
UVA URSI, 309
uterus(prolapsed), herbs for
burdock, 62
CHAMOMILE, 92
chaparral, 100
uva ursi, 209
uva ursi
history of, 309–11
influence and properties of, 308–9
nutrients in, 311
preparations and remedies, 312–13
safety and profile of, 313–15
uses for, 311–12

V

vaginal discharge, herbs for
blessed thistle, 51
comfrey, 113
juniper, 208
red raspberry, 275
slippery elm, 288
uva ursi, 309
yarrow, 340
yellow dock, 350
vaginal douches
alfalfa, 2
aloe, 13
COMFREY, 113, 116
garlic, 173
GOLDENSEAL, 189, 193, 197
juniper, 208, 212
red raspberry, 275, 278
slippery elm, 288

yarrow, 340
vaginitis, herbs for
  aloe, 13
  GOLDENSEAL, 189, 192
  red clover, 268
  red raspberry, 275
valerian
  history of, 318
  influence and properties, 316–17
  nutrients in, 318–19
  preparations and remedies, 321–22
  safety and profile of, 322–24
  uses for, 319–21
varicose veins, herbs for
  alfalfa, 1
  aloe, 12
  BILBERRY, 37
  CAPSICUM, 78
  yarrow, 344
vascular system, herbs for
  alfalfa, 1
  BILBERRY, 37, 40
  brigham tea, 58
  capsicum, 78
  garlic, 166–67
  ginger, 180–81
  hawthorn, 200
  kelp, 214
  LOBELIA, 231
vasoconstrictors
  brigham tea, 55, 58
  comfrey, 112
  eyebright, 144
venereal diseases, herbs for
  burdock, 62
  chaparral, 100
  goldenseal, 189
  slippery elm, 288
  uva ursi, 308, 312
  yellow dock, 350
varicose ulcers, herbs for
  St. John's wort, 298
varicose veins, herbs for
  milk thistle, 242
  yellow dock, 349
vermifuges. *See* worms, herbs to expel
vertigo, herbs for
  echinacea, 135
  valerian, 317
vomiting, herbs to induce
  blessed thistle, 50, 51, 54
  lobelia, 231, 233, 235, 237
  uva ursi, 308
  wild yam, 330
vomiting, herbs to stop
  catnip, 72
  GINGER, 176, 180
  PEPPERMINT, 257
  red raspberry, 274
  wild yam, 330
vulneraries
  capsicum, 79
  comfrey, 113
  GARLIC, 160
  mullein, 249
  slippery elm, 288
  St. John's wort, 297
  yarrow, 340

W
warmth, herbs for
  bilberry, 37
  CAPSICUM, 82–83, 85
  chamomile, 91
  echinacea, 130
  ginger, 177, 181
  licorice, 221
  peppermint, 258, 261
  wild yam, 330
warts, herbs for
  chaparral, 100
  dandelion, 123, 126
  GARLIC, 160
  slippery elm, 288
washes
  burdock, 67
  comfrey, 117
  red raspberry, 278
  slippery elm, 289
  valerian, 322
  yellow dock, 354
water retention. *See* diuretics
Watson, Sereno, 281
weakness(chronic), herbs for
  alfalfa, 1
weight loss, herbs for. *See also* obesity, herbs for
  brigham tea, 55, 59
  burdock, 64
  capsicum, 83

chaparral, 100
DANDELION, 123, 126
goldenseal, 189
kelp, 217
licorice, 224
uva ursi, 309
wheezing, herbs for
red clover, 270
whooping cough, herbs for
alfalfa, 2
BLACK COHOSH, 43
GARLIC, 160, 165
GINGER, 177
LOBELIA, 232
red clover, 267, 270, 272
saw palmetto, 280
slippery elm, 288
valerian, 316
wild lettuce, 325, 328
wild yam, 331
wild lettuce
history of, 326–27
influence and properties of, 325–26
nutrients in, 327
preparations and remedies, 328
safety and profile of, 328–29
uses for, 327–28
wild yam
history of, 332
influence and properties of, 330–32
nutrients, 333
preparations and remedies, 336–37
safety and profile of, 337–38
uses for, 333–36
women, herbs for. *See* breasts, herbs for the; fertility, herbs for; lactation, herbs for; menopause, herbs for; menstruation, herbs for; PMS (premenstrual syndrome), herbs for; pregnancy, herbs for; reproductive organs (female), herbs for
worms, herbs to expel. *See also* ringworm remedies
ALOE, 13, 18
black cohosh, 43
blessed thistle, 50, 53
catnip, 72, 74
chamomile, 91, 93, 94
CHAPARRAL, 99, 103
echinacea, 130

goldenseal, 188, 190
juniper, 207, 208, 211
kelp, 215
LOBELIA, 232
mullein, 249
slippery elm, 287, 291
ST. JOHN'S WORT, 297
valerian, 316
wild lettuce, 325
yellow dock, 349, 352
wounds, herbs for
alfalfa, 2
ALOE, 13, 15, 17
burdock, 61
capsicum, 79
chamomile, 92
chaparral, 99
COMFREY, 112, 115–16
echinacea, 130
GARLIC, 160, 164, 170
goldenseal, 194
lobelia, 232
red clover, 267
red raspberry, 274, 277
slippery elm, 291, 294
St. John's wort, 297, 301
WOUNDS, 189
yarrow, 340, 344, 352
yellow dock, 350

Y
yarrow
history of, 341–42
influence and properties of, 339–40
nutrients in, 342
preparations and remedies, 344–47
safety and profile of, 347–48
uses for, 342–44
yeast infection, herbs for. *See also* candida, herbs for
alfalfa, 2
COMFREY, 112, 116
dandelion, 122
garlic, 173
yarrow, 340, 344
yellow dock
history of, 351
influence and properties of, 349–50
nutrients in, 351
preparations and remedies, 353–54

safety and profile of, 354–55
uses for, 351–52

Common Names

Aaron's Rod: Mullein
African Bird Pepper: Cayenne
African Ginger: Ginger
All-heal: Valerian
Amantilla: Valerian
Amber: St. John's Wort
American Ephedra: Brigham Tea
American Peppermint: Peppermint
Arberry: Uva Ursi
Asthma Weed: Lobelia
Balm Mint: Peppermint
Barbados Aloe: Aloe
Barley Grass: Barley
Barren Myrtle: Uva Ursi
Bearberry: Uva Ursi
Bear's Grape: Uva Ursi
Beggars Buttons: Burdock
Begger's Blanket: Mullein
Bird Pepper: Cayenne
Bitter Thistle: Blessed Thistle
Black Ginger: Ginger
Black Peppermint: Peppermint
Black Root: Comfrey
Black Sampson: Echinacea
Black Snakeroot: Black Cohosh
Blacksnake Root: Black Cohosh
Black-tang: Kelp
Blackwort: Comfrey
Bladder Fucus: Kelp
Bladderpod: Lobelia
Bladderwrack: Kelp
Blaeberry: Bilberry
Blessed Cardus: Blessed Thistle
Bloodwort: Yarrow
Blowball: Dandelion
Blueberry: Bilberry

Boneset: Comfrey
Brandy Mint: Peppermint
Brown Raspberry: Goldenseal
Bruisewort: Comfrey
Buffalo Grass: Alfalfa
Buffalo Herb: Alfalfa
Bugbane: Black Cohosh
Bugwort: Black Cohosh
Bullock's Lungwort: Mullein
Bunny Ears: Mullein
Burn Aloe: Aloe
Camomile: Chamomile
Candlewick: Mullein
Cankerwort: Dandelion
Cape Aloes: Aloe
Capon's Tail: Valerian
Cardin: Blessed Thistle
Carpenter's Weed: Yarrow
Catmint: Catnip
Catnep: Catnip
Catrup: Catnip
Cat's Valerian: Valerian
Catswort: Catnip
Chaparro: Chaparral
Chasteberry: Chaste Tree
Chilean Clover: Alfalfa
China Root: Wild Yam
Clear Eye: Eyebright
Clove Garlic: Garlic
Clover Grass: Red Clover
Cockle Buttons: Burdock
Colic Root: Wild Yam
Common Flax: Flaxseed
Compass Plant: Wild Lettuce
Coneflower: Echinacea
Coralillo: Uva Ursi

Cow Grass: Red Clover
Cow's Lungwort: Mullein
Creosote Bush: Chaparral
Curled Dock: Yellow Dock
Curled Mint: Peppermint
Desert Tea: Brigham Tea
Devil's Bones: Wild Yam
Devil's Nettle: Yarrow
Dwarf Juniper: Juniper
Dwarf Palmetto: Saw Palmetto
Dyeberry: Bilberry
Elephant's Gall: Aloe
Elm Bark: Slippery Elm
English Chamomile: Chamomile
English Hawthorn: Hawthorn
English Valerian: Valerian
Englishman's Quinine: Yarrow
Ephedra: Brigham Tea
European Blueberry: Bilberry
Eye Balm: Goldenseal
Eye Root: Goldenseal
Eyebright: Lobelia
Eyewort: Eyebright
Father of All Foods: Alfalfa
Feltwort: Mullein
Field Balm: Catnip
First Aid Plant: Aloe
Flannel Flower: Mullein
Flannel Leaf: Mullein
Flax: Flaxseed
Fox Berry: Uva Ursi
Fox Cloth: Burdock
Garden Heliotrope: Valerian
Garden Patience: Yellow Dock
Garden Raspberry: Red Raspberry
General of Respiration: Brigham Tea
German Chamomile: Chamomile
Goatweed: St. John's Wort
Gobernadora: Chaparral
Gobo (Japan): Burdock
Golden Thread: Goldenseal
Gray Elm: Slippery Elm
Greasewood: Chaparral

Great Burr: Burdock
Green Endive: Wild Lettuce
Ground Apple: Chamomile
Ground Juniper: Juniper
Ground Raspberry: Goldenseal
Gum Plant: Comfrey
Hardhay: St. John's Wort
Hardock: Burdock
Hareburr: Burdock
Hawthorne: Hawthorn
Hindberry: Red Raspberry
Hindbur: Red Raspberry
Holy Thistle: Milk Thistle, Blessed Thistle
Horse Thistle: Wild Lettuce
Huckleberry: Bilberry
Hurr-bur: Burdock
Hydrastis: Goldenseal
Indian Dye: Goldenseal
Indian Elm: Slippery Elm
Indian Paint: Goldenseal
Indian Plant: Goldenseal
Indian Tobacco: Lobelia
Jacob's Staff: Mullein
Jamaica Ginger: Ginger
Jaundice Root: Goldenseal
Johns-Wort: St. John's Wort
Joint Fir: Brigham Tea
Juniper Berry: Juniper
Kelpware: Kelp
Kinnikinnick (Indian name): Uva Ursi
Klamath Weed: St. John's Wort
Knitback: Comfrey
Knitbone: Comfrey
Kombu: Kelp
Ladies' Mantle: Yarrow
Lamb Mint: Peppermint
Lammint: Peppermint
Lappa: Burdock
Licorice Root: Licorice
Lily of the Desert: Aloe
Linseed: Flaxseed
Lint Bells: Flaxseed
Lion's Tooth: Dandelion

COMMON NAMES — 417

Liver Root: Wild Yam
Lucerne: Alfalfa
Lucerne Grass: Alfalfa
Lungwort: Mullein
Macrotys: Black Cohosh
Manzanila: Chamomile
Marian Thistle: Milk Thistle
May Bush: Hawthorn
Mayblossom: Hawthorn
Mayflower: Hawthorn
Meadow Clover: Red Clover
Medicine Plant: Aloe
Mealberry: Uva Ursi
Mexican Wild Yam: Wild Yam
Milfoil: Yarrow
Miner's Tea: Brigham Tea
Monk's Pepper: Chaste Tree
Moose Elm: Slippery Elm
Mormon Tea: Brigham Tea
Mountain Box: Uva Ursi
Mountain Cranberry: Uva Ursi
Mullein Dock: Mullein
Myrtle Blueberry: Bilberry
Narrow Dock: Yellow Dock
Nipbone: Comfrey
Northern Mint: Peppermint
Nose-bleed: Yarrow
Old Man's Pepper: Yarrow
Opium Lettuce: Wild Lettuce
Orange Root: Goldenseal
Our Lady's Thistle: Milk Thistle
Pearl Barley: Barley
Pearled Barley: Barley
Philanthropium: Burdock
Phu: Valerian
Pipo: Cayenne
Poor Man's Opium: Wild Lettuce
Poor Man's Treacle: Garlic
Pot Barley: Barley
Prickly Lettuce: Wild Lettuce
Priest's Crown: Dandelion
Puffball: Dandelion
Pukeweed: Lobelia

Purple Clover: Red Clover
Purple Coneflower: Echinacea
Purple Medic: Alfalfa
Quickset: Hawthorn
Rattleroot: Black Cohosh
Rattlesnake Root: Black Cohosh
Rattleweed: Black Cohosh
Red Elm: Slippery Elm
Red Eyebright: Eyebright
Red Pepper: Cayenne
Rheumatism Root: Wild Yam
Richweed: Black Cohosh
Rock Elm: Slippery Elm
Rockberry: Uva Ursi
Roman Chamomile: Chamomile
Rudbeckie: Echinacea
Rumex: Yellow Dock
Sabal: Saw Palmetto
Salsify: Comfrey
Sampson Root: Echinacea
Sawtooth Palm: Saw Palmetto
Scotch Barley: Barley
Seal-all: Goldenseal
Seaweed: Kelp
Seawrack: Kelp
See Bright: Eyebright
Setewale: Valerian
Setwall: Valerian
Shepherd's Club: Mullein
Shrub Palmetto: Saw Palmetto
Silybin: Milk Thistle
Slippery Root: Comfrey
Snake Root: Echinacea
Snakeroot: Black Cohosh
Soldier's Woundwort: Yarrow
Sour Dock: Yellow Dock
Spotted Thistle: Blessed Thistle
Sprouted Barley: Barley
Sprouted Barley Malt: Barley
Squaw Root: Black Cohosh
Squaw Tea: Brigham Tea
St. Benedict Thistle: Blessed Thistle
St. John's Grass: St. John's Wort

St. John's Wort: St. John's Wort
St. Mary's Thistle: Milk Thistle
Staunchweed: Yarrow
Sticky Bob: Burdock
Stinking Rose: Garlic
Stinkweed: Chaparral
Sweet Elm: Slippery Elm
Sweet Root: Licorice
Sweet Wood: Licorice
Tangleweed: Kelp
Thorny Burr: Burdock
Thousand Seed: Yarrow
Thousand-leaf: Yarrow
Tipton Weed: St. John's Wort
Torch Weed: Mullein
Trefoil: Red Clover
True Aloe: Aloe
Turkey Burrseed: Burdock
Turmeric Root: Goldenseal
Vandal Root: Valerian
Velvet Dock: Mullein
Velvet Leaf: Mullein
Vitex: Chaste Tree
Vomitwort: Lobelia
Wallwort: Comfrey
Wand of Heaven: Aloe
Warnera: Goldenseal
White Peppermint: Peppermint
Whitethorn: Hawthorn
Whortleberry: Bilberry
Wild Chamomile: Chamomile
Wild Clover: Red Clover
Wild Curcuma: Goldenseal
Wild Endive: Dandelion
Wild Tobacco: Lobelia
Windmill Palm: Saw Palmetto
Winged Elm: Slippery Elm
Woundwort: Comfrey
Yarroway: Yarrow
Yellow Puccoon: Goldenseal
Yellow River: Brigham Tea
Yellow Root: Goldenseal
Yuma: Wild Yam

Latin Names (Scientific Names)

Achillea millefolium: Yarrow
Actaea racemosa: Black Cohosh
Allium sativum: Garlic
Aloe barbadensis: Aloe
Aloe vera: Aloe
Arctium lappa: Burdock
Arctostaphylos uva ursi: Uva Ursi
Capsicum annum: Cayenne
Chamaemelum nobile: Chamomile
Cimicifuga racemosa: Black Cohosh
Cnicus benedictus: Blessed Thistle
Crataegus laevigata: Hawthorn
Dioscorea villosa: Wild Yam
Echinacea angustifolia: Echinacea
Echinacea pallida: Echinacea
Echinacea purpurea: Echinacea
Ephedra nervadensis: Brigham Tea
Ephedra viridis: Brigham Tea
Euphrasia officinalis: Eyebright
Fucus vesiculosus: Bladderwrack (Kelp)
Glycyrrhiza glabra: Licorice
Hordeum vulgare: Barley
Hydrastis canadensis: Goldenseal
Hypericum perforatum: St. John's Wort
Juniperus communis: Juniper

Lactuca virosa: Wild Lettuce
Laminaria digitata: Kelp
Larrea divaricata: Chaparral
Larrea tridentata: Chaparral
Linum usitatissimum: Flaxseed
Lobelia inflata: Lobelia
Matricaria rectita: Chamomile
Medicago sativa: Alfalfa
Mentha pipertita: Peppermint
Nepeta cataria: Catnip
Rubus idaeus: Red Raspberry
Rumex crispus: Yellow Dock
Serenoa repens: Saw Palmetto
Silybum marianum: Milk Thistle
Symphytum officinale: Comfrey
Taraxacum officinale: Dandelion
Trifolium pratense: Red Clover
Ulmus rubra: Slippery Elm
Vaccinium myrtillus: Bilberry
Valeriana officinalis: Valerian
Verbascum thapsus: Mullein
Vitex Agnus-Castus: Chaste Tree
Zingiber officinale: Ginger

Key Components

For an excellent review of how individual minerals, vitamins, and their co-factors affect the body's daily function, growth and healing capacities, see 'The How to Herb Book' by Velma J. Keith and Monteen Gordon

Vitamins and Co-Factors

A. Alfalfa 3, 5; Alfalfa Sprouts 8; Aloe 15; Barley Grass 31; Black Cohosh 46; Burdock 64; Catnip 74; Cayenne 81; Chamomile 92; Comfrey 115; Dandelion 124; Echinacea 133; Eyebright 143; Garlic 164; Ginger 179; Goldenseal 191; Kelp 218; Mullein 255; Peppermint 263; Red Clover 272; Red Raspberry 279; Saw Palmetto 286; Yarrow 347; Yellow Dock 356

Carotenes *(easily transforms in the body to Vitamin A):* Alfalfa 8; Cayenne 81

Lutein *(yellow carotenoid pigment):* Cayenne 81; Garlic 164

B1 (thiamine): Alfalfa 3; Alfalfa Sprouts 8; Barley Grain 29; Barley Grass 31; Burdock 64; Catnip 74; Cayenne 81; Dandelion 124; Eyebright 143; Flaxseed 151; Garlic 164, 168-9; Ginger 179; Goldenseal 191; Hawthorn 203; Kelp 218; Licorice 227; Mullein 255; Red Clover 272; Red Raspberry 279

B2 (riboflavin): Alfalfa 3; Alfalfa Sprouts 8; Barley Grain 29; Barley Grass 31; Catnip 74; Cayenne 81; Dandelion 124; Eyebright 143; Flaxseed 151; Garlic 164; Ginger 179; Goldenseal 191; Hawthorn 203; Kelp 218; Licorice 227; Mullein 255; Red Clover 272

B3 (niacin): Alfalfa 3; Alfalfa Sprouts 8; Barley Grain 29; Burdock 64; Catnip 74; Cayenne 81; Dandelion 124; Eyebright 143; Flaxseed 151; Garlic 164; Ginger 179; Goldenseal 191; Hawthorn 203; Kelp 218; Licorice 227; Mullein 255; Red Clover 272; Red Raspberry 279

B5 (pantothenic acid): Alfalfa 3; Barley Grain 29; Barley Grass 31; Black Cohosh 46; Burdock 64; Catnip 74; Cayenne 81; Dandelion 124; Eyebright 143; Flaxseed 151; Garlic 164; Ginger 179; Goldenseal 191; Hawthorn 203; Licorice 227; Red Clover 272

B6 (pyridoxine): Alfalfa 4; Barley Grain 29; Barley Grass 31; Burdock 64; Catnip 74; Cayenne 81; Dandelion 124; Eyebright 143; Flaxseed 151; Garlic 164, 166; Ginger 179; Goldenseal 191; Hawthorn 203; Kelp 218; Licorice 227; Mullein 255; Red Clover 272

B9 (folic acid): Alfalfa 4; Aloe 15; Barley Grain 29; Barley Grass 31; Burdock 64; Catnip 74; Cayenne 81; Dandelion 124; Eyebright 143; Flaxseed 151; Ginger 179; Goldenseal 191; Hawthorn 203; Kelp 218; Licorice 227; Mullein 255; Red Clover 272

B12 (cobalamin): Alfalfa 4; Aloe 15; Barley Grass 31; Burdock 64; Catnip 74; Cayenne 81; Comfrey 115; Dandelion 124; Eyebright 143; Ginger 179; Goldenseal 191; Hawthorn 203; Kelp 218; Licorice 227; Mullein 255; Red Clover 272

Biotin *(part of the B-complex,*

essential to the metabolism of carbohydrates, proteins, and fats): Alfalfa 4; Burdock 64; Catnip 74; Cayenne 81; Dandelion 124; Eyebright 143; Ginger 179; Goldenseal 191; Hawthorn 203; Kelp 218; Licorice 227; Mullein 255; Red Clover 272

Choline (recently recognized as an essential nutrient of the diet, a member of the B complex, is a component of the fatty constituent lecithin and the neurotransmitter acetylcholine): Alfalfa 4; Aloe 15; Burdock 64; Catnip 74; Cayenne 81; Dandelion 124; Eyebright 143; Garlic 164; Ginger 179; Goldenseal 191; Hawthorn 203; Kelp 218; Licorice 227; Mullein 255; Red Clover 272; St. John's Wort 304; Yarrow 347

Inositol (part of the B-complex, a component of the outer linings of all cells, particularly the heart and brain): Alfalfa 4; Burdock 64; Catnip 74; Cayenne 81; Dandelion 124; Eyebright 143; Ginger 179; Goldenseal 191; Hawthorn 203; Kelp 218; Licorice 227; Mullein 255; Red Clover 272

PABA (Para-Amino Benzoic Acid, a member of the B-complex family, it is one of the the basic parts of folic acid): Alfalfa 4; Burdock 64; Catnip 74; Cayenne 81; Dandelion 124; Eyebright 143; Ginger 179; Goldenseal 191; Hawthorn 203; Kelp 218; Licorice 227; Mullein 255; Red Clover 272

C (Ascorbic Acid): Alfalfa 4, 7; Alfalfa Sprouts 8; Aloe 15; Barley Grain 29; Barley Grass 31; Bilberry 39; Burdock 64; Catnip 74; Cayenne 81, 84, 86; Chaparral 101; Comfrey 115; Dandelion 124; Echinacea 133; Eyebright 143; Flaxseed 151; Garlic 164, 166-8; Ginger 179; Goldenseal 191; Hawthorn 203; Juniper 210; Kelp 218; Peppermint 263; Red Clover 272; Red Raspberry 279; Yarrow 347; Yellow Dock 356

Bioflavonoids (Substances that are often found with Vitamin C and are known to improve life): Alfalfa 5; Burdock 64; Cayenne 81; Dandelion 124; Red Clover 272; Slippery Elm 294

D: Alfalfa 4; Dandelion 124; Eyebright 143; Mullein 255; Red Raspberry 279

E: Alfalfa 4; Alfalfa Sprouts 8; Aloe 15; Barley Grass 31; Burdock 64;

Vitamin E (continued) Cayenne 81; Comfrey 115; Dandelion 124; Echinacea 133; Eyebright 143; Flaxseed 151-2; Garlic 164, 166-7; Goldenseal 191; Kelp 218; Licorice 227; Milk Thistle 247; Red Raspberry 279; Slippery Elm 294; Yarrow 347

K: Alfalfa 4, 7; Alfalfa Sprouts 8; Cayenne 81; Garlic 164; Slippery Elm 294; Yarrow 347

Minerals
Aluminum: Chaparral 101, Garlic 164
Barium: Chaparral 101
Boron: Dandelion 124
Calcium: Alfalfa 4; Alfalfa Sprouts 8; Aloe 15; Barley Grain 29; Barley Grass 31-2; Black Cohosh 46; Burdock 64; Cayenne 81; Chamomile 92; Comfrey 115-6; Dandelion 124; Flaxseed 151; Garlic 164; Ginger 180; Goldenseal 191; Kelp 218-9; Licorice 227; Lobelia 237; Red Clover 272; Red Raspberry 279; Slippery Elm 294; Valerian 323-4

Chlorine: Chaparral 101; Garlic 164; Kelp 218-9
Chromium: Aloe 15; Bilberry 39; Kelp

218; Licorice 227

Cobalt: Dandelion 124; Juniper 210; Kelp 218; Lobelia 237; Red Clover 272

Copper: Alfalfa 9; Aloe 15; Barley Grain 29; Barley Grass 31; Burdock 64; Comfrey 115; Dandelion 124; Echinacea 133; Eyebright 143; Flaxseed 151; Garlic 164; Goldenseal 191; Juniper 210; Kelp 218; Lobelia 237; Peppermint 263; Red Clover 272; Slippery Elm 294; Valerian 323; Yarrow 347

Fluorine: Alfalfa 4, 6; Kelp 218

Germanium: Garlic 164, 168

Iodine: KELP 216, 218-20

Iron: Alfalfa 4, 7; Alfalfa Sprouts 8; Aloe 15; Barley Grain 29; Barley Grass 31; Black Cohosh 46; Burdock 64; Catnip 74; Cayenne 81; Chamomile 92; Comfrey 115; Dandelion 124; Echinacea 133; Eyebright 143; Flaxseed 151; Garlic 164; Ginger 180; Goldenseal 191; Hawthorn 203; Kelp 218; Lobelia 237; Mullein 255; Peppermint 263; Red Clover 272; Red Raspberry 279-80; Slippery Elm 294; Yarrow 347; Yellow Dock 355-9

Magnesium: Alfalfa 4; Alfalfa Sprouts 8; Aloe 15; Barley Grain 29, 30; Barley Grass 31-2; Black Cohosh 46; Catnip 74; Cayenne 81; Chamomile 92; Comfrey 115; Dandelion 124; Flaxseed 151; Garlic 164; Ginger 180; Kelp 218-9; Licorice 227; Mullein 255; Peppermint 263; Red Clover 272; Red Raspberry 279; Valerian 323-4

Manganese: Aloe 15; Barley Grain 29; Barley Grass 31; Catnip 74; Chamomile 92; Dandelion 124; Flaxseed 151; Garlic 164, 166; Goldenseal 191; Kelp 218; Licorice 227; Red Clover 272; Red Raspberry 279; Yarrow 347; Yellow Dock 356

Molybdenum: Red Clover 272, 275

Phosphorous: Alfalfa 4; Barley Grain 29; Barley Grass 31; Black Cohosh 46; Brigham Tea 59; Catnip 74; Cayenne 81; Comfrey 115-6; Dandelion 124; Flaxseed 151; Garlic 164; Ginger 180; Goldenseal 191; Hawthorn 203; Kelp 218; Red Raspberry 279; Slippery Elm 294

Potassium: Alfalfa 4; Alfalfa Sprouts 8; Aloe 15; Barley Grain 29; Barley Grass 31-2; Black Cohosh 46; Burdock 64; Cayenne 81; Chamomile 92; Chaparral 101; Comfrey 115; Dandelion 124-5; Echinacea 133; Flaxseed 151; Garlic 164; Ginger 180; Goldenseal 191; Kelp 218-9; Lobelia 237; Mullein 255; Peppermint 267; Red Raspberry 283; Slippery Elm 294; Valerian 323; Yellow Dock 356

Selenium: Alfalfa Sprouts 8; Aloe 15; Barley Grain 29, 30; Flaxseed 151; Garlic 164, 166-8; Kelp 218; Lobelia

Selenium (continued)
237; Red Clover 272; Red Raspberry 279; Slippery Elm 294

Silicon: Alfalfa 4; Chaparral 101; Dandelion 124

Sodium: Alfalfa 4; Aloe 15; Barley Grass 31-2; Catnip 74; Chaparral 101; Dandelion 124; Flaxseed 151; Garlic 164; Ginger 180; Hawthorn 203; Kelp 218; Lobelia 237; Red Raspberry 279; Slippery Elm 294

Sulfur: Alfalfa 4; Burdock 64; Catnip 74; Cayenne 81; Chaparral 101; Comfrey 115; Dandelion 124; Echinacea 133; Garlic 164; Juniper 210; Kelp 218; Lobelia 237; Mullein 255; Peppermint 263; Red Raspberry 279

Tin: Chaparral 101

Vanadium: Kelp 218

Zinc: Alfalfa Sprouts 8; Aloe 15; Barley

Grain 29; Barley Grass 31; Burdock 64; Chamomile 92; Comfrey 115; Dandelion 124; Eyebright 143; Flaxseed 151; Garlic 164; Ginger 180; Goldenseal 191; Hawthorn 203; Kelp 218; Licorice 227; Slippery Elm 294

Trace Minerals: Alfalfa 4; Barley Grass 31; Black Cohosh 46; Burdock 64; Chaparral 101; Dandelion 124; Eyebright 143; Hawthorn 203; Juniper 210; Kelp 218; Lobelia 237; Peppermint 263; Red Clover 272; Valerian 323; Yellow Dock 356

Selected 'Other' Key Components

Algin (thickening agent): Kelp 218, 220-1

Alkaloids (various organic compounds that contain nitrogen and have alkaline properties; exhibits a physiological effect on nervous and circulatory systems): Alfalfa 4; Comfrey 115; Goldenseal 191; St. John's Wort 304; Wild Yam 338; Yarrow 347

Allantoin (promotes tissue growth): Comfrey 115; Uva Ursi 316

Allicin: Garlic 164, 166-8

Bitters: Aloe Vera 13; Blessed Thistle 53; Burdock 62, 64; Catnip 72, 74; Chamomile 90, 92; Chaparral 99, 101; Comfrey 112, 115; Dandelion 122, 124; Eyebright 143; Goldenseal 188, 191, 195; Juniper 210; Milk Thistle 247, 249; St. John's Wort 304; Wild Lettuce 330, 332-3; Wild Yam 335, 338; Yarrow 344, 347; Yellow Dock 354, 356

Capsaicin: Cayenne 81

Chlorophyll: Alfalfa 4-7; Alfalfa Sprouts 8; Barley Grass 31-2; Comfrey 115

Coumarins (a vanilla-scented constituent that reduces blood clotting): Alfalfa 4; Red Clover 272

Enzymes: Alfalfa 4, 7; Alfalfa Sprouts 8; Aloe 15; Barley Grass 31; Garlic 164

Ephedrine - Pseudo-ephedrine: Brigham Tea 59

Flavonoids (Any of a large group of water-soluble plant pigments that have antioxidant qualities and are beneficial to health): Chaste Tree 109; Eyebright 143; Hawthorn 203; Juniper 210; Milk Thistle 250; St. John's Wort 304, 311; Yarrow 347

Hormone-like Compounds (including Isoflavones, Lignans, Phytoestrogens, Phytosterin, Phytosterols, Saponins, Sterols, and others): Alfalfa 4, 6; Aloe 15; Barley 30; Black Cohosh 46-7; Cayenne 81; Echinacea 136; Flaxseed 151, 154; Licorice 227, 229; Red Clover 271-2, 274; Saw Palmetto 286; Wild Yam 337-8, 340

Inulin (low calorie starch): Burdock 64; Dandelion 124

Linoleic Acid (essential, unsaturated fatty acid): Slippery Elm 294; Yarrow 347

Mannitol (sweetener): Kelp 218-9

Menthol: Peppermint 263-4

Mucilage (gelatinous substance that protects mucous membranes and inflamed tissues): Comfrey 112, 115-6; Dandelion 124; Echinacea 133, 136; Flaxseed 149; Kelp 218; Milk

Mucilage (continued) Thistle 247, 249; Mullein 255; Slippery Elm 294, 296

NDGA (Nordihydro guaiaretic acid, a powerful antioxidant): Chaparral 101

Omega-3 Fatty Acids: Flaxseed 151-3

Pectin: Red Raspberry 279; St. John's Wort 304

Salicylic Acid (aspirin precursor):

Black Cohosh 46; Yarrow 347

Tannins *(a group of phenol and flavonoid compounds that exhibit astringent qualities): Bilberry 39; Black Cohosh 46; Blessed Thistle 53; Brigham Tea 59; Catnip 74; Eyebright 143; Juniper 210; Red Raspberry 279-80; St. John's Wort 304; Uva Ursi 316; Yarrow 347; Yellow Dock 356*

Studies

Arthritis: Ginger 182; Wild Yam 339
Asthma: Barley 30
Blood Thinning: Ginger 181, 186
Blood Vessels:
Arteriosclerosis – Hardening of the Arteries: Garlic 166-7; Ginger 181; Red Clover 273
Blood Pressure: Catnip 74; Flaxseed 153; Hawthorn 204
Cholesterol – Blood Lipids: Aloe 19; Flaxseed 153; Garlic 167; Ginger 181; Licorice 229; Red Clover 273; Wild Yam 338-9
Varicose Veins: Bilberry 41
Cancer: Alfalfa 7; Flaxseed 154; Garlic 168; Kelp 220; Milk Thistle 249; Saw Palmetto 288
Tumors: Chaparral 103; Garlic 168
Diabetes: Alfalfa 6; Aloe 19; Barley 30; Bilberry 40; Flaxseed 152; Juniper 213; Milk Thistle 249
Digestive Tract: Flaxseed 152
Abdominal Cramps: Peppermint 264
Digestion:
Saw Palmetto 285
Irritable Bowel Syndrome (IBS): Peppermint 264
Nausea: Ginger 179-80
Ulcerative Colitis: Aloe 18
Ulcers: Licorice 227
Eyes: Bilberry 39-40
Female:
Child Birth – Labor: Red Raspberry 280
Hormone Balance: Black Cohosh 47
Menopause: Black Cohosh 47-8; Flaxseed 154
Menstruation: Chaste Tree 109; Kelp 221
Morning Sickness: Ginger 180
Pre-Menstrual Syndrome (PMS): *Chaste Tree 110*
First Aid:
Accelerated Healing: Barley Grass 33; Chamomile 94
Burns: Aloe 15
Heart:
Circulation: Bilberry 40; Hawthorn 205
Disease: Aloe 19; Garlic 167; Hawthorn 205-6
Immune System: Aloe 20
Infections: Aloe 16; Comfrey 116; Echinacea 132; Garlic 165; Uva Ursi 317
Anti-Fungal: Echinacea 134
Inflammation: Bilberry 40; Chamomile 94
Liver: Milk Thistle 248-9
Cirrhosis: Milk Thistle 248
Male - Prostate Health: Saw Palmetto 287-8
Mouth:
Cankers: Aloe 19
Gingivitis: Aloe 19
Nervous System:
Alzheimer's: Flaxseed 153; Ginger 181
Anxiety: Valerian 324
Depression: Licorice 229; St. John's Wort 305-6
Osteoporosis: Alfalfa 7; Red Clover 274
Skin:
Dermatitis: Licorice 229
Eczema: Chamomile 93
Psoriasis: Aloe 19
Seborrheic Dermatitis: Aloe 17
Skin Disease – Accelerated Healing: Barley Grass 33
Sleep: Valerian 323, 325
Toxic Conditions – Radiation: Kelp 221
Weight: Barley 30

Acknowledgments

Much can be said about our selfless friend, researcher, editor, and writer, Connie Meagher; thank you for your tenacity in researching, writing, and completing this book. Without you and your daughter, Jenny, this would be a very plain, ordinary book. Instead, it is full of every detail we could find about each of these fantastic herbs. You made it wonderful! Thank you.

A special thank you to my dear friend and master herbalist, Becky Boyd. Her overwhelming excitement for this herb knowledge and her willingness to help facilitate teaching **The Top 40 Herbs of North America** workshops helped make this dream a reality. She truly lives what she preaches.

I am so grateful to the Wilen Sisters, Joan and Lidia, my mentors and muses. These wonderful authors, researchers and friends launched me into the world of writing and teaching about these healing herbs. Thank you for teaching and mentoring me. You truly changed the projection for my life.

My mom was my first Herbalist. She taught me to be a fearless herbalist. She is still my inspiration today. Thank you for helping me be a "brave" herbalist. I love my mom.

My dad, without question, is the guy who is willing to take as many herbs as I will give him to get well. From him I have learned dedication to my craft. He has taught me to have joy in any moment. I love my dad.

My children sacrificed healthy home cooked meals and time with me so you can have these herbs in your life too. My children fanned my passion and drive to write this book so this knowledge would be passed down for generations to come. I love you each with all my heart. You are the reason I am an Herbalist.

The Top 40 Herbs of North America wouldn't have come to life without the devotion and dedication of my sweet husband, Curtiss. He always believed in me, my "gut" feelings, and dreams of a healthy healed world. Thank you for that undying faith. Together we can accomplish just about anything. I love you.

About The Author

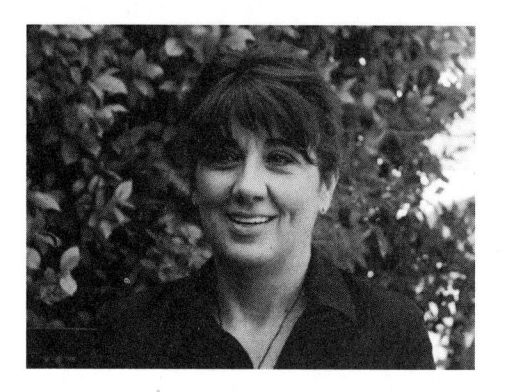

Angela Harris

As a fifth-generation herbalist, using herbs for health has always been a part of my life. Just like my mother and those who came before her, I found solutions to everyday problems using herbs for myself and my young family. While pregnant with my sixth child, I was diagnosed with life-threatening illnesses that produced a grim outlook for my future. Allopathic medical practices offered nothing in the way of hope for a long and healthy life. With limited options, I tapped into the generations of herbal heritage from which I hailed, prompting an extensive search into nature's herbal bounty. What I found was nothing less than miraculous. Herbs are made for healing! Since discovering for myself the amazing medicinal properties of these God-given plants, my family and I have dedicated the past 30 years of our lives to teaching this increasingly endangered knowledge by promoting herbal living and helping countless others employ the use of herbs for health and nutrition.

In 2004, our family opened Herbally Grounded, a natural health-food store that not only filled our needs for reliable, quality herbs but those of other herbalists as well. Due to ever increasing government restrictions, we could not see a way in which we could teach the history of herbs and continue to sell them at the same time. This led my husband, Curtiss and I to give up our beloved store and create HerbU.org, a free educational platform where people could not only gain knowledge in the lost art of herbalism but implement it as well. Our health ministry continues to grow within the Harris family and with every new herbalist inspired by the divinity of these incredible plants.